RESILIENCE IN CHILDREN

ANNALS OF THE NEW YORK ACADEMY OF SCIENCES
Volume 1094

RESILIENCE IN CHILDREN

Edited by Barry M. Lester, Ann S. Masten, and Bruce McEwen

Published by Blackwell Publishing on behalf of the New York Academy of Sciences
Boston, Massachusetts
2006

Library of Congress Cataloging-in-Publication Data

Resilience in children / edited by Barry M. Lester, Ann S. Masten, and Bruce McEwen.
p. ; cm. – (Annals of the New York Academy of Sciences, ISSN 0077-8923 ; v. 1094)
Includes bibliographical references.
ISBN-13: 978-1-57331-643-9 (paper: alk. paper)
ISBN-10: 1-57331-643-1 (paper: alk. paper)
1. Resilience (Personality trait) in children–Congresses. I. Lester, Barry M. II. Masten, Ann S. III. McEwen, Bruce S. IV. New York Academy of Sciences. V. Series.
[DNLM: 1. Adaptation, Psychological–Congresses. 2. Adolescent. 3. Child Development–Congresses. 4. Child. W1 AN626YL v.1094 2006 / WS 105.5.A8 R4335 2006]

BF723.R46R475 2006
155.4'1824–dc22

2006038320

The *Annals of the New York Academy of Sciences* (ISSN: 0077-8923 [print]; ISSN: 1749-6632 [online]) is published 28 times a year on behalf of the New York Academy of Sciences by Blackwell Publishing, with offices located at 350 Main Street, Malden, Massachusetts 02148 USA, PO Box 1354, Garsington Road, Oxford OX4 2DQ UK, and PO Box 378 Carlton South, 3053 Victoria Australia.

Information for subscribers: Subscription prices for 2006 are: Premium Institutional: $3850.00 (US) and £2139.00 (Europe and Rest of World).
Customers in the UK should add VAT at 5%. Customers in the EU should also add VAT at 5% or provide a VAT registration number or evidence of entitlement to exemption. Customers in Canada should add 7% GST or provide evidence of entitlement to exemption. The Premium Institutional price also includes online access to full-text articles from 1997 to present, where available. For other pricing options or more information about online access to Blackwell Publishing journals, including access information and terms and conditions, please visit www.blackwellpublishing.com/nyas.

Membership information: Members may order copies of the *Annals* volumes directly from the Academy by visiting www.nyas.org/annals, emailing membership@nyas.org, faxing 212-298-3650, or calling 800-843-6927 (US only), or +1 212-298-8640 (International). For more information on becoming a member of the New York Academy of Sciences, please visit www.nyas.org/membership.

Journal Customer Services: For ordering information, claims, and any inquiry concerning your institutional subscription, please contact your nearest office:
UK: Email: customerservices@blackwellpublishing.com; Tel: +44 (0) 1865 778315; Fax +44 (0) 1865 471775
US: Email: customerservices@blackwellpublishing.com; Tel: +1 781 388 8599 or 1 800 835 6770 (Toll free in the USA); Fax: +1 781 388 8232
Asia: Email: customerservices@blackwellpublishing.com; Tel: +65 6511 8000; Fax: +61 3 8359 1120
Members: Claims and inquiries on member orders should be directed to the Academy at email: membership@nyas.org or Tel: +1 212 838 0230 (International) or 800-843-6927 (US only).

Mailing: The *Annals of the New York Academy of Sciences* are mailed Standard Rate. **Postmaster:** Send all address changes to *Annals of the New York Academy of Sciences*, Blackwell Publishing, Inc., Journals Subscription Department, 350 Main Street, Malden, MA 01248-5020. Mailing to rest of world by DHL Smart and Global Mail.

Annals are available to subscribers online at the New York Academy of Sciences and also at Blackwell Synergy. Visit www.annalsnyas.org or www.blackwell-synergy.com to search the articles and register for table of contents e-mail alerts. Access to full text and PDF downloads of *Annals* articles are available to nonmembers and subscribers on a pay-per-view basis at www.annalsnyas.org.

The paper used in this publication meets the minimum requirements of the National Standard for Information Sciences Permanence of Paper for Printed Library Materials, ANSI Z39.48_1984.

ISSN: 0077-8923 (print); 1749-6632 (online)
ISBN-10: 1-57331-643-1 (paper); ISBN-13: 978-1-57331-643-9 (paper)

A catalogue record for this title is available from the British Library.

Digitization of the *Annals of the New York Academy of Sciences*

An agreement has recently been reached between Blackwell Publishing and the New York Academy of Sciences to digitize the entire run of the *Annals of the New York Academy of Sciences* back to volume one.

The back files, which have been defined as all of those issues published before 1997, will be sold to libraries as part of Blackwell Publishing's Legacy Sales Program and hosted on the Blackwell Synergy website.

Copyright of all material will remain with the rights holder. Contributors: Please contact Blackwell Publishing if you do not wish an article or picture from the *Annals of the New York Academy of Sciences* to be included in this digitization project.

Dedicated to Norman Garmezy in recognition of his extraordinary leadership in pioneering research on resilience in children

ANNALS OF THE NEW YORK ACADEMY OF SCIENCES

Volume 1094
December 2006

RESILIENCE IN CHILDREN

Editors
BARRY M. LESTER, ANN S. MASTEN, AND BRUCE MCEWEN

This volume is the result of a conference entitled **Resilience in Children**, sponsored by the New York Academy of Sciences and Brown Medical School, held on February 26–28, 2006 in Arlington, Virginia.

CONTENTS

Issues

Prevention

Part II. Neurobiological Processes

Emotion Regulation

Genetics

Neuroendocrine Processes

Neuroscience and Intervention

Part III. Integration and Wrap-Up

Part IV. Short Papers

We gratefully acknowledge the support of the National Institute on Drug Abuse, the National Institute of Mental Health, and the National Institute of Child Health & Human Development.

Preface

A landmark interdisciplinary conference on Resilience in Children was held February 26–28, 2006, in Arlington, Virginia, sponsored by the New York Academy of Sciences and Brown Medical School. This volume of the *Annals* contains the proceedings of that conference that ushered in a new era in the study of resilience. This conference brought together a highly distinguished group of scientists to discuss the neurobiology of resilience together with its behavioral aspects.

We started with an old question that has intrigued researchers for more than 30 years: Why is it that some children grow up in adverse circumstances and still have a relatively positive psychological outcome? Many children experience conditions such as war, poverty, maltreatment, chronic illness, catastrophic life events, and parental mental illness or substance abuse, yet manage to overcome hardship and grow into functioning and caring adults.

Resilience research emerged in the 1970s, with the mission of exploring the individual and contextual influences that protect children growing up in adverse conditions against poor outcomes. A large body of research has accumulated on these protective factors, including cognitive and personality attributes, family dynamics, relationships with friends and adults, and the broader social environment.

The resilience field has generated a tremendous amount of excitement in the scientific community because it provides another window to understanding developmental processes in atypical as well as typically developing children. Resilience research has also been vital to the development of prevention programs, which provide targeted interventions to help high-risk children thrive. Additionally, resilience science has matured beyond the identification of resilience predictors, toward the study of dynamic processes that explain successful adaptation, despite having experienced adversity.

Until very recently, however, the complex questions of resilience were addressed primarily from a behavioral and psychosocial perspective, with less attention to biological influences. Advances in neuroscience now afford the opportunity to integrate neurobiology in the study of resilience and to ask if there are specific neurobiological processes and mechanisms that can contribute to our understanding of resilience. Neurobiological processes, including neural plasticity, gene–environment interplay, and neuroendocrine factors may play crucial roles in helping a child overcome adversity.

We felt that the field of resilience research was poised for an important step in its evolution—the examination of potential biological mechanisms of

Ann. N.Y. Acad. Sci. 1094: xiii–xv (2006). © 2006 New York Academy of Sciences.
doi: 10.1196/annals.1376.001

resilience in relation to behavioral development. An important focus of this conference was the potential of neurobiological processes to substantially advance the field of resilience. The objectives of the conference were to examine evidence concerning both behavioral–psychosocial and neurobiological aspects of resilience and the potential for integrating these two perspectives.

This volume begins with a keynote address by Sir Michael Rutter on resilience concepts and how they inform our scientific understanding. The volume is then divided into four parts.

In Part I, Behavioral and Psychosocial Processes are discussed. In the opening section, Ann Masten and Jelena Obradović highlight the contributions from behavior research on adaptive systems and Theodore Wachs examines studies of temperament in children, with both articles serving as guides to "hot spots" for integrating the study of resilience across multiple levels of analysis. Richard Lerner discusses their articles in the context of developmental systems theory. The next section features articles on family, relationship, and broader environmental factors. These include gene–environment interactions in rhesus monkeys by Stephen Suomi and human capital by Pamela Klebanov and Jeanne Brooks-Gunn. Edward Tronick discusses these articles from the perspective of the stress of normal interactions. Issues critical to psychosocial resilience research are discussed in the following section, including conceptual issues by Suniya Luthar and psychosocial risk factors by Arnold Sameroff and Katherine Rosenblum. Part I concludes with a section on prevention. Thomas Dishion and Arin Connell focus on self-regulatory processes, long implicated as playing a central role in resilience, while Mark Greenberg examines the interface of preventive intervention with neuroscience. Karol Kumpfer and Julia Franklin-Summerhays comment and expand on these prevention papers, examining additional cognitive precursors of resilience.

In Part II, we turn to Neurobiological Processes. In the section entitled Emotion Regulation, Marc Lewis discusses the neural mechanisms related to aggression. Linda Mayes provides a discussion of this article and considers the role of the medial amygdala in arousal regulation. In the Genetics section, Mary-Anne Enoch discusses the role of genetic and environmental factors in the development of alcoholism. In the subsequent section entitled Neuroendocrine Processes, changes in the adolescent brain and HPA activity are discussed by Russell Romeo and Bruce McEwen, and in another article, Philip Fisher, Megan Gunnar, Mary Dozier, Jacqueline Bruce, and Katherine Pears show that intervention can alter HPA axis function in children placed in foster care. These articles and psychobiological stress and coping processes are discussed by Bruce Compas. Finally, on the theme of Neuroscience and Intervention, Kiki Chang discusses advances in the prevention of pediatric bipolar disorder.

In Part III, Dante Cicchetti and Jennifer Blender provide an Integration and Wrap-up for this conference. They suggest a multiple-levels-of-analysis approach to integrate biology into the study of resilience. In his discussion of this article, Myron Hofer considers similarities between resilience and vulnerability from an evolutionary perspective.

In Part IV, we present a collection of short papers based on the poster session held at the conference. These papers were selected to represent the range of topics discussed at the meeting and indicate future directions for resilience research.

This volume brings together a unique set of articles from the first conference focused on integrating neurobiological and psychosocial approaches to resilience research. We hope it serves as an organizing force for a surge of science on the biology of resilience, at the same time that it serves an integrating role in linking this new type of resilience research with the knowledge that has been gained on the psychosocial aspects of resilience. We believe this volume will help generate a new research agenda that, as seamlessly as possible, incorporates the biology of resilience into existing conceptual models of resilience.

Financial support for this conference was provided through an NIH conference grant from the National Institute on Drug Abuse, the National Institute on Child Health and Human Development, and the National Institute of Mental Health. We are very grateful for their support and interest. We also wish to thank the staff members at the New York Academy of Sciences for their hard work in helping to bring the conference and this volume to fruition.

We hope you enjoy this volume (as much as we enjoyed bringing it to you) and look forward to this new wave of research that will facilitate the integration of behavioral and neurobiological approaches to the study of resilience. This transdisciplinary collaboration will enhance our understanding of resilience and lead to the development of public health preventive interventions for children at risk.

BARRY M. LESTER
Director, Brown Center for the Study of Children at Risk
Professor, Psychiatry and Human Behavior and Pediatrics
Brown Medical School
Women and Infants Hospital
Providence, Rhode Island 02912

ANN S. MASTEN
Distinguished McKnight University Professor
Institute of Child Development
University of Minnesota
Minneapolis, Minnesota 55455

BRUCE S. MCEWEN
Alfred E. Mirsky Professor
Harold and Margaret Milliken Hatch
Laboratory of Neuroendocrinology
The Rockefeller University
New York, New York 10021

Implications of Resilience Concepts for Scientific Understanding

MICHAEL RUTTER

Developmental Psychopathology, SGDP Centre, Institute of Psychiatry, De Crespigny Park, Denmark Hill, London, United Kingdom

ABSTRACT: Resilience is an interactive concept that refers to a relative resistance to environmental risk experiences, or the overcoming of stress or adversity. As such, it differs from both social competence positive mental health. Resilience differs from traditional concepts of risk and protection in its focus on individual variations in response to comparable experiences. Accordingly, the research focus needs to be on those individual differences and the causal processes that they reflect, rather than on resilience as a general quality. Because resilience in relation to childhood adversities may stem from positive adult experiences, a life-span trajectory approach is needed. Also, because of the crucial importance of gene–environment interactions in relation to resilience, a wide range of research strategies spanning psychosocial and biological methods is needed. Five main implications stem from the research to date: (1) resistance to hazards may derive from controlled exposure to risk (rather than its avoidance); (2) resistance may derive from traits or circumstances that are without major effects in the absence of the relevant environmental hazards; (3) resistance may derive from physiological or psychological coping processes rather than external risk or protective factors; (4) delayed recovery may derive from "turning point" experiences in adult life; and (5) resilience may be constrained by biological programming or damaging effects of stress/adversity on neural structures.

KEYWORDS: gene–environment interactions; individual differences; stress/adversity; coping processes; turning point experiences; biological effects

INTRODUCTION

The term *resilience* is used to refer to the finding that some individuals have a relatively good psychological outcome despite suffering risk experiences that would be expected to bring about serious sequelae.[1] In other words, it implies

Address for correspondence: Prof. Michael Rutter, Developmental Psychopathology, PO 80, MRC SGDP Centre, Institute of Psychiatry, De Crespigny Park, Denmark Hill, London SE 5 8AF, UK. Voice: 020-7848-0882; fax: 020-7848-0866.
e-mail: j.wickham@iop.kcl.ac.uk

**Ann. N.Y. Acad. Sci. 1094: 1–12 (2006). © 2006 New York Academy of Sciences.
doi: 10.1196/annals.1376.002**

relative resistance to environmental risk experiences, or the overcoming of stress or adversity.[2–4] It is not, however, just social competence[5] or positive mental health.[6] Both of them are important concepts but they refer to something different from resilience. Essentially, resilience is an interactive concept that is concerned with the combination of serious risk experiences and a relatively positive psychological outcome despite those experiences.

There are two sets of research findings that provide a background to the resilience notion. First, there is the universal finding of huge individual differences in people's responses to all kinds of environmental hazard.[1] Before inferring resilience from these individual differences in response there are two major methodological artifactual possibilities that have to be considered. To begin with, apparent resilience might be simply a function of variations in risk exposure. This possibility means that resilience can only be studied effectively when there is both evidence of environmentally mediated risk and a quantitative measure of the degree of such risk. The other possible artifact is that the apparent resilience might be a consequence of measuring too narrow a range of outcomes. The implication is that the outcome measures must cover a wide range of possibly adverse sequelae. The details of the research strategies that need to be employed for these purposes are considered in Rutter[1] and Rutter.[7]

Second, there is the evidence that, in some circumstances, the experience of stress or adversity sometimes *strengthens* resistance to later stress[8]—a so-called "steeling" effect. Although the research literature is much more sparse than that on individual differences in response to environmental hazards, there are some empirically based examples of stress experiences increasing resistance to later stress.[9] For example, it has been shown that experimental stress in rodents leads to structural and functional effects on the neuroendocrine system that are associated with greater resistance to later stress.[9] Similarly, repeated parachute jumping by humans leads to physiological adaptation associated with both a change in the timing and nature of the anticipatory physiological response and also the reduced subjective feeling of stress.[8] It is well known, of course, that exposure to infections (either by natural exposure or through vaccination or immunization) leads to relative immunity to later exposure to the same infectious agents. The experience of happy separations in early childhood may also possibly lead to a better adaptation to hospital admission.[10] Older children's experience of coping successfully with family poverty seemed, in the Californian studies of the Great Depression, to lead to greater psychological strengths later.[11] It is important to question what are the circumstances that lead stress/adversity to result in steeling effects rather than sensitization. There is a paucity of good research data on this matter but it seems that probably the key element is some form of successful coping with the challenge or stress or hazard. This is likely to involve physiological adaptation, psychological habituation, a sense of self-efficacy, the acquisition of effective coping strategies, and/or a cognitive redefinition of the experience.

DOES RESILIENCE ADD TO RISK AND PROTECTION CONCEPTS?

Whenever a new term becomes fashionable, it is always necessary to consider whether it is simply a new way of repackaging old material or whether it introduces some new perspective. In other words, is resilience just a fancy way of reinventing concepts of risk and protection? It is not, because risk and protection both start with a focus on variables, and then move to outcomes, with an implicit assumption that the impact of risk and protective factors will be broadly similar in everyone, and that outcomes will depend on the mix and balance between risk and protective influences. By contrast, resilience starts with a recognition of the huge individual variation in people's responses to the same experiences, and considers outcomes with the assumption that an understanding of the mechanisms underlying that variation will cast light on the causal processes and, by so doing, will have implications for intervention strategies with respect to both prevention and treatment.

Does that mean that resilience concepts reject the traditional study of risk and protective factors? Certainly not, because there is an abundance of evidence that much of the variation in psychopathological outcomes can be accounted for by the summative effects of risk and protective factors. Also, and more importantly, resilience is an interactive concept that can only be studied if there is a thorough measurement of risk and protective factors. In short, resilience requires the prior study of risk and protection but adds a different, new dimension.

A second possibility that has to be considered is that because resilience is an inference based on evidence of an interaction, this means that it can be adequately assessed through finding a statistically significant multiplicative interaction. At first sight, it sounds obvious that that must be the case, but in fact it is wrong. That is because a statistical interaction requires variation in both variables and not just one and because synergistic interactions may involve either an additive or a multiplicative interaction.[12,13] The point about statistical interaction requiring variation in both variables is that there are quite common circumstances in which there clearly is an interaction in a biological sense, but yet this is not reflected in the statistical interaction term. For example, there are major individual differences in people's responses to malaria, and something is known about the genes that moderate this. This will not result in a statistical interaction in areas where malaria is endemic because everyone will have been exposed to more or less the same degree of risk of infection. Similarly, there are big individual differences, again genetically influenced, in atopy. Thus, some people respond to the spring pollens by the development of hay fever, whereas others do not show this response. But, in ordinary circumstances everyone living in the same area is exposed to much the same level of pollens. Accordingly, there will be no statistical interaction, despite the obvious evidence of a biological interaction.

A further possibility that has to be considered is the assumption that it should be possible to measure resilience directly as an observed trait, rather than having to rely on an inference based on some kind of interaction, however, assessed. Numerous researchers and clinicians are searching for such questionnaire or interview measures of this postulated trait. It is a fallacious approach, however, because resilience is not a single quality. People may be resilient in relation to some sort of environmental hazards but not others. Equally they may be resilient in relation to some kinds of outcomes but not others. In addition, because context may be crucial, people may be resilient at one time period in their life but not at others.

GENE–ENVIRONMENT INTERACTION (G × E)

Some of these issues are well illustrated by considering findings on gene–environment interactions (G × E) in relation to some environmental risk influence, as investigated with respect to some psychopathological outcome. For a long time, behavioral geneticists tended to argue that such interactions were sufficiently rare and so minor in their effects that they could be ignored in most genetic analyses. It is clear that this was a mistaken assumption.[14,15] G × E relies on studying an environmental risk factor for which there is good evidence of substantial risk, and of environmental mediation of that risk, as well as heterogeneity in outcome. In other words, despite conventional wisdom suggesting the opposite, the implication is that, in the present state of knowledge, the starting point has to be the study of environmental risk, and not identification of genetic risk.[15–17]

Three key findings from the Dunedin study well illustrate the phenomenon. FIGURES 1, 2, and 3 show the pattern. FIGURE 1 deals with variations in response to childhood maltreatment in terms of the outcome of antisocial behavior, according to moderation by the allelic variation in the gene that regulates MAOA activity. Considered in quantitative terms there was no main effect of genes, there was a small, significant effect of childhood maltreatment, but the big effect came from the interaction. Childhood maltreatment had a rather small effect on the individuals with high MAOA activity but it had a very big effect in relation to those with low MAOA activity. FIGURE 2 shows a comparable pattern with respect to the serotonin transporter gene again with maltreatment as the risk variable, but this time with depression as the outcome. FIGURE 3 shows the findings in relation to the valine variant of the COMT gene in relation to the effects of early heavy use of cannabis, schizophrenia being the outcome variable. In both these latter examples, there was the same overall pattern of no genetic main effect, a significant environmental effect, but with the biggest effect coming from the interaction between the identified gene and the measured risk environment. Each of these findings has now been replicated in one way or another and the serotonin transporter gene finding also has a much broader

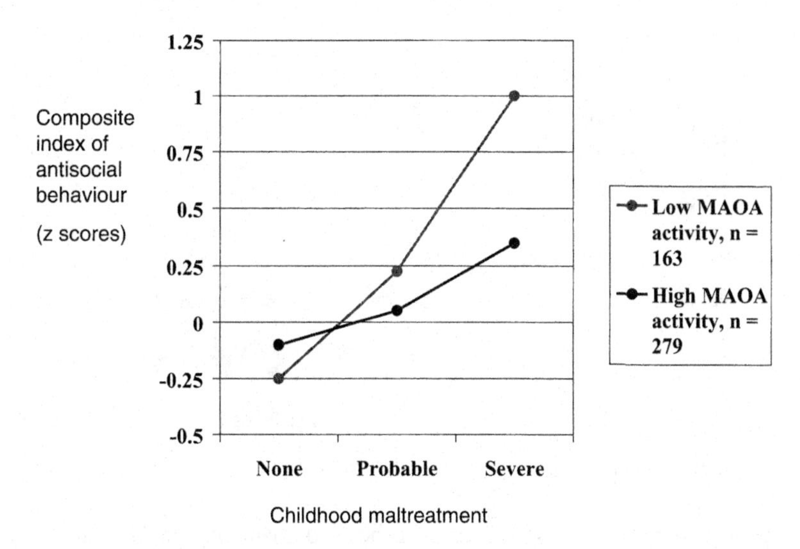

FIGURE 1. Antisocial behavior as a function of MAOA activity and a childhood history of maltreatment.[28]

body of biological research using a range of research strategies including imaging studies of response to stress, rearing studies in rhesus monkeys, and animal models of other kinds.[15] There are a series of quite important methodological checks that need to be undertaken before inferring a G $\times$ E but such steps were undertaken in a thorough and resolute fashion by the Dunedin study team and the results are compelling in showing that the interaction is valid, and not artefactual.

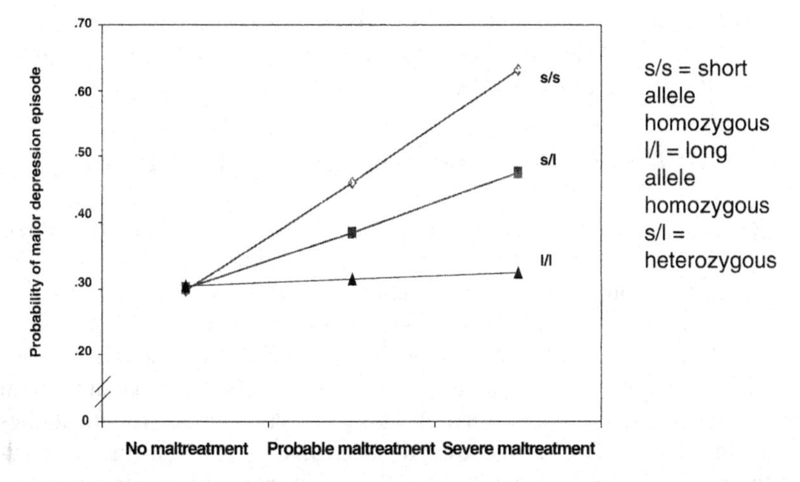

FIGURE 2. Effect of maltreatment in childhood on liability to depression moderated by 5-HTT gene.[29]

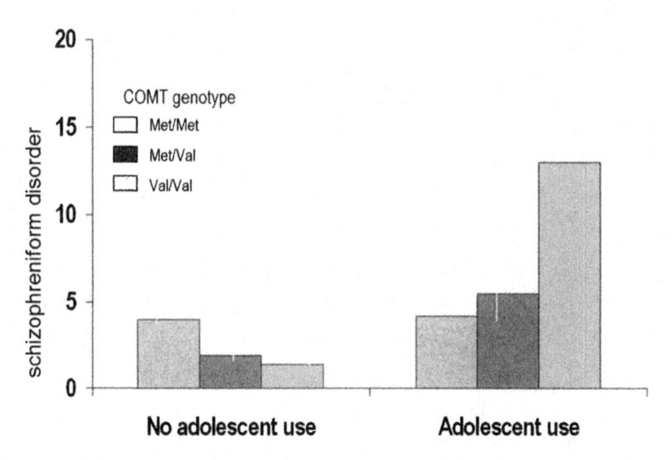

FIGURE 3. Schizophrenia spectrum disorder: cannabis use interacts with genotype.[30]

There are four main lessons from the body of research on G × E. First, as in the three Dunedin study examples, the influence of the genes was only shown through demonstration of the interaction with the environmental hazard. Second, in each case, the G × E was specific to a particular psychopathological outcome. The finding underlines the fact that there is not, and cannot be, a single universally applicable resilience trait. Third, the implication of the G × E is that both the G and the E share the same causal pathophysiological pathway. Of course, that suggestion needs to be tested. Nevertheless, the point is that the resilience finding has causal process implications for both genes and environment. Fourth, the genetic variant is neither a risk nor a protective factor in itself. That is, there is little or no effect on psychopathology in the absence of the environmental risk factor. There could scarcely be any better example of the value of a resilience concept in studying causal processes because it identified a significant and important genetic effect that would not have been detected in the absence of studying the interaction.

OTHER LESSONS FROM RESILIENCE FINDINGS

Obviously, resilience is not just a feature of G × E. There are numerous other circumstances in which resilience is evident. The findings from such studies bring out four more important lessons for scientific understanding. First, resistance to environmental hazards may come from *exposure* to risk in controlled circumstances, rather than *avoidance* of risk. This is best demonstrated, of course, in the natural immunity to infections and that brought about by immunization and vaccination. It is also evident in the rodent studies of stress to which reference has already been made. The Californian studies of the great economic depression[11] provide an interesting example of the benefits of adolescents coping successfully, the contrast being with the findings of adverse effects in younger children who were not able to cope in the same way. Treatment studies of fears and phobias have also shown that exposure is an important (although not necessarily essential) element in their successful treatment.[18,19] Avoidance of the feared object is the action most likely to lead to persistence of the fear. It has to be said that there is a paucity of good evidence on the protective effect of controlled exposure to stress/adversity in relation to psychopathological outcomes, and clearly there is a need to consider both physiological mediation and cognitive/affective mediation. Nevertheless, the parallels with internal medicine are sufficiently compelling to indicate that it is quite likely that there are psychological parallels to the immunity example.

Second, protection may derive from circumstances that are either neutral or risky in the absence of the key environmental hazard. For example, it is apparent in the protection against malaria provided by heterozygote sickle-cell status.[20] Being a carrier of the sickle-cell is not in itself a good thing but it happens to be protective against malaria. It has no particular benefits for people living in a malaria-free area but it has important benefits for those in areas where malaria is endemic. Adoption may well constitute a psychological example. Adoption is an experience that probably carries some risks (albeit small ones) that stem from it being atypical in all societies. If children who are adopted come from a low-risk background, there are no particular advantages to being adopted. By sharp contrast, however, for children who have been exposed in early life to parental abuse or neglect, adoption can be highly advantageous.[21]

FIGURE 4 illustrates the point in a somewhat different way by its indication that actions that are protective in depriving circumstances may be of no particular benefit in advantageous conditions. Quinton and Rutter[22] showed that the

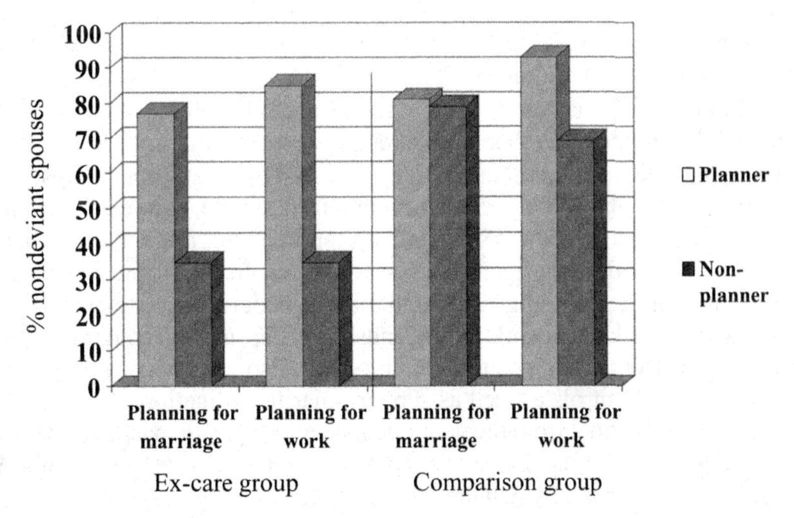

FIGURE 4. Planning and nondeviant spouses.[22]

phenomenon of planning (meaning no more than taking considered decisions rather than acting impulsively) made it much more likely that young people who had been reared in institutions would marry a nondeviant spouse. Moreover, this effect was evident, not just with respect to planning for marriage, but also planning as evident in the work context. By contrast, the planning tendency made no significant difference in a comparison population sample. The point is that the peer group for the children who had been raised in residential group homes was largely a deviant one and when they left the institutions and returned to discordant families there was considerable pressure to marry to get out of the arena of conflict. This did not apply in the comparison group who, if they married entirely by random selection, were most likely to land up with a nondeviant spouse and their circumstances provided no particular pressure to marry in haste.

The third message, therefore, is that protection may derive from what people do to deal with stress or adversity. That is, the notion of resilience focuses attention on coping mechanisms, mental sets, and the operation of personal agency. In other words, it requires a move from a focus on external risks to a focus on *how* these external risks are dealt with by the individual. More generally, this means that resilience, unlike risk and protective factor approaches, forces attention on dynamic *processes*, rather than static factors that act in summative fashion. Such processes may involve neurotransmitters as in the G $\times$ E example, neuroendocrine effects as seen in stress adaptation, or cognitive/emotional mechanisms. It should be noted that the study of cognitive/emotional mechanisms may require qualitative methods to generate hypotheses (although quantitative measures will still be required to test the hypothesis so generated). Thus, Hauser *et al.*,[23] in their study of resilience in young people who had had a prolonged psychiatric hospitalization, found that three features were strongly characteristic of resilience (as compared with average outcomes). These were: personal agency and a concern to overcome adversity; a self-reflective style; and a commitment to relationships.

Fourth, protection may derive from circumstances that come about long after the risk experience. In other words, resilience may sometimes reflect later recovery, rather than an initial failure to succumb. Thus, Laub and Sampson,[24] in their follow-up of the Gluecks' institutionalized sample, showed that a beneficial turning point effect was seen with a supportive marriage. It might have been supposed that the beneficial effect derived solely from a secure attachment relationship, but their findings indicated that the benefits also stemmed from the new extended kin network and friendship group that marriage brought, providing hitherto lacking positive role models. Also, the spouses frequently exerted informal controls as well as support, marital obligations often cut off the antisocial individual from the delinquent peer group, and marriage brought expectations of providing financial support (so that regular employment also provided social controls). Much the same complex mix of influences was seen with the parallel finding of the turning point effect of armed services for young people from a severely disadvantaged background.[25] It was not that serving in the armed services was of itself beneficial but, rather, it provided opportunities for continuing education in a more adult environment. It brought a widening of the peer group and it often delayed marriage until careers were more effectively managed.

IS RESILIENCE UNLIMITED?

Resilience notions have generally been interpreted as conveying great optimism regarding the possibility of surviving adversity. Such optimism is well justified but it is necessary to ask whether resilience is limited. Findings indicate that it is. Thus, our follow-up study of children from profoundly depriving residential institutions in Romania, who were adopted into well-functioning UK families, showed remarkable persistence of adverse sequelae even after more than 7.5 years in the adoptive home.[26,27] As FIGURE 5 indicates, there were no persisting sequelae that could be detected when the children had left the institutions before the age of 6 months but there was then a marked increase in multiple impairments that occurred even within the group of children spending just 6 to 12 months in depriving institutions. Curiously, there was no further increase in risk with persistence of the depriving circumstances beyond the 6-month period (at least up to the age of 42 months). The implication seems to be that the pervasively depriving circumstances took some months to have an effect but when they lasted beyond the age of 6 months, they tended to have effects that endured many years. The inference is that there may have been some form of intraorganismic change—either neural damage or biological programming of some kind.

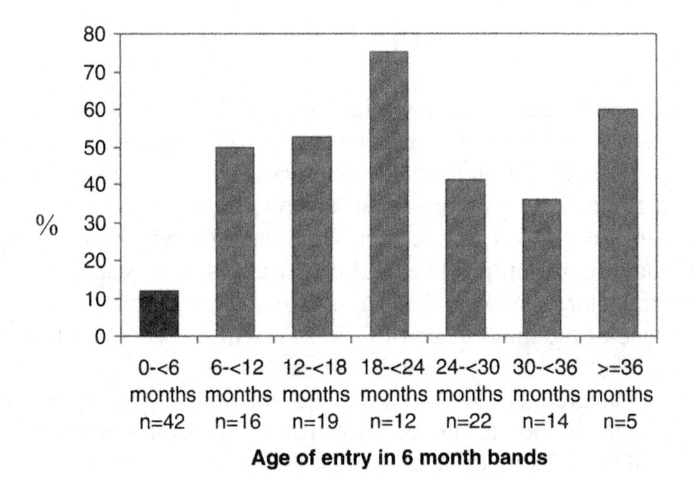

FIGURE 5. Rates of children with 2+ impairments by age of entry pooled in 6-month bands (institution-reared Romanian adoptees) (from Kreppner *et al.*, submitted).

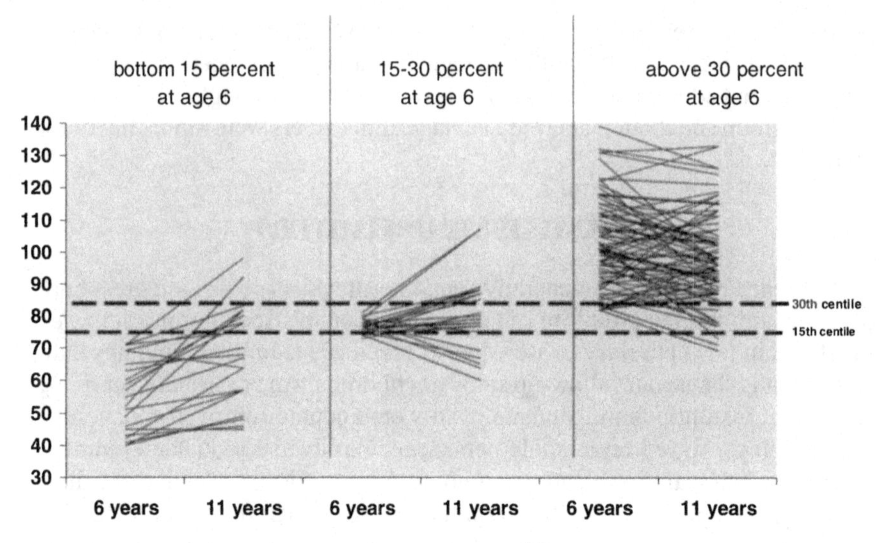

FIGURE 6. Change in IQ between ages 6 and 11.[26]

On the other hand, although the effects were remarkably persistent, there was change between 6 and 11 years as illustrated in FIGURE 6 showing a line scattergram for cognitive change between 6 and 11 years. It is notable that the changes, however, were largely confined to the group that was most impaired at 6 years. Also, it is striking that there was huge heterogeneity in outcome with some children showing superior cognitive functioning despite the prolonged institutional deprivation. Factors promoting resilience in the face of this extraordinarily pervasive and profound deprivation remain unclear.

CONCLUSIONS

There are three broad research implications that derive from resilience findings. Because resilience is not a general quality that represents a trait of the individual, research needs to focus on the processes underlying individual differences in response to environmental hazards, rather than resilience as an abstract entity. Second, because resilience in relation to adverse childhood experiences may stem from positive adult experiences, it is necessary to adopt a life-span trajectory approach that can investigate later turning point effects. Third, because of the importance of G $\times$ E, it will be necessary to combine psychosocial and biological research approaches and to use a diverse range of research strategies. These should include functional imaging of cognitive processing, neuroendocrine studies, investigation of mental sets and models, and the use of animal studies of various kinds.

Resilience findings also provide five key implications for scientific understanding of substantive effects. First, resistance to hazards may derive from controlled exposure to risk (rather than its avoidance). Second, resistance may derive from traits or circumstances that are either risky or neutral in the absence of the relevant environmental hazard. Third, resistance may derive from physiological or psychological coping processes, rather than external risk or protective factors. Fourth, delayed recovery may derive from "turning point" effects in adult life. Fifth, resilience may be constrained by biological programming or by the damaging effects of stress/adversity on neural structures.

REFERENCES

1. Rutter, M. 2006. The promotion of resilience in the face of adversity. *In* Families Count: Effects on Child and Adolescent Development. A. Clarke-Stewart & J. Dunn, Eds.: 26–52. Cambridge University Press. New York & Cambridge. In press.
2. Cicchetti, D., F.A. Rogosch, M. Lynch & K.D. Holt. 1993. Resilience in maltreated children: processes leading to adaptive outcome. Dev. Psychopathol. **5:** 629–648.
3. Luthar, S. 2003. Resilience and Vulnerability: Adaptation in the Context of Childhood Adversities. Cambridge University Press. New York.
4. Masten, A.S. 2001. Ordinary magic: resilience processes in development. Am. Psychol. **56:** 227–238.
5. Masten, A.S. 2006. Competence and psychopathology in development. *In* Developmental Psychopathology. Vol. 3: Risk, disorder and psychopathology, 2nd ed. D. Cicchietti & D. Cohen, Eds.: 696–738. J. Wiley & Sons. New York.
6. Layard, R. 2005. Happiness: Lessons from a New Science. Allen Lane. London.
7. Rutter, M. Proceeding from correlation to causal inference: the use of natural experiments. Submitted.
8. Rutter, M. 1981. Stress, coping and development: some issues and some questions. J. Child Psychol. Psychiatry **22:** 323–356.
9. Hennessey, J.W. & S. Levine. 1979. Stress, arousal, and the pituitary-adrenal system: a psychoendocrine hypothesis. *In* Progress in Psychobiology and Physiological Psychology. J.M. Sprague & A.N. Epstein, Eds.: 133–178. Academic Press, New York.
10. Stacey, M., R. Dearden, R. Pill & D. Robinson. 1970. Hospitals, children and their families: the report of a pilot study. Routledge & Kegan Paul. London.
11. Elder, G.H. 1974. Children of the Great Depression. University of Chicago Press. Chicago.
12. Rutter, M. 1983. Statistical and personal interactions: facets and perspectives. *In* Human Development: An Interactional Perspective. D. Magnusson & V. Allen, Eds.: 295–319. Academic Press. New York.
13. Rutter, M. 2006. Genes and Behavior: Nature-Nurture Interplay Explained. Blackwell Publishing. Oxford.
14. Rutter, M. & J. Silberg. 2002. Gene-environment interplay in relation to emotional and behavioral disturbance. Annu. Rev. Psychol. **53:** 463–490.
15. Rutter, M., T.E. Moffitt & A. Caspi. 2006. Gene-environment interplay and psychopathology: multiple varieties but real effects. J. Child Psychol. Psychiatry **47:** 226–261.

16. MOFFITT, T.E., A. CASPI & M. RUTTER. 2005. Strategy for investigating interactions between measured genes and measured environments. Arch. Gen. Psychiatry **62:** 473–481.
17. MOFFITT, T.E., A. CASPI & M. RUTTER. 2006. Measured gene-environment interactions in psychopathology: concepts, research strategies, and implications for research, intervention, and public understanding of genetics. Perspectives on Psychological Science: **1:** 5–27.
18. MARKS, I.M. 1987. Fears, Phobias, and Rituals: Panic, Anxiety and Their Disorders. Oxford University Press. Oxford.
19. RACHMAN, S.J. 1990. Fear and Courage. W.H. Freeman, New York.
20. ROTTER, J.I. & J.M. DIAMOND. 1987. What maintains the frequencies of human genetic diseases? Nature **329:** 289–290.
21. DUYME, M., A-C. DUMARET & S. TOMKIEWICZ. 1999. How can we boost IQs of "dull children"?: A late adoption study. Proc. Natl. Acad. Sci. USA **96:** 8790–8794.
22. QUINTON, D. & M. RUTTER. 1988. Parenting breakdown: The making and breaking of inter-generational links. Avebury. Aldershot.
23. HAUSER, S., J. ALLEN, E. GOLDEN. 2006. Out of the Woods: Tales of Resilient Teens. Harvard University Press. Cambridge, MA.
24. LAUB, J. & R. SAMPSON. 2003. Shared Beginnings, Divergent Lives: Delinquent Boys to Age 70. Harvard University Press. Cambridge, MA.
25. ELDER, G.H. JR. 1986. Military times and turning points in men's lives. Dev. Psychol. **22:** 233–245.
26. BECKETT, C., B. MAUGHAN, M. RUTTER, *et al.* 2006. Do the effects of early severe deprivation on cognition persist into early adolescence? Findings from the English and Romanian Adoptees Study. Child Dev. **77:** 696–711.
27. KREPPNER, J.M., M. RUTTER, C. BECKETT, *et al.* (submitted). Normality and impairment following profound early institutional deprivation. A longitudinal follow-up into early adolescence.
28. CASPI, A., J. MCCLAY, T.E. MOFFITT, *et al.* 2002. Role of genotype in the cycle of violence in maltreated children. Science **297:** 851–854.
29. CASPI, A., K. SUGDEN, T.E. MOFFITT, *et al.* 2003. Influence of life stress on depression: Moderation by a polymorphism in the 5-HTT gene. Science **301:** 386–389.
30. CASPI, A., T.E. MOFFITT, M. CANNON, *et al.* 2005. Moderation of the effect of adolescent-onset cannabis use on adult psychosis by a functional polymorphism in the COMT gene: Longitudinal evidence of a gene-environment interaction. Biol. Psychiatry **57:** 1117–1127.

Competence and Resilience in Development

ANN S. MASTEN AND JELENA OBRADOVIĆ

Institute of Child Development, University of Minnesota, Twin Cities, Minneapolis, Minnesota, USA

ABSTRACT: The first three waves of research on resilience in development, largely behavioral in focus, contributed a compelling set of concepts and methods, a surprisingly consistent body of findings, provocative issues and controversies, and clues to promising areas for the next wave of resilience research linking biology and neuroscience to behavioral adaptation in development. Behavioral investigators honed the definitions and assessments of risk, adversity, competence, developmental tasks, protective factors, and other key aspects of resilience, as they sought to understand how some children overcome adversity to do well in life. Their findings implicate fundamental adaptive systems, which in turn suggest hot spots for the rising fourth wave of integrative research on resilience in children, focused on processes studied at multiple levels of analysis and across species.

KEYWORDS: development; risk; biobehavioral processes; resilience

INTRODUCTION

This volume of the *Annals* heralds a new era in research on resilience and its applications, bringing together scientists and disciplines to chart the course toward a fully integrated, multilevel understanding of resilience in development. The conference on which it is based, *Resilience in Children*, held in February 2006, marked the rise of the fourth wave of research on developmental resilience. In this article, contributions from the first three waves of behavioral research on resilience in children are highlighted, with an eye toward informing the goals and strategies of the fourth wave.

The first three waves of research on resilience in development were behavioral in focus.[1,2] The origins of research on resilience have deep roots in the history of medicine, psychology, and education.[3,4] It was around 1970, however, that the systematic study of resilience emerged within the broader context

Address for correspondence: Ann S. Masten, University of Minnesota, Institute of Child Development, 51 East River Road, Minneapolis, MN 55455-0345, USA. Voice: 612-624-0215; fax: 612-624-6373.

e-mail: amasten@umn.edu

Ann. N.Y. Acad. Sci. 1094: 13–27 (2006). © 2006 New York Academy of Sciences.
doi: 10.1196/annals.1376.003

of *developmental psychopathology*, the study of behavioral health and adaptation from a developmental perspective.[5,6] In the first wave of work, pioneering behavioral scientists in search of knowledge about the etiology of serious mental disorders recognized the significance of children who appeared to develop well under risky conditions. These pioneers set out to identify the correlates and markers of good adaptation among young people expected to struggle because of their genetic or environmental risk. The initial work was largely descriptive, but ambitious in ultimate objective: to ascertain what makes a difference in the lives of such children, in order to guide efforts to improve the life chances of children at risk for problems due to hazardous experiences and vulnerabilities. A "short list" of potential assets or protective factors associated with resilience in children and youth emerged from the first wave and this list continues to be corroborated in diverse studies.[1,6,7] The second wave of resilience research has been focused on uncovering the processes and regulatory systems that account for the short list, a formidable agenda that is still under way.[6,8] The third wave, characterized by efforts to promote resilience through prevention, intervention, and policy, rose from a sense of urgency for the welfare of children growing up with adversities and vulnerabilities, who could not wait for a complete elucidation of resilience. Resilience intervention efforts were spurred by the concomitant rise of prevention science, which underscored the importance of promoting competence as a strategy for preventing or ameliorating behavioral and emotional problems.[4,9,10] The initial waves of resilience research, largely led by scientists in clinical psychology, psychiatry, and human development, have contributed a compelling set of concepts and methods, and a surprisingly consistent body of findings, as well as issues, controversies, and cautionary notes. These contributions provide intriguing clues to "hot spots" for integrating research across levels of analysis and also pitfalls to avoid in the excitement of a fourth wave of research.

THEORY AND CONCEPTS: COMPETENCE, RISK, AND RESILIENCE IN DEVELOPMENTAL CONTEXT

Resilience is a broad conceptual umbrella, covering many concepts related to positive patterns of adaptation in the context of adversity. The conceptual family of resilience encompasses a class of phenomena where the adaptation of a system has been threatened by experiences capable of disrupting or destroying the successful operations of the system. The idea of resilience can be applied to any functional system, but in developmental science it has been applied most frequently to individuals as living systems and less often to higher level social systems, including families,[11] classrooms,[12] and schools.[13] Resilience is quintessentially inferential: to judge the resilience of a system requires criteria for identifying whether the system is doing whatever it is supposed to be doing, and also whether there is or has been a potential threat to the system. Thus, if one identifies a child as resilient, two judgments have been made: this child meets expectations for positive adaptation and there has been a significant threat to the adaptation of the child.[4,8]

Lois Murphy[14] noted long ago that the adaptive quality of a living system has two aspects: adapting to the environment, what she called Coping I, and maintaining internal integration, termed Coping II. In the lives of children, there have been many criteria for external adaptation, ranging from school achievement to getting along with peers; and also criteria for internal adaptation, such as psychological well-being or physical health.

One of the most important contributions of the early resilience researchers in behavioral sciences was their attention to the criteria for judging positive adaptation. The Project Competence group, initially led by Norman Garmezy and later by the first author, focused on competence criteria for positive adaptation in their studies of resilience and particularly on competence in age-salient developmental tasks.[15] These investigators built an evolving conceptual framework for defining positive adaptation in children that focused on manifestly effective behavior expected for children in multiple domains of achievement; these expectations varied over the course of development, as well as across cultural and historical contexts.[1,9] This *developmental task* approach focused on external adaptation from a developmental perspective, rather than internal well-being. This group did not ignore emotional health, which they studied in relation to competence in developmental tasks. However, resilience was operationally defined in terms of successful adaptation to the environment in age-salient developmental tasks, rather than happiness or symptoms related to internal well-being. Other investigators of resilience chose to include emotional health in their defining criteria.[8]

Developmental task theory, which emerged in the mid 20th century, has been refined as a result of this recent attention, and a number of its propositions put to empirical test.[9,16] Among the conclusions supported by this body of research are the following:

1. Adaptation is multidimensional and developmental in nature.
2. Success in salient tasks of particular developmental periods forecast success in future age-salient tasks, even in new domains.
3. Competence and symptoms are related within and across time for multiple reasons, including: (*a*) symptoms undermining competence; (*b*) failures (or perceived failures) in competence increasing symptoms in various ways; (*c*) a common cause contributing both to competence problems and symptoms; and, (*d*) transactional or sequential combinations of these reasons.
4. Success or failure in multiple developmental task domains can have cascading consequences that lead to problems in other domains of adaptation, both internal and external.
5. Interventions to promote success in these tasks have preventive effects on behavioral and emotional problems.

Defining resilience also required judgments about the nature of threats to a system's adaptation. A wide range of risk factors and challenges have been the focus of study, including cumulative life events (tallies of negative experiences over time) and specific experiences (e.g., divorce, bereavement, war, natural disasters, etc.), acute trauma and chronic adversities, and well-established "risk factors" that statistically forecast later developmental difficulties in the general population, such as low birth weight.

MODELS AND METHODS: OPERATIONALIZING RESEARCH ON RESILIENCE

Testing concepts of competence and resilience required the development of models and methods, including new measures and strategies of analysis. Before the pioneers motivated the first wave of research on resilience, little attention was given to models or measures incorporating positive predictors or outcomes. It was necessary for the early investigators to develop strategies of assessment and analysis of competence, assets, resources, promotive, and protective factors, and the diagnosis of resilience in addition to psychopathology, risks, vulnerabilities, and stressors.[17] Investigators pursued variable-focused as well as person-focused approaches to resilience.[18]

Variable-focused models and analyses, using multivariate statistics with increasing sophistication, were well-suited to testing hypotheses about the multidimensional nature of adaptation within and across time, how positive aspects of adjustment are related to problems and symptoms over time, and the cumulative effects of co-occurring risks as manifested in "risk gradients." Interaction findings (adversity X a moderating variable) highlighted the striking exception of individuals with high adversity scores whose adaptive success appeared to be "off the gradient" (better than predicted by their level of risk; see FIG. 1). Multivariate findings hinted at the potential role of combined predictors, mediators, and moderators of good outcomes in the context of risk or adversity. Multidimensional models of competence were corroborated,[19] and later investigators began to test more complex cascade and transactional models linking distinct domains of behavior across time, where one domain of adjustment predicts changes in another domain over time.[9,20] Rarely, however, have these multidimensional models tested for interactions across multiple levels of analysis, as proposed by developmental theorists.[21]

Although it was rare for resilience investigators to study linkages extending from the level of genetic or neural activity to behavior or family levels of functioning, they did test for the effects of parenting quality or parent–child relationships as mediators and moderators of adversity, capturing individual and family dynamics to a limited degree.[22] Intervention studies in the third wave of work provide some of the most compelling evidence for the power of the family environment for individual resilience. These include quasi-experimental

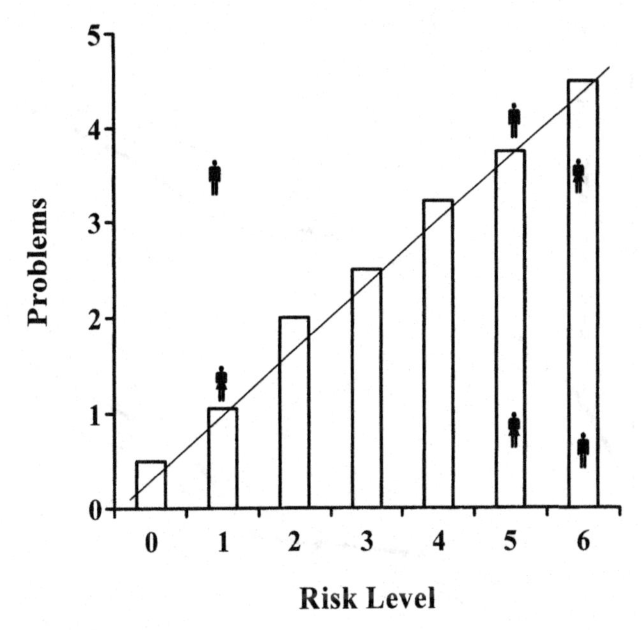

FIGURE 1. A risk gradient illustrating how average levels of problems rise as a function of rising risk level, and also showing how individuals can be "on" (near the average predicted level) or "off-gradient" (doing much worse or much better than predicted for a given level of risk).

interventions to dramatically improve the rearing environment and randomized clinical trials of interventions to promote child adaptation by helping parents function more effectively during difficult times. An example of the former is provided by the studies of Romanian orphans adopted internationally after regime change in the early 1990s, where marked improvements have been observed in many of the children moved from severe privation to adequate families, particularly for children adopted prior to 6 months of age.[23,24] Examples of the latter are prevention experiments showing that interventions targeting parent functioning resulted in better adjusted children in families following divorce.[25,26]

Recent developments in multivariate research signify that the fourth wave is under way. For example, recent gene–environment interaction studies[27] suggest that measurable genetic polymorphisms (e.g., 5-HTTLPR) moderate the association of adverse experiences (e.g., maltreatment) with behavioral outcomes. At a more intermediate level of multilevel interaction and analysis, spanning individual differences in temperament or personality traits, there is growing interest in altering self-regulation to promote better adaptation among children growing up in stress-laden environments.[28]

Person-focused studies also have a long history in resilience research, beginning with compelling single-case portraits of resilience, and now moving

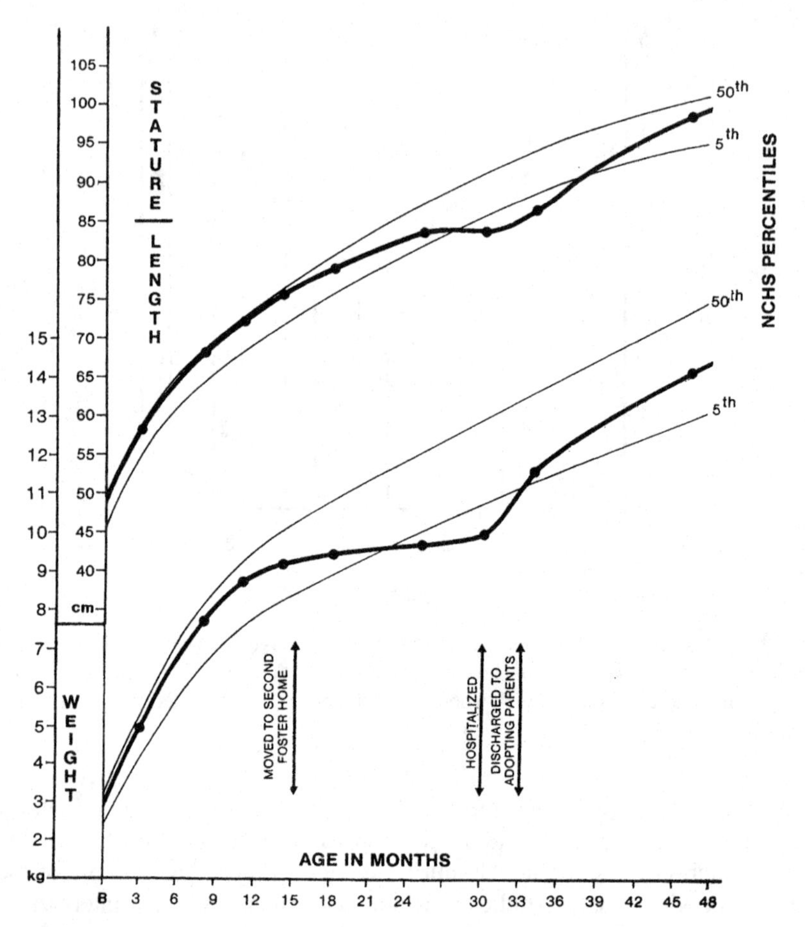

FIGURE 2. Growth chart from the case study of "Sara," illustrating a dramatic slowing of growth rate after catastrophic loss of caregivers shortly after 12 months of age, and dramatic recovery to normative growth following hospitalization and adoption by a loving family around 30 months of age. Originally appearing in the case report by Masten & O'Connor[29] in the *Journal of the American Academy of Child and Adolescent Psychiatry* (1989, *28* [2], p. 276), and reproduced with permission of LIPPINCOTT WILLIAMS & WILKINS.

rapidly toward very sophisticated statistical models of growth and developmental trajectories. Single case studies can serve as powerful heuristic and communication tools, illustrating dramatic turning points in development. The growth chart of "Sara" shown in FIGURE 2 (from the case report by Masten & O'Connor[29]) is illustrative: Sara's growth rate (as well as her social development) plummeted following a catastrophic loss of caregiving and recovered following adoption into a loving and well-matched family environment. Such cases, compelling as they may be, rarely can be generalized to other cases because of their unique features. Therefore, person-focused work moved toward case aggregation and the detection of repeated life patterns in more representative samples of children. Classic studies of resilience often identified a large risk group and then compared a subgroup of individuals doing well across multiple criteria of positive adaptation to another subgroup in the sample that shares similar high-risk levels but is doing poorly in multiple ways.[30] This approach has been extended to include cases of low-risk individuals who are doing well (meet competence criteria but have low exposure to risk or adversity), along with resilient cases (competent + high risk), and maladaptive or impaired competence cases (failing to meet competence criteria in multiple domains + high risk). Comparisons of this nature often find strong similarities in the high competence groups, despite divergent adversity exposure, and striking differences between the resilient and maladaptive groups, despite shared risks or adversity exposure, as illustrated in FIGURE 3 (see Masten *et al.*[31,32]). As levels of adversity levels increase, the differences in the resources of resilient versus maladaptive individual can be even greater, as illustrated by the stars in FIGURE 3, which show the means for the subset of children within each high adversity group who have histories of catastrophic level lifetime adversity.[33] There is also a notably "empty cell" effect in such studies, suggesting that cases of low risk and poor adaptation (suggesting great vulnerability or a non-normal organism) are much less common than cases

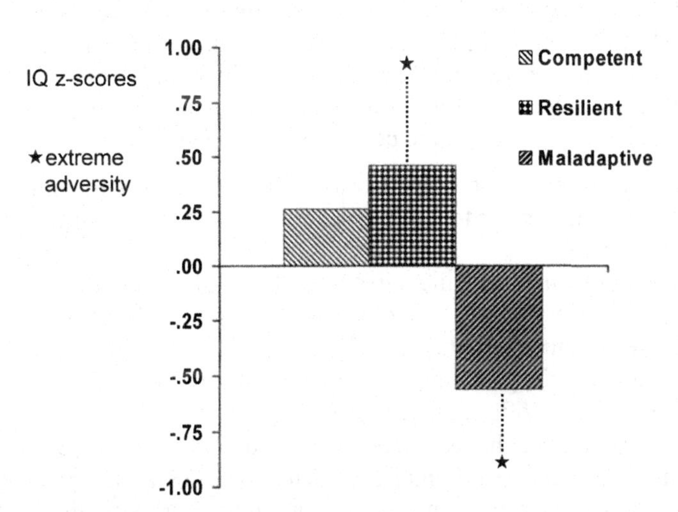

FIGURE 3. A comparison of three groups of youth "diagnosed" around the age of 20 years as *competent* (good adaptation and low adversity history), *resilient* (good adaptation and high adversity history), and *maladaptive* (poor adaptation and high adversity history). Mean IQ scores from childhood (measured 10 years earlier) are shown for the three groups.[31] Means for the subgroups of resilient and maladaptive youth with extremely high lifetime adversity are shown by stars.[33]

of high risk and good adaptation, perhaps indicating the adaptive and self-righting bias of development in a species shaped by eons of natural and cultural selection.

Recent advances in person-oriented studies hint that the next wave of work will use powerful new statistical tools for identifying subgroups pertinent to understanding resilience, such as group-based modeling of developmental trajectories;[34] (see the example provided by Obradović, Burt & Masten, this issue). It should be possible to identify positive pathways of development or recovery among groups of individuals who have experienced very high adversity exposure or trauma.

Multiple levels of analysis in person-focused studies are exceedingly rare to date. It should become feasible, once particular gene–environment findings become well established, to study subgroups who defy expected patterns in order to learn more about protective processes at many levels of interaction. It is clearly not the case that 100% of individuals with a particular and common polymorphism become ill or maladaptive in the face of a particular form of adversity. Moreover, adversity itself comes in many forms, contexts, and timings. There are bound to be processes that moderate gene–environment effects.

ISSUES AND CONTROVERSIES

Behavioral studies focused on competence, adversity, and resilience engendered much useful criticism about concepts, measures, methods, and gaps in knowledge that served (though sometimes slowly in the eyes of critics) to advance the thinking and quality of work on resilience in development. Challenging questions were raised, including the following:[2,5,8,35–39]

1. Who decides or defines the criteria for judging good adaptation?
2. Does resilience refer to positive internal adaptation, positive external adaptation, or both?
3. Can an individual be resilient in one context and not another, at one time and not another, for one kind of stressor and not another, for one kind of adaptive domain and not another?
4. How can knowledge be aggregated if the criteria for defining and analyzing resilience often vary across studies?
5. Is a concept of resilience necessary or is this just a positive way of renaming the same underlying phenomenon of vulnerability and risk?
6. Does the focus on resilience distract us from addressing the burden of risk in the lives of children?
7. Does resilience research "blame the victim" when children do not overcome adversity?
8. What do we know about resilience in non-Western cultures and the developing world?

9. What are the processes behind the promotive or protective "factors" descriptively associated with resilience?
10. What is the role of neuroscience in the study of resilience?

Discussion of such issues by behavioral and developmental scientists served to sharpen subsequent research and is now shaping a future research agenda.

SURPRISINGLY CONSISTENT FINDINGS: CLUES TO ADAPTIVE SYSTEMS IN HUMAN DEVELOPMENT

Despite the growing number of well-deserved criticisms directed at the early waves of resilience research and the variability in definitions, measures, situations, and cultures studied, findings have continued to show a striking consistency.[1,18] Recurring attributes of person, relationships, and context emerge as predictors or correlates of resilience across diverse situations, implicating a "short list" of probable and rather general factors associated with good adaptation or recovery during or following significant adversity. This list in turn suggests that there are fundamental but common and ordinary adaptive systems that play a crucial role in resilience, and also more broadly in human development.[1,18] When these adaptive systems (see TABLE 1) are available and operating normally, individual resilience is common. The most devastating threats to children and child development occur when these systems are damaged, destroyed, or develop abnormally as a result of adversity. Moreover, many of these systems relate to the self-regulatory capacity of the human brain as

TABLE 1. Adaptive systems implicated in the world literature on resilience

Learning systems of the human brain
—problem solving, information processing
Attachment system
—close relationships with caregivers, friends, romantic partners, spiritual figures
Mastery motivation system
—self-efficacy processes, reward systems related to successful behavior
Stress response systems
—alarm and recovery systems
Self-regulation systems
—emotion regulation, executive functioning, activation and inhibition of attention or behavior
Family system
—parenting, interpersonal dynamics, expectations, cohesion, rituals, norms
School system
—teaching, values, standards, expectations
Peer system
—friendships, peer groups, values, norms
Cultural and societal systems
—religion, traditions, rituals, values, standards, laws

it learns and develops, and the social regulatory capacity embedded in human relationships and ties to cultural traditions.

There is extensive, though often fragmented research, on the development, functioning, and dysfunction of many of these adaptive systems in the lives of individuals, such as attachment relationships or executive functioning. Other systems, consistently implicated in resilience studies, have been relatively neglected until quite recently, such as the mastery motivation system and religious beliefs and practices. In either case, this list provides important clues for integrating biological and behavioral approaches to resilience. Some domains already have been investigated at multiple levels of analysis, as well as across species (e.g., executive functioning has been studied at the levels of observed behavior, neuropsychological test performance, and neural function, through tests and functional magnetic resonance imaging of rats, monkeys, and people) and these approaches could be integrated in studies of resilience. Other areas of work seem ripe for multilevel integration in studies of resilience, including the up- or down-regulation of arousal and response tendencies by prosocial or deviant peers[40] and the regulatory or relational functions of cultural systems embedded in religion and faith.[41]

CAUTIONARY NOTES

Beyond the issues and controversies that have hounded and also informed the research agenda on resilience, the first three waves of work produced a set of important cautions for fourth wave investigators to keep in mind. These include the following:[36,41–45]

1. Resilience is a complex family of concepts that always requires careful conceptual and operational definition.
2. Resilience is not a single trait or process—many attributes and processes are involved.
3. There are multiple pathways to resilience.
4. Resilience definitions are embedded in cultural, developmental, and historical contexts, even if these contexts are assumed rather than made explicit.
5. Resilience definitions always have a time frame and it is quite possible for the picture to look quite different in a shorter or longer time frame, and there are likely to be cases of adaptive trade-offs, with risk and benefits in the short and long term.
6. It is easy to make the mistake of blaming the victim when resilience does not occur, if one assumes that resilience arises only from internal capacities.
7. The evidence strongly implicates the roles of transactional processes and adaptive capacity arising external to the organism in resilience.

8. Adaptive systems that are operating in normal ways can be "hijacked" for goals and purposes disapproved by society or damaging to development (e.g., by drug addiction or by savvy gang leaders recruiting young people for antisocial goals).
9. There are no magic bullets for producing resilience.
10. There are no invulnerable children.
11. There are levels of risk and adversity so overwhelming that resilience does not occur and recovery is extraordinarily rare or impossible.
12. And, finally, in the enthusiasm for understanding and promoting resilience, it is important to remember that many sources of threat to child development are preventable (e.g., land mines, premature birth, many injuries, homelessness, war), and far less costly to prevent than to address once they begin to erode development and the adaptive tools for life.

FOURTH WAVE RISING

The *Resilience in Children* conference signaled a sea change and the rise of the fourth wave in resilience research, focused on integrating the study of resilience across levels of analysis, across species, and across disciplines. Of course, this surge is part of a larger transformation in all the sciences concerned with genes, brain function, and development, made possible by dramatic advances in technologies for studying biobehavioral processes (e.g., brain imaging, noninvasive assaying, statistic modeling of complex dynamics), advancing strategies for studying measured genes in relation to measured behavior and environments, and new animal models for behavioral phenomena, a transformation quite evident in this issue of the *Annals*. The tools are at hand for venturing across levels of analysis and mapping the processes in development that account for the diverse phenomena described as resilience in the lives of children. Integrative research promises to open new avenues for basic and applied research, but this work is likely to require a new level of collaboration among scientists, each equipped with expertise in the concepts and methods of their disciplinary training, but also equipped with the skills, motivation, and funding required for cooperative multilevel research. Transdisciplinary training experiences would facilitate this kind of collaboration.

The fourth wave offers intriguing possibilities for a much deeper understanding of how processes work within and across levels to produce resilience in children. The first three waves of research, which focused on individual and family systems for the most part, suggest "hot spots" for integration, where theory and data to date point to important processes amenable to study at multiple levels and across species. Some of these spots include the core adaptive systems implicated by the short list at the level of child, relationships, family, and other systems (e.g., effortful control; goal-directed behavior in the context of affectively arousing conditions; the motivation to adapt and succeed; parenting under stress; up- and down-regulation of affect by media, peers, parents, and religious practices). Many of these hot spots involve human and social capital and reward systems that serve positive regulatory functions in the presence of threat. It is also important to remember that resilience in children depends on resilience across interconnected systems in which human development unfolds, such as families, schools, and neighborhoods. During major disasters (natural and by human design), systems may collapse at multiple levels, with reverberating effects across diverse domains of functioning.[46]

The integrated agenda of the fourth wave also promises to overturn some long-held assumptions of early work on resilience, particularly on the plasticity of adaptive functioning itself. This conference suggested the tantalizing possibility that fundamental adaptive systems that develop within the individual child, once thought to be enduring attributes, may be "reprogrammable" to a degree unimagined by the pioneers in resilience. Examples include attention-regulation[47] and stress-regulation[48] systems that may have developed in nonoptimal ways due to early experiences. A wave of creative new interventions is beginning to appear on the horizon just behind the rise of research that integrates neuroscience, molecular genetics, and behavioral development in the study of resilience in children.

ACKNOWLEDGMENTS

The authors are indebted to the past and present Project Competence research team and study participants. Project Competence studies of resilience have been supported by grants from the William T. Grant Foundation, the National Institute of Mental Health, the National Science Foundation, and the University of Minnesota to Ann Masten, Norman Garmezy, and Auke Tellegen.

REFERENCES

1. MASTEN, A.S. 2004. Regulatory processes, risk and resilience in adolescent development. Ann. N.Y. Acad. Sci. **1021:** 310–319.
2. WRIGHT, M.O.D. & A.S. MASTEN. 2005. Resilience processes in development: fostering positive adaptation in the context of adversity. *In* Handbook of Resilience in Children. S. Goldstein & R. Brooks, Eds.: 17–37. Kluwer Academic/Plenum. New York.
3. MASTEN, A.S. 1989. Resilience in development: implications of the study of successful adaptation for developmental psychopathology. *In* The Emergence of a Discipline: Rochester Symposium on Developmental Psychopathology. D. Cicchetti, Ed.: 261–294.Vol 1. Lawrence Erlbaum Associates. Hillsdale, NJ.
4. MASTEN, A.S. & J.D. COATSWORTH. 1998. The development of competence in favorable and unfavorable environments: lessons from research on successful children. Am. Psychol. **53:** 205–220.
5. CICCHETTI, D. & W.J. CURTIS. 2006. The developing brain and neural plasticity: implications for normality, psychopathology, and resilience. *In* Developmental

Psychopathology: Developmental Neuroscience. D. Cicchetti & D.J. Cohen, Eds.: 1–64. Vol 2. Second edition. Wiley. Hoboken, NJ.
6. MASTEN, A.S. 2006. Developmental psychopathology: pathways to the future. Int. J. Behav. Dev. **31:** 46–53.
7. MASTEN, A.S. & A.H. GEWIRTZ. 2006. Vulnerability and resilience in early child development. *In*: Handbook of Early Childhood Development. K. McCartney & D.A. Phillips, Eds.: Blackwell. 22–43. Malden, MA.
8. LUTHAR, S.S. 2006. Resilience in development: a synthesis of research across five decades. *In* Developmental Psychopathology: Risk, Disorder, and Adaptation. D. Cicchetti & D.J. Cohen, Eds.: Vol 3. Second edition. Wiley. New York.
9. MASTEN, A.S., K. BURT & J.D. COATSWORTH. 2006. Competence and psychopathology in development. *In* Developmental Psychopathology. D. Ciccheti & D. Cohen, Eds.: Second edition. Wiley. New York.
10. WEISSBERG, R.P., K.L. KUMPFER & M.E.P. SELIGMAN. 2003. Prevention that works for children and youth: an introduction. Am. Psychol. **58:** 425–432.
11. PATTERSON, J. 2002. Understanding family resilience. J. Clin. Psychol. **58:** 233–246.
12. DOLL, B., S. ZUCKER & K. BREHM. 2006. Resilient Classroom: Creating Health Environments for Learning. Guilford. New York.
13. WANG, M.C. & E.W. GORDON. 1994. Educational Resilience in Inner-City America: Challenges and Prospects. Lawrence Erlbaum Associates. Hillsdale, NJ.
14. MURPHY, L.B. 1962. The Widening World of Childhood: Paths Toward Mastery. Basic Books. New York.
15. MASTEN, A.S. & J.L. POWELL. 2003. A resilience framework for research, policy, and practice. *In* Resilience and Vulnerability: Adaptation in the Context of Childhood Adversities. S.S. Luthar, Ed.: 1–25. Cambridge University Press. New York.
16. ROISMAN, G.I., A.S. MASTEN, J.D. COATSWORTH & A. TELLEGEN. 2004. Salient and emerging developmental tasks in the transition to adulthood. Child Dev. **75:** 1–11.
17. MASTEN, A.S. & M-G.J. REED. 2002. Resilience in development. *In* Handbook of Positive Psychology. C.R. Snyder & S.J. Lopez, Eds.: 74–88. Oxford University Press. London.
18. MASTEN, A.S. 2001. Ordinary magic: resilience processes in development. Am. Psychol. **56:** 227–238.
19. MASTEN, A.S., J.D. COATSWORTH, J. NEEMANN, *et al.* 1995. The structure and coherence of competence from childhood through adolescence. Child Dev. **66:** 1635–1659.
20. MASTEN, A.S., G. ROISMAN, J.D. LONG, *et al.* 2005. Developmental cascades: linking academic achievement, externalizing and internalizing symptoms over 20 years. Dev. Psychol. **41:** 733–746.
21. GOTTLIEB, G. 1998. The significance of biology for human development: a developmental psychobiological systems view. *In* Handbook of Child Psychology. W. Damon & R.M. Lerner, Eds.: 233–273.Vol 1. Fifth edition. John Wiley & Sons. New York.
22. MASTEN, A.S., A. SHAFFER. 2006. How families matter in child development: reflections from research on risk and resilience. *In* Families Count: Effects on Child and Adolescent Development. A. C-S & J. Dunn, Eds.: 5–25. Cambridge University Press. Cambridge.

23. BECKETT, C., B. MAUGHAN, M. RUTTER, *et al.* 2006. Do the effects of early deprivation on cognition persist into early adolescence? Findings from the English and Romanian Adoptees Study. Child Dev. **77:** 696–711.
24. RUTTER, M., TEAM TEARAES. 1998. Developmental catch-up, and deficit, following adoption after severe global early privation. J. Child Psychol. Psychiatry **39:** 465–476.
25. FORGATCH, M.S. & D.S. DEGARMO. 1999. Parenting through change: an effective prevention program for single mothers. J. Consult. Clin. Psychol. **67:** 711–724.
26. WOLCHIK, S., I. SANDLER, R.E. MILLSAP, *et al.* 2002. Six-year follow-up of preventive interventions for children of divorce. A randomized controlled trial. J. Am. Med. Assoc. **288:** 1874–1881.
27. MOFFITT, T.E., A. CASPI & M. RUTTER. 2006. Measured gene-environment interactions in psychopathology: concepts, research strategies, and implications for research, intervention, and public understanding of genetics. Pers. Psychol. Sci. **1:** 5–27.
28. GREENBERG, M.T., N.R. RIGGS & C. BLAIR. 2007. The role of preventive interventions in enhancing neurocognitive functioning and promoting competence in adolescence. *In* Adolescent Psychopathology and the Developing Brain: Integrating Brain and Prevention Science. D. Romer & E. Walker, Eds.: 441–461. Oxford University Press. New York.
29. MASTEN, A.S. & M.J. O'CONNOR. 1989. Vulnerability, stress, and resilience in the early development of a high risk child. J. Am. Acad. Child Adol. Psychiatry **28:** 274–278.
30. WERNER, E.E. & R.S. SMITH. 1982. Vulnerable but Invincible: A Study of Resilient Children. McGraw-Hill. New York.
31. MASTEN, A.S., J.J. HUBBARD, S.D. GEST, *et al.* 1999. Competence in the context of adversity: pathways to resilience and maladaptation from childhood to late adolescence. Dev. Psychopathol. **11:** 143–169.
32. MASTEN, A.S., J. HUBBARD, S.D. GEST, *et al.* 1999. Adversity, resources and resilience: pathways to competence from childhood to late adolescence. Dev. Psychopathol. **11:** 143–169.
33. HUBBARD, J.J. & A.S. MASTEN. 1997. Trauma and adaptation through time in a normative sample of children. Paper presented at the biennial meeting of the Society for Research on Child Development, April; Washington, DC.
34. NAGIN, D.S. 2005. Group-Based Modeling of Development. Harvard University Press. Cambridge, MA.
35. LUTHAR, S.S., Ed.: 2003. Resilience and Vulnerability: Adaptation in the Context of Childhood Adversities. Cambridge University Press. New York.
36. RUTTER, M. 2000. Resilience reconsidered: conceptual considerations, empirical findings, and policy implications. *In* Handbook of Early Intervention. J.P. Shonkoff & S.J. Meisels, Eds.: 651–681. Second edition. Cambridge University Press. New York.
37. LUTHAR, S., D. CICCHETTI & B. BECKER. 2000. The construct of resilience: a critical evaluation and guidelines for future work. Child Dev. **71:** 543–562.
38. MASTEN, A.S. 1999. Resilience comes of age: reflections on the past and outlook for the next generation of research. *In* Resilience and Development: Positive Life Adaptations. M.D. Glantz, J.Johnson, & L. Huffman, Eds.: 289–296. Plenum. New York.

39. Boelcke, K.A. & A.S. Masten. 2001. How do Young Adults versus Developmental Psychologists Judge Competence? Poster session presented at the annual meeting of the American Psychological Association, August; San Francisco, CA.
40. Dishion, T.J. & T.F. Piehler. Peer dynamics in the development and change of child and adolescent problem behavior. *In* Multilevel Dynamics in Developmental Psychopathology: Pathways to the Future: Minnesota Symposia on Child Psychology. A.S. Masten, Ed.: Vol 34. University of Minnesota. Minneapolis. MN. In press.
41. Crawford, E., M.O.D. Wright & A.S. Masten. 2006. Resilience and spirituality in youth. *In* The Handbook of Spiritual Development in Childhood and Adolescence. P.L. Benson, E.C. Roehlkepartain, P.E. King, L. Wagener, Eds.: 355–370. Sage. Newbury Park, CA.
42. Masten, A.S. & J.R. Riley. 2005. Resilience in context. *In* Resilience in Children, Families, and Communities: Linking Context to Practice and Policy R.D. Peters, B. Leadbeater, R.J. McMahon, Eds.: 13–25. Kluwer Academic/Plenum. New York.
43. Riley, J.R. & A.S. Masten. 2005. Resilience in context. *In* Resilience in Children, Families, and Communities: Linking Context to Practice and Policy. R.D. Peters, B. Leadbeater & R. McMahon, Eds.: 13–25. Kluwer Academic/Plenum. New York.
44. Yates, T.M. & A.S. Masten. 2004. Fostering the future: resilience theory and the practice of positive psychology. *In* Positive Psychology in Practice. P.A. Linley & S. Joseph, Eds.: Wiley. Hoboken, NJ.
45. Sameroff, A. 2006. Identifying risk and protective factors for healthy child development. *In* Families Count: Effects on Child and Adolescent Development. A. Clark-Stewart & J. Dunn, Eds.: 53–76. Cambridge University Press. New York.
46. Pine, D.S., J. Costello & A.S. Masten. 2005. Trauma, proximity, and developmental psychopathology: the effects of war and terrorism on children. Neuropsychopharmacology **30:** 1781–1792.
47. Rueda, M.R., M.K. Rothbart, L. Saccomanno & M.I. Posner. 2007. Modifying brain networks underlying self-regulation. *In* Adolescent Pspychopathology and the Developing Brain: Integrating Brain and Prevention Science. D. Romer & E. Walker, Eds.: Oxford University Press. New York. 401–418.
48. Gunnar, M. 2006. Social regulation of stress in early child development. *In* Blackwell Handbook of Early Childhood Development. K. McCartney & D. Phillips, Eds.: 106–125. Blackwell. Malden, MA.

Contributions of Temperament to Buffering and Sensitization Processes in Children's Development

THEODORE D. WACHS

Department of Psychological Sciences, Purdue University, W. Lafayette, Indiana, USA

ABSTRACT: Temperament refers to relatively stable, early appearing, biologically rooted individual differences in behavioral traits. Individual differences in temperament are multidetermined encompassing both biological and experiential influences. Evidence indicates that certain temperament traits, such as impulsivity, inhibition, and negative emotionality, can serve as developmental risk factors. Evidence also indicates that other temperament traits, such as flexible self-regulation, sociability, and task orientation, can serve to increase children's resilience. Five potential mechanisms through which individual differences in temperament can increase vulnerability or facilitate resilience are presented: (1) Differential treatment of children with different temperaments by caregivers or teachers (reactive covariance). (2) Children with different temperament styles seeking out environments that may increase risk or promote resilience (active covariance). (3) Goodness or poorness of fit between child temperament characteristics and environmental demands. (4) Children with different temperaments reacting to similar levels or types of stress in different ways. (5) Different coping strategies used by children with different temperaments.

KEYWORDS: stress; temperament; resilience; self-regulation

INTRODUCTION

While there are multiple definitions of *temperament,* a working definition often used by a majority of researchers in this area refers to temperament as: "Biologically rooted individual differences in behavior tendencies that are present early in life and are relatively stable across various kinds of situations and over the course of time."[1] It is important to understand that individual differences in temperament should not be regarded as unvarying across time or

Address for correspondence: Prof. Theodore D. Wachs, Department of Psychological Sciences, Purdue University, W. Lafayette, Indiana 47907-1364, USA. Voice: 765-494-6992; fax: 765-496-1264.
e-mail: wachs@psych.purdue.edu

Ann. N.Y. Acad. Sci. 1094: 28–39 (2006). © 2006 New York Academy of Sciences.
doi: 10.1196/annals.1376.004

place. Rather than complete stability researchers view temperament as *predisposing individual characteristics* that have the potential to both quantitatively and qualitatively change over time as the child develops, and which can manifest themselves in different ways in response to the nature of the context within which the individual is functioning.[2] For example, even highly inhibited children may react in the same way as less inhibited children when the situation is familiar to the child. It is only in unfamiliar situations that we would see differences between more and less inhibited children.

Behavior tendencies that are considered to fall within the domain of temperament include negative and positive emotionality (now regarded as distinct dimensions), soothability, activity level, adaptability, approach to new situations or persons, sensitivity, sociability, attentional patterns, persistence in task situations, and behavioral rhythmicity. There have also been a number of conceptual approaches for organizing these separate dimensions into a higher-order framework. The most well-known of these approaches are the Chess and Thomas[3] classification of easy, difficult, and slow to warm-up temperaments, and the conceptual framework developed by Rothbart[4] wherein individual differences in temperament dimensions reflect underlying differences in reactivity and self-regulation.

In terms of biological roots it is clear that individual differences in temperament reflect individual differences in central nervous system function and structure.[5,6] There is also a consistent body of evidence documenting the contribution of genotype to individual differences in temperament.[7] However, it is also becoming increasingly apparent that individual differences in temperament are multidetermined reflecting not only genetic and brain contributions but also the contribution of bioecological influences (e.g., nutrition[8]) and environmental characteristics involving both parenting styles[9,10] and the nature of the home context.[11] Given evidence on the sensitivity of the central nervous system to environmental input,[12] contextual characteristics may influence both the behavioral and neural aspects of individual differences in temperament.

At a functional level certain dimensions of temperament, such as negative emotionality, inhibition, low adaptability, or the combination of low self-regulation and high reactivity, have been shown to act as a developmental risk, increasing the likelihood of children's developing behavioral problems or reduced social and academic competence.[13–15] Available evidence also indicates that the contributions of temperament to developmental risk are significantly stronger when children displaying risk temperament dimensions live in dysfunctional families, in families under stress, or in families where parents use high levels of negative disciplinary techniques.[16–18] It seems clear that certain dimensions of temperament can act to increase children's developmental risk. Can temperament also promote resilience in children?

TEMPERAMENT AND RESILIENCE

Resilient children are those who show age-appropriate developmental competencies in spite of repeated exposures to biological and psychosocial developmental risk factors.[19] It is clear that individual differences in resilience are multidetermined by a variety of individual, family, and contextual influences.[20,21] Temperament has been proposed as one domain of individual characteristics that may act to promote resilience in children.[22,23] If temperament can promote resilience, a critical question is which specific dimensions of temperament are linked to the development of resilience. The age range in the studies reviewed goes from infancy through adolescence. The environmental risks encountered by the children in the studies reviewed include living in poverty, exposure to major life event stresses, family conflict and divorce, and exposure to violence or parent and peer substance abuse.

In interpreting findings from this body of literature there are methodological issues that need to be noted. For example, results have been found to vary by reporting source,[24] outcome measures used,[25] child gender,[21] and presence or absence of certain maternal characteristics, such as depression[26] or self-efficacy.[27] Keeping these methodological issues in mind, what dimensions of temperament have been linked to resilience in children?

Easy–Difficult Temperament

Compared to children with difficult temperament, children characterized as having an easy temperament were found to have significantly *lower levels of behavior problems*,[28–31] *higher levels of social competence*,[21,29,32] and *higher levels of adaptive behavior at school* [31,33] and *at home*.[34]

Emotionality

While there is some evidence showing greater resilience for children with overall lower levels of emotional reactivity,[35] the majority of studies report that the nature of the emotional reaction to stress is critical. Specifically, results indicate that for at-risk children a temperament pattern characterized as *high in positive emotional reactivity* is linked to resilience, as manifest in higher levels of social and emotional competence,[32] lower rates of behavioral–emotional problems,[25,36] and lower levels of substance abuse.[24] Conversely, a temperament pattern characterized as *high in negative emotional reactivity* is linked to reduced resilience, as manifest in higher rates of behavior problems[26] and lower ratings of school competence for children under stress.[37]

Sociability/Approach

For conceptual reasons I am integrating studies where children are characterized as showing high or low levels of sociability or approach to new or complex situations.[2] Results show significantly lower levels of behavior problems[35] and higher than expected levels of cognitive performance[38] and social–emotional competence[21,32] for children experiencing stress who are high in sociability as compared to children with lower levels of sociability. Similarly, significantly lower levels of behavior problems are found for children under stress who are high in the temperament dimension of approach, as compared to children who are low in approach.[28,39,40]

Self-Regulation

For conceptual reasons I also am integrating studies directly measuring self-regulation, as well as studies using related dimensions of temperament, such as flexibility/adaptability and level of impulsivity. Children who are higher in flexibility or adaptability show significantly fewer behavior problems than children who are temperamentally rigid or unadaptable.[39,40] Children under stress who are rated by themselves and their parents as higher in self-regulation also show a significantly lower level of internalizing behavior problems than children rated as lower in self-regulation.[41] Similarly, for children with physiological markers of increased self-regulation (high vagal tone) there is no relation of family stress to either adjustment or health, whereas for children with physiological markers of poor self-regulation (low vagal tone) family stress is linked to both poorer adjustment and health.[42,43] Not surprisingly children under stress who are high in impulsivity, which can denote poor self-regulation, show a higher level of externalizing behavior problems than children who are low in impulsivity.[25]

Attention–Task Orientation

While individual differences in attention/orientation are often considered to be dimensions of self-regulation, I view these aspects of temperament as "hybrid traits" encompassing both the temperament and cognitive domains.[44] For these reasons I treat attention/orientation separately from self-regulation. Similar to what is found for self-regulation children of divorce or children exposed to high levels of family conflict who are rated as higher in task orientation[24,39] or attention focusing[36] have significantly lower levels of behavior problems or problems with substance abuse than children with lower levels of these traits. Given that persistence is also regarded as a dimension of attention–task orientation[15] it is not surprising to also find that adolescents who were previously rated by parents as high in task persistence were more resilient (significantly fewer behavior problems) following loss of a parent than adolescents who were previously rated as low in persistence.[28]

PROCESSES UNDERLYING LINKS BETWEEN TEMPERAMENT AND RESILIENCE

While the available literature is relatively small it is also surprisingly consistent. Across a wide range of ages, life stressors and outcome variables more resilient children are those with easy temperaments, or who have higher levels of positive emotionality, sociability/approach, are more flexible, or possess more optimal levels of self-regulation and higher levels of attention focusing and task orientation. Given these patterns of findings a critical issue involves the processes or mechanisms through which individual differences in temperament translate into higher levels of resilience.

Because the qualities that define child competence are highly similar to the qualities that characterize "resilient" children[21,45] I chose to focus on underlying processes that are involved in explaining the contributions of individual differences to normal developmental competence.[46] Five potential mechanisms will be considered. Two of these mechanisms involve temperament–environment *covariance.* The remaining three mechanisms involve different forms of temperament–environment *interaction.*

Reactive Covariance

Reactive covariance refers to differential treatment of children with different individual characteristics.[46] While the fundamental assumption that temperament influences parenting is correct in a broad sense it is also clear that the influence of child temperament on parenting is moderated by a variety of nontemperament factors including child age, gender, parental personality, or adjustment and characteristics of the home environment.[44,46,47] While the path from child temperament to parenting is more complex than a simple main effect, within a reactive covariance framework we would expect a greater likelihood of resilience to occur when children have temperament patterns that elicit more positive and supporting parenting, which in turn helps to buffer the child when the family or child encounters major life stresses or disruptions.[48]

There are a number of studies that support the operation of reactive covariance processes underlying temperament–resilience links. Parents of children high in negative emotionality or difficult temperament show decreasing involvement with their child, either in terms of reduced attempts to develop their child's regulatory capacities[49] or in terms of providing less positive discipline and adequate monitoring.[48] This decreasing involvement with the child can lead to even greater vulnerability when children encounter subsequent stresses. Conversely, more sociable infants elicit more positive responses and support from their parents and other adults than unsociable infants, which in turn promotes resilience.[21] Evidence also indicates that parents of shy inhibited children are less likely to try to promote a sense of independence by their child, which only increases their child's initial inhibitory tendencies.[50] This decreases the likelihood that these children will become involved with and learn from peers, which again is likely to increase the child's vulnerability to subsequent stress. In terms of physiological measures Katz and Gottman[43] report that 24-month-old children with vagal tone patterns indicating better self-regulation received more parental support and positive parental interactions in the areas of emotional expression and emotional regulation than less regulated children. In turn, the children with better self-regulation and more supportive parenting had better cognitive, behavioral, and social outcomes following parental divorce.

Active Covariance

Active covariance refers to a process wherein children with different individual characteristics selectively gravitate to environments that are compatible with their characteristics.[46] If active covariance processes are occurring, children with certain temperament patterns would be more likely to select environments that do not expose the individual to environmental risk factors, or which allow the child to structure their world to compensate for deficits in certain skills.[48] In terms of promoting vulnerability, evidence indicates that difficult to manage children are more likely to encounter negative life events[51] and have higher rates of physical injury than more tractable children.[52] In terms of resilience, low activity levels in adolescents have been shown to predict higher levels of self-control, which in turn predict less association with peers who are substance abusers.[53] Similarly, the path from peer substance abuse to adolescent substance abuse is significantly lower for individuals who are high in task orientation and positive emotionality.[24] These results suggest that specific dimensions of temperament have the potential to both reduce the child's exposure to major risk factors in their environment and increase the child's ability to resist peer pressure to engage in risky behaviors.

Interaction: Goodness-of-Fit

The concept of goodness-of-fit is derived from the writings of Chess and Thomas[3] who hypothesized that positive development occurs when child temperament characteristics are congruent with the interaction styles, values, and goals of the child's caregivers, such as parents or teachers. Put within a temperament–resilience framework, parents or teachers are more likely to function as a support for children under stress when child temperament characteristics fit what adults value in a child.[3] While a theoretically compelling concept with some validating research, in a recent review of this area my conclusion was that empirical support for the operation of goodness-of-fit processes for both normal and abnormal development was inconsistent at best.[54] One major reason for inconsistent findings may be that goodness-of-fit may depend upon other factors besides child temperament and parent values and rearing styles. For example, using a sample of depressed mothers with difficult temperament infants Teti and Gelfand[27] report that a good mother–infant fit is more likely to occur for depressed women with a high level of maternal self-efficacy beliefs than for depressed women with a low sense of maternal self-efficacy beliefs.

Interaction: Differential Reactivity

Differential reactivity refers to a process wherein children with different individual characteristics are more or less reactive to the same level and type of environmental input.[46] Vulnerable children should be highly reactive to environmental stressors or less reactive to environmental supports. Children high in fearfulness,[17] difficult temperament,[34,55,56] and negative emotionality[16] have been shown to be more reactive to environmental stressors than less fearful, less difficult, or less negative children. Resilient children should be less reactive to environmental stressors or more reactive to environmental supports. Lower reactivity to environmental stressors has been shown for children high in positive emotionality[36] or low in negative emotionality.[57] These data, while supporting the operation of differential reactivity, are only a first step. As Rutter[23] has emphasized it is critical to begin defining what mechanisms underlie differential reactivity. One suggested mechanism for differential reactivity involves temperament-driven differential sensitivity to reward and punishment cues in the environment.[58,59]

Interaction: Differential Coping

It has also been hypothesized that temperament differences predispose to children's utilization of different coping mechanisms to deal with stress, and that the type of coping mechanisms used can lead either to vulnerability or resilience.[60] Evidence suggests that under stress conditions inhibited children are more likely to practice avoidant coping strategies, such as expression of negative emotions and proximity seeking to adults.[61] The child's use of nonproductive avoidance strategies in dealing with early stresses is not likely to promote the child's coping with later stresses (sensitization). In contrast, under stress children high in self-regulation are better able to redirect their attention as needed[62] and are more likely to respond in adaptive and flexible ways depending upon the nature of the stressor.[39,49] Evidence also indicates that children who are high in the temperament dimensions of positive emotionality, approach, and activity level are more likely to use active coping mechanisms to deal with stress, while children low in these temperament dimensions are more likely to try to cope with stress by using avoidant strategies.[36,39,63] Children who use more active, flexible coping strategies when faced with stress are more likely to successfully cope with stress and thus show what we would describe as resilience. Further, the child's ability to successfully deal with early stresses through use of active flexible coping strategies may predispose the child to use active flexible coping when faced with stress later in life (buffering).[23]

SUMMARY AND CONCLUSIONS: PROCESS MECHANISMS AND FUTURE DIRECTIONS

Clearly, there is far more evidence available on dimensions of temperament that promote or inhibit resilience than on the processes underlying how individual differences in temperament translate into vulnerability or resilience. In terms of available evidence, reactive covariance and differential coping processes have the most support. While there is also evidence in support of the operation of differential reactivity, more research is needed on exactly what leads to children with specific temperaments being more or less sensitive to environmental risk. Goodness-of-fit has conceptual elegance, but its utility as an explanatory mechanism is severely limited by inconsistent results. At present far too little is known about active covariance to determine if this can also serve as a process underlying resilience. Looking at development across time there are existing research models describing processes through which early temperament risk factors can translate into later deficits in cognitive and social–emotional competence sensitization.[64] However, far less is known about the processes through which early protective temperaments, as described in this article, may translate into later resilience in the face of stress (steeling).

What is also not known is the generalizability of our findings and theories on resilience in general, and temperament and resilience in particular, to the vast majority of the world's children who live in developing countries, and who encounter multiple and chronic life stresses that are far more severe than those encountered by children in developed countries (e.g., malnutrition, severe chronic infection, refugee status as a result of religious or political violence[65]). With a few exceptions,[66] the overwhelming majority of research and theorizing on resilience involves children from developed countries. A paper on temperament and resilience may seem a strange venue for raising this issue except for the fact that what little research is available indicates that temperament plays a part in both risk exposure[67] and competence of children from developing countries.[68] Extending the study of resilience to children living in developing countries seems an important step, both for testing the generalizability of our theories and findings on resilience, and for designing intervention strategies to promote resilience in the all too many children across the world who are currently exposed to multiple severe risks that threaten developmental competence.

REFERENCES

1. Bates, J. 1989. Concepts and measures of temperament. *In* Temperament in Childhood. G. Kohnstamm, J. Bates & M. Rothbart, Eds.: 3–26. Wiley. New York.

2. ROTHBART, M. & J. BATES. 1998. Temperament. *In* Handbook of Child Psychology: Vol. 3, Social, Emotional, and Personality Development, Fifth edition. W. Damon, Series Ed. & N. Eisenberg, Vol. Ed.: 105–176. Wiley. New York.
3. CHESS, S. & A. THOMAS. 1991. Temperament and the concept of goodness of fit. *In* Explorations in Temperament. J. Strelau & A. Angleitner, Eds.: 15–28. Plenum. New York.
4. ROTHBART, M. 1989. Biological processes in temperament. *In* Temperament in Childhood. G. Kohnstamm, J. Bates & M. Rothbart, Eds.: 77–110. Wiley. New York.
5. FOX, N. *et al.* 2005. Behavioral inhibition: linking biology and behavior within a developmental framework. Annu. Rev. Psychol. **56:** 235–262.
6. NELSON, C. 1994. Neural basis of infant temperament. *In* Temperament: Individual Difference at the Interface of Biology and Behavior. J. Bates & T.D. Wachs, Eds.: 47–82. American Psychological Association. Washington, DC.
7. DILALLA, L. & S. JONES. 2000. Genetic and environmental influences on temperament in preschoolers. *In* Temperament and Personality Development Across the Life Span. V. Molfese & D. Molfese, Eds.: 33–54. Erlbaum. Mahwah, NJ.
8. WACHS, T.D. 2000. Linking nutrition and temperament. *In* Temperament and Personality Development Across the Life Span. V. Molfese & D. Molfese, Eds.: 57–84. Erlbaum. Mahwah, NJ.
9. ARCUS, D. 2001. Inhibited and uninhibited children: Biology in the social context. *In* Temperament in Context. T.D. Wachs & G. Kohnstamm, Eds.: 43–60. Lawrence Erlbaum Associates, Publishers. Mahwah, NJ.
10. PAULI-POTT, U., B. MERTESACKER & D. BECKMANN. 2004. Predicting the development of infant emotionality from maternal characteristics. Dev. Psychopathol. **16:** 19–42.
11. MATHENY, A. & K. PHILLIPS. 2001. Temperament and context: Correlates of home environment with temperament continuity and change, newborn to 30 months. *In* Temperament in Context. T.D. Wachs & G. Kohnstamm, Eds.: 81–102. Erlbaum. Hillsdale, NJ.
12. NELSON, C. 1999. Neural plasticity and human development. Curr. Dir. Psychol. Sci. **8:** 42–45.
13. BATES, J. & G. PETTIT. Temperament, parenting and socialization. *In*: Handbook of Socialization. J. Grusec & P. Hastings, Eds. Guilford. New York. In press
14. EISENBERG, N. & R. FABES. 2006. Emotion regulation and children's socioemotional development. *In* Child Psychology: A Handbook of Contemporary Issues. L. Balter & C. Tamis-LeMonda, Eds.: 357–384. Psychology Press. New York.
15. GUERIN, D. *et al.* 2003. Temperament: Infancy Through Adolescence. Kluwer Academic Press. New York.
16. BELSKY, J., K. HSIEH & K. CRNIC. 1998. Mothering, fathering, and infant negativity as antecedents of boys' externalizing problems and inhibition at age 3 years: differential susceptibility to rearing experience? Dev. Psychopathol. **10:** 301–319.
17. COLDER, C., J. LOCHMAN & K. WELLS. 1997. The moderating effects of children's fear and activity level on relations between parenting practices and childhood symptomatology. J. Abnorm. Child Psychol. **25:** 251–263.
18. MURRAY-HARVEY, R. & P.T. SLEE. 1998. Family stress and school adjustment: predictors across the school years. Early Child Dev. Care **145:** 133–149.
19. LUTHAR, S., D. CICCHETTI & B. BECKER. 2000. The construct of resilience: a critical evaluation and guidelines for future work. Child Dev. **71:** 543–562.

20. MASTEN, A. & J. POWELL. 2003. A resilience framework for research, policy, and practice. *In* Resilience and Vulnerability: Adaptation in the Context of Childhood Adversities. S. Luthar, Eds.: 1–25. Cambridge University Press. New York.
21. WERNER, E. & R. SMITH. 1992. Overcoming the Odds. Cornell University Press. Ithaca, New York.
22. COMPAS, B. *et al.* 2001. Coping with stress during childhood and adolescence: problems, progress, and potential in theory and research. Psychol. Bull. **127:** 87–127.
23. RUTTER, M. 1987. Psychosocial resilience and protective mechanisms. Am. J. Orthopsychiat. **57:** 316–331.
24. WILLS, T. *et al.* 2001. Family risk factors and adolescent substance use: moderation effects for temperament dimensions. Dev. Psychol. **37:** 283–297.
25. LENGUA, L. *et al.* 2000. The additive and interactive effects of parenting and temperament in predicting problems of children of divorce. J. Clin. Child Psychol. **29:** 232–244.
26. OWENS, E. & D. SHAW. 2002. Predicting growth curves of externalizing behavior across the preschool years. J. Abnorm. Psychol. **31:** 575–590.
27. TETI, D. & D. GELFAND. 1991. Behavioral competence among mothers of infants in the first year: the mediational role of maternal self-efficacy. Child Dev. **62:** 918–929.
28. RUSCHENA, E. *et al.* 2005. A longitudinal study of adolescent adjustment following family transitions. J. Child Psychol. Psychiatry **46:** 353–363.
29. SMITH, J. & M. PRIOR. 1995. Temperament and stress resilience in school-age children: a within-families study. J. Am. Acad. Child Adolesc. Psychiatry **34:** 168–179.
30. TSCHANN, J. *et al.* 1996. Resilience and vulnerability among preschool children: family functioning, temperament, and behavior problems. J. Am. Acad. Child Adolesc. Psychiatry **35:** 184–192.
31. WYMAN, P. *et al.* 1999. Caregiving and developmental factors differentiating young at-risk urban children showing resilient versus stress-affected outcomes: a replication and extension. Child Dev. **70:** 645–659.
32. WERNER, E. & R. SMITH. 1982. Vulnerable but Invincible. McGraw Hill. New York.
33. WYMAN, P. *et al.* 1991. Developmental and family milieu correlates of resilience in urban children who have experienced major life stress. Am. J. Community Psychol. **19:** 405–426.
34. HETHERINGTON, E. 1989. Coping with family transitions. Child Dev. **60:** 1–14.
35. O'KEEFE, M. 1994. Adjustment of children from maritally violent homes. Fam. Soc. **75:** 403–415.
36. LENGUA, L. *et al.* 1999. Emotionality and self-regulation, threat appraisal, and coping in children of divorce. Dev. Psychopathol. **11:** 15–37.
37. KILMER, R., E. COWEN & P. WYMAN. 2001. A micro-level analysis of developmental, parenting, and family milieu variables that differentiate stress-resilient and stress-affected children. J. Community Psychol. **29:** 391–416.
38. KIM-COHEN, J. *et al.* 2004. Genetic and environmental processes in young children's resilience and vulnerability to socioeconomic deprivation. Child Dev. **75:** 651–668.
39. LENGUA, L. & I. SANDLER. 1996. Self-regulation as a moderator of the relation between coping and symptomatology in children of divorce. J. Abnorm. Child Psychol. **24:** 681–701.

40. LOSEL, F. & T. BLIESENER. 1994. Some high-risk adolescents do not develop conduct problems: a study of protective factors. Int. J. Behav. Dev. **17:** 753–777.
41. LENGUA, L. & A. LONG. 2002. The role of emotionality and self-regulation in the appraisal-coping process: tests of direct and moderating effects. J. Appl. Dev. Psychol. **23:** 471–493.
42. EL-SHEIKH, M., J. HARGER & S. WHITSON. 2001. Exposure to interparental conflict and children's adjustment and physical health: the moderating role of vagal tone. Child Dev. **72:** 1617–1636.
43. KATZ, L. & K. GOTTMAN. 1997. Buffering children from marital conflict and dissolution. J. Clin. Child Psychol. **26:** 157–171.
44. WACHS, T.D. 2006. The nature, etiology and consequences of individual differences in temperament. *In* Child Psychology: A Handbook of Contemporary Issues. Second edition. T. LeMonda & L. Balter, Eds.: 27–52. Garland. New York.
45. MASTEN, A. 2001. Ordinary magic: resilience processes in development. Am. Psychol. **56:** 227–238.
46. WACHS, T.D. 2000b. Necessary but not sufficient: the respective roles of single and multiple influences on human development. American Psychological Association Press. Washington, DC.
47. PUTNAM, S., A. SANSON & M. ROTHBART. 2002. Child temperament and parenting. *In* Handbook of parenting: Vol. 1: Children and parenting, Second edition. M. Bornstein, Eds.: 255–277. Lawrence Erlbaum Associates. Mahwah, NJ.
48. WILLS, T. & T. DISHION. 2004. Temperament and adolescent substance use: a transactional analysis of emerging self-control. J. Clin. Child Adolesc. Psychol. **33:** 69–81.
49. FRICK, P. & A. MORRIS. 2004. Temperament and developmental pathways to conduct problems. J. Clin. Child Adolesc. Psychol. **33:** 54–68.
50. RUBIN, K. *et al.* 1999. The transaction between parents' perceptions of their children's shyness and their parenting styles. Int. J. Behav. Dev. **23:** 937–958.
51. KARRAKER, K., M. LAKE & T. PARRY. 1994. Infant coping with everyday stressful events. Merrill Palmer Q. **40:** 171–189.
52. MATHENY, A. 1986. Injuries among toddlers. J. Pediatr. Psychol. **11:** 161–176.
53. WILLS, T., M. WINDLE & S. CLEARY. 1998. Temperament and novelty seeking in adolescent substance use: convergence of dimensions of temperament with constructs from Cloninger's theory. J. Pers. Soc. Psychol. **74:** 387–406.
54. WACHS, T.D. 2005. Person-environment "fit" and individual development. *In* Handbook of Research Methods in Developmental Science. D. Teti, Ed.: 443–466. Blackwell. Oxford, UK.
55. CROCKENBERG, S. 1987. Predictors and correlates of anger toward and punitive control of toddlers by adolescent mothers. Child Dev. **58:** 964–975.
56. WACHS, T.D. 1987. Specificity of environmental action as manifest in environmental correlates of infant's mastery motivation. Dev. Psychol. **23:** 782–790.
57. MORRIS, A. *et al.* 2004. Temperamental vulnerability and negative parenting as interacting predictors of child adjustment. J. Marriage Fam. **64:** 461–471.
58. COLDER, C., J. MOTT & A. BERMAN. 2002. The interactive effects of infant activity level and fear on growth trajectories of early childhood behavior problems. Dev. Psychopathol. **14:** 1–23.
59. DERRYBERRY, D., M. REED & C. PILKENTON-TAYLOR. 2003. Temperament and coping: advantages of an individual differences perspective. Dev. Psychopathol. **15:** 1049–1066.

60. COMPAS, B., J. CONNOR-SMITH & S. JASER. 2004. Temperament, stress reactivity, and coping: implications for depression in childhood and adolescence. J. Clin. Child Adolesc. Psychol. **33:** 21–31.
61. PARRITZ, R. 1996. A descriptive analysis of toddler coping in challenging circumstances. Infant Behav. Dev. **19:** 171–180.
62. LONIGAN, C. *et al.* 2004. Temperament, anxiety, and the processing of threat-relevant stimuli. J. Clin. Child Adolesc. Psychol. **33:** 8–20.
63. CARSON, D. & M. BITTNER. 2001. Temperament and school-aged children's coping abilities and responses to stress. J. Genet. Psychol. **155:** 289–302.
64. MOFFITT, T. 1993. The neuropsychology of conduct disorder. Dev. Psychopathol. **5:** 135–151.
65. UNICEF. 2004. The State of the World's Children 2005: Childhood Under Threat. UNICEF. New York.
66. ZEITLIN, M. 1991. Nutritional resilience in a hostile environment. Nutr. Rev. **49:** 259–268.
67. SCHEPER-HUGHES, N. 1987. Culture, scarcity and maternal thinking. *In* Child Survival. N. Scheper-Hughes, Ed.: 187–208. Reidel. Dordrecht.
68. DURBROW, E., B. SCHAEFER & S. JIMERSON. 2000. Learning behaviours, attention and anxiety in Caribbean children: beyond the "usual suspects" in explaining academic performance. Sch. Psychol. Int. **21:** 242–251.

Resilience as an Attribute of the Developmental System

Comments on the Papers of Professors Masten & Wachs

RICHARD M. LERNER

Tufts University, Medford, Massachusetts, USA

ABSTRACT: When conceptualized within a developmental systems theoretical framework, resilience involves mutually beneficial, reciprocally influential relations between a person and his or her context. The key features of developmental systems theory, which stress the plasticity of these relations, lead to an optimistic view of the possibility of promoting positive human development (PHD) across the life span. The results of recent longitudinal research about adolescent development allow this period to serve as a sample case of how positive development is associated with the alignment of the strengths of individuals with ecological resources for healthy growth.

KEYWORDS: developmental systems theory; plasticity; adolescence; positive development

INTRODUCTION

Resilience is an attribute of the developing, bidirectional, person ←→ context system, a point made clear by both Masten (this volume) and Wachs (this volume) as well by other contributors to the present volume (e.g., Rutter, this volume; Sameroff, this volume). Resilience describes person ←→ context exchanges that are mutually beneficial for the individual and his or her setting. Identifying a relationship within the developmental system as indicative of resilience means that, despite whatever challenges to adaptive or healthy functioning that may impinge on the person at a given point in time, and that may threaten his or her expression of positive behaviors in a setting (and that thus may diminish the "quality of life" in that setting), the person manifests

Address for correspondence: Richard M. Lerner, Institute for Applied Research in Youth Development, 301 Lincoln-Filene Building, Tufts University, Medford, MA 02155. Voice: 617-627-5558; fax: 617-627-5596.
e-mail: richard.lerner@tufts.edu

Ann. N.Y. Acad. Sci. 1094: 40–51 (2006). © 2006 New York Academy of Sciences.
doi: 10.1196/annals.1376.005

behaviors that are linked to positive functioning either within that time frame and/or across time.[1–4]

As a dynamic attribute of a relationship within the multilevel and integrated developmental system, and not a characteristic of either component of the relationship (i.e., resilience is not an attribute of the person or of the context), resilience should be studied within a nonreductionist theoretical frame and through the use of change-sensitive and multilevel (and hence multivariate) developmental methods (e.g., longitudinal designs that involve measurement models that are change and diversity sensitive[5,6]). To approach the conceptualization and study and measurement of resilience in this manner suggests the use of contemporary developmental systems theoretical models of human development, which—today—are at the cutting-edge of developmental science.[7,8]

Indeed, the scientific study of resiliency within the developmental system is an excellent sample case of the utility of such theoretical models as frames for the elucidation of the basic, relational processes of human development and, as well, for the application of developmental science to promote positive human development (PHD) (Masten, this volume; Wachs, this volume). Accordingly, to understand the nature and significance for basic and applied facets of developmental science of the study of resilience, it is useful to specify the features of current developmental systems models. This discussion will afford specification of the dynamic, relational character of resilience.

THE DEVELOPING CONTEXT OF THE CONCEPT OF DEVELOPMENT

Developmental psychology has been transformed into developmental science. As richly illustrated by the chapters across the four volumes of the *Handbook of Child Psychology*, 6th edition,[9] as well as in other major publications in the field, (e.g., [10,11]) the study of human development has evolved from focusing on either a psychogenic or a biogenic approach to conceptualizing and studying the life span to a multidisciplinary approach that seeks to integrate variables from biological through cultural and historical levels of organization into a synthetic, co-actional system.[12–20] As such, reductionist accounts of development, ones that adhere to a Cartesian dualism and that thus split apart facets of the integrated developmental system—for instance, splitting concepts, such as nature versus nurture, continuity versus discontinuity, or stability versus instability—are eschewed; in turn, postmodern, relational models stressing the integration of levels of organization are forwarded as means to understand and to study life-span human development.[21]

Thus, as exemplified by the focus of inquiry in the contemporary study of resilience, (e.g., Masten [this volume], Rutter [this volume])[2,3,22–25] the theoretical emphasis of developmental systems models is placed on conceptualizing the nature of mutually influential, individual ←→ context relations, that is, of developmental regulations engaging individual and context in mutually influential (and, in adaptive instances, in mutually beneficial) relations.[1,7,26] TABLE 1 summarizes the set of defining features of developmental systems models.

To summarize the developmental systems perspective, then, we may note that the possibility of adaptive developmental relations between individuals and their contexts and the potential plasticity of human development that is a defining feature of ontogenetic change within the dynamic, developmental system[12,16,20] stand as distinctive features of this approach to human development. As well, these core features of developmental systems models provide a rationale for making a set of methodological choices that differ in design, measurement, sampling, and data analytic techniques from selections made by researchers using split or reductionist approaches to developmental science.[27,28] Moreover, the emphasis on how the individual acts on the context to contribute to the plastic relations with it, relations that regulate adaptive development,[26] fosters an interest in person-centered (as compared to variable-centered) approaches to the study of human development.[17,18,21]

Furthermore, given that the array of individual and contextual variables involved in these relations constitute a virtually open set (e.g., there are more than 70 trillion potential human genotypes and each of them may be coupled across life with an even larger number of life course trajectories of social experiences[29]), the diversity of development becomes a prime, substantive focus for developmental science.[1,9] This diversity may be approached with the expectation that positive changes can be promoted across all instances of this variation, as a consequence of health-supportive alignments between people and settings.[20] If this stance is adopted, then diversity becomes the necessary subject of developmental science inquiry.

It is in the linkage between the ideas of plasticity and diversity that a basis exists for the extension of developmental systems thinking to form an optimistic view about the application of developmental science to promote person ←→ context exchanges that may reflect and/or promote health and positive, successful development[1,27] or, in other words, that may reflect resilience. Accordingly, employing a developmental systems frame for the application of developmental science affords a basis for forging a new, strength-based vision of and vocabulary about the nature of human development. In short, the plasticity-diversity linkage within developmental systems theory and method provides the basis for the formulation of a PHD perspective, one where the potential for human resilience is ubiquitous across the life span.

KEY FACETS OF A PHD PERSPECTIVE

The key feature of a view of PHD predicated on developmental systems theory is an emphasis on individual strengths (e.g., the possession of relative plasticity across the life span). Given the ubiquity of plasticity across the life span,[12,30] the PHD perspective posits that all individuals have the potential to develop more positively (by enhancing adaptive, that is, mutually beneficial, developmental regulations). All people have the potential to be in relations with their setting that reflect resilience.

Such mutually influential person ←→ context relations occur when the strengths of individuals are aligned with those resources present in the ecology of human development that maximize the probability that individual strengths are instantiated as positive functioning or healthy developmental outcomes.[31,32] These resources may be termed "developmental assets,"[30] and a key idea within the PHD perspective is that individuals are embedded in contexts (e.g., families, schools, and communities) that possess such assets. Accordingly, within the PHD perspective, as well as within developmental systems models that give rise to this view of human development, the ubiquity of both human strengths and contextual developmental assets means that both individuals and their ecologies are active contributors to the developmental process and to the possible promotion of healthy human development.[7,26] Resilience, then, is a key sample case of the adaptive developmental regulations that involve the mutually interactive contribution of person and setting to PHD.

The PHD perspective has been instantiated in research across the life span. Arguably, the richest and most innovative research program, to date, which exemplifies this approach to describing, explaining, and optimizing human development has been conducted by Baltes and his colleagues in regard to the assessment of the individual and contextual bases of successful aging.[12] More than a quarter century of research (e.g., in regard to the Berlin Study of Aging, Baltes, *et al.*[12]) has demonstrated convincingly that gains in psychosocial functioning, and not just losses, can characterize the development of people into even the 10th and 11th decades of life.

In addition, within the study of the second decade of life—of adolescence[11]—a second sample case of the PHD perspective has arisen within the last 10 to 15 years.[27,33] The research supporting this instance of the PHD—what has been termed the positive youth development (PYD) perspective—speaks more closely than does the study of aging to the understanding of the focal interest in the present volume, that is, resilience in children. As such, the PYD perspective may be used to illustrate the positive, strength-based approach to human behavior and development that is brought to the fore by a developmental systems perspective.

THE SAMPLE CASE OF ADOLESCENCE: THE PYD PERSPECTIVE

Beginning in the early 1990s, and burgeoning in the first half decade of the twenty-first century, a new vision and vocabulary for discussing young people

TABLE 1. Defining features of developmental systems theories

A relational meta-theory:

Predicated on a postmodern philosophical perspective that transcends Cartesian dualism, developmental systems theories are framed by a relational meta-theory for human development. There is, then, a rejection of all splits between components of the ecology of human development, e.g., between nature- and nurture-based variables, between continuity and discontinuity, or between stability and instability. Systemic syntheses or integrations replace dichotomizations or other reductionist partitions of the developmental system.

The integration of levels of organization:

Relational thinking and the rejection of Cartesian splits are associated with the idea that all levels of organization within the ecology of human development are integrated, or fused. These levels range from the biological and physiological through the cultural and historical.

Developmental regulation across ontogeny involves mutually influential individual ←→ context relations:

As a consequence of the integration of levels, the regulation of development occurs through mutually influential connections among all levels of the developmental system, ranging from genes and cell physiology through individual mental and behavioral functioning to society, culture, the designed and natural ecology and, ultimately, history. These mutually influential relations may be represented generically as Level 1 ←→ Level 2 (e.g., Family ←→ Community) and, in the case of ontogeny may be represented as individual ←→ context.

Integrated actions, individual ←→ context relations, are the basic unit of analysis within human development:

The character of developmental regulation means that the integration of actions—of the individual on the context and of the multiple levels of the context on the individual (individual ←→ context)—constitute the fundamental unit of analysis in the study of the basic process of human development.

Temporality and plasticity in human development:

As a consequence of the fusion of the historical level of analysis—and therefore temporality—within the levels of organization comprising the ecology of human development, the developmental system is characterized by the potential for systematic change, by plasticity. Observed trajectories of intraindividual change may vary across time and place as a consequence of such plasticity.

Plasticity is relative:

Developmental regulation may both facilitate and constrain opportunities for change. Thus, change in individual ←→ context relations is not limitless, and the magnitude of plasticity (the probability of change in a developmental trajectory occurring in relation to variation in contextual conditions) may vary across the life span and history. Nevertheless, the potential for plasticity at both individual and contextual levels constitutes a fundamental strength of all human's development.

Intraindividual change, interindividual differences in intraindividual change, and the fundamental substantive significance of diversity:

The combinations of variables across the integrated levels of organization within the developmental system that provide the basis of the developmental process will vary at least in part across individuals and groups. This diversity is systematic and lawfully produced by idiographic, group differential, and generic (nomothetic) phenomena. The range of interindividual differences in intraindividual change observed at any point in time is evidence of the plasticity of the developmental system, and makes the study of diversity of fundamental substantive significance for the description, explanation, and optimization of human development.

Continued.

TABLE 1. Continue

Optimism, the application of developmental science, and the promotion of PHD:
The potential for and instantiations of plasticity legitimate an optimistic and proactive search for characteristics of individuals and of their ecologies that, together, can be arrayed to promote PHD across life. Through the application of developmental science in planned attempts (i.e., interventions) to enhance (e.g., through social policies or community-based programs) the character of humans' developmental trajectories, the promotion of PHD may be achieved by aligning the strengths (operationalized as the potentials for positive change) of individuals and contexts.
Multidisciplinarity and the need for change-sensitive methodologies:
The integrated levels of organization comprising the developmental system require collaborative analyses by scholars from multiple disciplines. Multidisciplinary knowledge and, ideally, interdisciplinary knowledge is sought. The temporal embeddedness and resulting plasticity of the developmental system requires that research designs, methods of observation and measurement, and procedures for data analysis be change sensitive and able to integrate trajectories of change at multiple levels of analysis.

has emerged. These innovations were framed by the developmental systems theories that were engaging the interest of developmental scientists. The focus on plasticity within such theories led in turn to an interest in assessing the potential for change at diverse points across ontogeny, ones spanning from infancy through the "old old," 10th and 11th decades of life.[12] Moreover, these innovations were propelled by the increasingly more collaborative contributions among adolescent development researchers,[1,30,33,34] practitioners in the field of youth development,[35–37] and policy makers concerned with improving the life chances of diverse youth and their families.[38,39] These interests converged in the formulation of a set of ideas that enabled youth to be viewed as resources to be developed, and not as problems to be managed.[40,41]

These ideas may be discussed in regard to several key hypotheses. In addition, recent reviews[1,27,30,33] have summarized the burgeoning data in support of these ideas. Accordingly, to illustrate the links between the developmental systems notion of resilience and the PYD perspective, only a summary of the set of ideas constituting the current status of the PYD perspective is presented.

A first hypothesis is based on the idea that the potential for systematic intraindividual change across life (i.e., for plasticity) represents a fundamental strength of human development. Accordingly, the hypothesis was generated that, if the strengths of youth are aligned with resources for healthy growth present in the key contexts of adolescent development—the home, the school, and the community—then enhancements in positive functioning within time and the promotion of positive development across time can be achieved. Resilience in the face of challenges to positive development would, then, be likely through the aligning of individual strengths and contextual resources for healthy development.

Within the PYD perspective, a hypothesis subsidiary to the first, "alignment" notion is that there exist, across the key settings of youth development (i.e., families, schools, and communities), at least some supports for the promotion of PYD, that is, there exist "developmental assets."[30] In addition, a related hypothesis is that resources for positive development are present in youth development programs,[34,42,43] for example, in the programs of organizations, such as 4-H, Boys and Girls Clubs, Scouting, Big Brothers/Big Sisters, YMCA, or Girls, Inc. There are data suggesting that, in fact, developmental assets associated with youth development programs (i.e., programs that adopt the ideas associated with the PYD perspective),[40,41] are linked to indices of PYD. This finding raises the question of what are in fact the indicators of PYD. Addressing this question involves the second key hypothesis of the PYD perspective.

Based on both the experiences of practitioners and on reviews of the adolescent development literature,[1,34,41] "Five Cs"—Competence, Confidence, Connection, Character, and Caring—have been hypothesized as a way of conceptualizing PYD (and of integrating all the separate indicators of it, such as academic achievement or self-esteem). Recent reports from the 4-H Study of Positive Youth Development[28,44,45] confirm the presence of these Cs, as first-order latent variables and, as well, of their convergence on a second-order latent variable of "PYD."

A subsidiary hypothesis to the one postulating the Five Cs is that there should be an inverse relation within and across development between indicators of PYD and behaviors indicative of risk behaviors or internalizing and externalizing problems. Data from the 4-H Study lend some support to this idea as well.[28,32,46] Thus, in at least the early portions of the adolescent period assessed to date within the 4-H Study, evidence exists that greater levels of positive development (and thus, by inference here, a greater history of person ←→ context exchanges that may be characterized as resilient) have some covariation with lower likelihoods of behaviors indicative of engagement in risk behaviors (e.g., substance use) or in manifestations of problems of development (e.g., depression).

In sum, replacing what has been the historically prototypic deficit view of adolescence,[47–49] the PYD perspective sees all adolescents as having strengths (by virtue, at least, of their potential for change). The perspective suggests that positive development, and that person ←→ context relations reflecting resilience, are possible for all youth through aligning the strengths of young people with the developmental assets present in their social and physical ecology. Thus, the relational processes thought to be involved in the developmental system in the promotion of PYD are the very same, health-supporting person ←→ context linkages discussed by Masten (this volume) and Wachs (this volume) in regard to the development of resilience.

CONCLUSIONS: THE WORK OF MASTEN AND WACHS AS EXEMPLARS OF CONTEMPORARY APPROACHES TO DEVELOPMENTAL SCIENCE

The work of both Masten (this volume) and Wachs (this volume) reflects the use of concepts associated with developmental systems models of human development. For instance, Masten (this volume) focuses on competence (strength), and on the potential for positive outcomes across a young person's development, by framing her work within a relational model that stresses individual differences in biology, context, and—most important—individual ←→ context relations. Indeed, the scholarship of both Masten (this volume) and Wachs (this volume) reflects a concern with the linkages between individual actions, contextual resources (or affordances), and adaptive developmental regulations.

Both scholars share as well a concern with the substantive importance of developmental diversity, with the questions of interindividual differences in intraindividual change that afford multidirectionality in developmental trajectories and, as well therefore, with understanding the histories of person ←→ context relations that result in either multifinality or equifinality across development. Reflecting this interest in plasticity, and thus with the use of information about the diversity of person ←→ context exchanges for understanding the basic, relational character of resilience and, as well, for applications that can enhance the probability that person ←→ context exchanges will move individuals to healthier outcomes, there is strategic focus discernable in their work on a complex, multilevel, and multivariate set of questions: What attributes, of what individuals, at what points in their development, and in what contexts, will result in what immediate and what long-term features of development?

Answering this multitiered question will provide the knowledge of person ←→ contexts relations needed to promote resilience across the life span and throughout the world. Indeed, a clear interest in both the work of Masten (this volume) and Wachs (this volume) is to applying developmental science to foster resilience and to promote PYD. For instance, Masten (this volume) calls for "... a new surge of ideas for explaining and intervening to influence adaptive processes that foster resilience, both early and later in development" and, in turn, Wachs (this volume) underscores the significance in developmental science of "Time linked approaches ... [and] The importance of testing models of risk/resilience with children from developing countries."

In essence, then, the scholarship of Masten (this volume) and Wachs (this volume) reflects the full range of conceptual orientations to understanding and applying knowledge about the developmental system that, today, sits at the cutting-edge of developmental science.[8] Their work does more than use developmental systems thinking to understand and enhance resilience in children. The broad vision of PYD found in the work of these two scholars, a vision that includes the diverse array of people and contexts that constitute the global community, has the potential to enable the application of developmental systems approaches to resilience to be instruments promoting well-being and social justice within diverse settings in the United States and abroad. To my mind, there is no better use to be had for the conduct of good science.

ACKNOWLEDGMENTS

The writing of this article was supported in part by grants from the National 4-H Council and from the John Templeton Foundation.

REFERENCES

1. LERNER, R.M. 2004. Liberty: thriving and civic engagement among American youth. Sage. Thousand Oaks, CA.
2. MASTEN, A.S. 2001. Ordinary magic: resilience processes in development. Am. Psychol. **56:** 227–238.
3. MASTEN, A.S. 2004. Regulatory processes, risk and resilience in adolescent development. Ann. N. Y. Acad. Sci. **1021:** 310–319.
4. MASTEN, A.S. & M.G. REED. 2002. Resilience in development. *In* Handbook of Positive Psychology. C. R. Snyder & S. J. Lopez, Eds.: 74–88. Oxford University Press. London.
5. BALTES, P.B., H.W. REESE & J.R. NESSELROADE. 1977. Life-span developmental psychology: introduction to research methods. Brooks/Cole. Monterey, CA.
6. LERNER, R.M., E. DOWLING & J. CHAUDHURI. 2005. Methods of contextual assessment and assessing contextual methods: a developmental contextual perspective. In Handbook of Research Methods in Developmental Science. D.M. Teti, Ed.:183–209. Blackwell. Cambridge, MA.
7. LERNER, R.M. 2002. Concepts and theories of human development. Third edition. Erlbaum. Mahwah, NJ.
8. LERNER, R.M. 2006. Developmental science, developmental systems, and contemporary theories. *In* Theoretical Models of Human Development. Volume 1 of Handbook of Child Psychology. Sixth edition. R.M. Lerner, Vol. Ed., W. Damon & R.M. Lerner, Editors-in-chief.: 1–17. Wiley. Hoboken, NJ.
9. DAMON, W. & R.M. LERNER, Eds. 2006. Handbook of Child Psychology. Sixth edition. Wiley. Hoboken, NJ.
10. BORNSTEIN, M.H. & M.E. LAMB, Eds. 2005. Developmental Science: An Advanced Textbook. Erlbaum. Mahwah, NJ.
11. LERNER, R.M. & L. STEINBERG, Eds. 2004. Handbook of Adolescent Psychology, Second edition. Wiley. Hoboken, NJ.
12. BALTES, P.B., U. LINDENBERGER & U.M. STAUDINGER. 2006. Lifespan Theory in Developmental Psychology. *In* Theoretical Models of Human Development. Volume 1 of Handbook of Child Psychology, Sixth edition. R.M. Lerner, Vol. Ed., W. Damon & R.M. Lerner, Editors-in-chief.: 569–664. Wiley. Hoboken, NJ.

13. BRONFENBRENNER, U. & P.A. MORRIS. 2006. The bioecological model of human development. *In* Theoretical models of human development. Volume 1 of Handbook of Child Psychology. Sixth edition. R.M. Lerner, Vol. Ed., W. Damon & R.M. Lerner, Editors-in-chief.: 793–828. Wiley. Hoboken, NJ.
14. ELDER, G.H., JR. & M.J. SHANAHAN. 2006. The life course and human development. *In* Theoretical models of human development. Volume 1 of Handbook of Child Psychology. Sixth ed. R.M. Lerner, Vol. Ed., W. Damon & R.M. Lerner, Editors-in-chief.: 665–715. Wiley. Hoboken, NJ.
15. FISCHER, K.W. & T.R. BIDELL. 2006. Dynamic Development of Action, Thought, and Emotion. *In* Theoretical Models of Human Development. Volume 1 of Handbook of Child Psychology. Sixth edition. R.M. Lerner, Vol. Ed., W. Damon & R.M. Lerner, Editors-in-chief.: 313–399. Wiley. Hoboken, NJ.
16. GOTTLIEB, G., D. WAHLSTEN & R. LICKLITER. 2006. The significance of biology for human development: a developmental psychobiological systems view. *In* Theoretical Models of Human Development. Volume 1 of Handbook of Child Psychology. Sixth edition. R.M. Lerner, Vol. Ed., W. Damon & R.M. Lerner, Editors-in-chief.: 210–257. Wiley. Hoboken, NJ.
17. MAGNUSSON, D. & H. STATTIN. 2006. The person in the environment: towards a general model for scientific inquiry. *In* Theoretical Models of Human Development. Volume 1 of Handbook of Child Psychology. Sixth edition. R.M. Lerner, Vol. Ed., W. Damon & R.M. Lerner, Editors-in-chief.: 400–464. Wiley. Hoboken, NJ.
18. RATHUNDE, K. & M. CSIKSZENTMIHALYI. 2006. The developing person: an experiential perspective. *In* Theoretical Models of Human Development. Volume 1 of Handbook of Child Psychology. Sixth edition. R.M. Lerner, Vol. Ed., W. Damon & R.M. Lerner, Editors-in-chief.: 465–515. Wiley. Hoboken, NJ.
19. SPENCER, M.B. 2006. Phenomenological variant of ecological systems theory (PVEST): a human development synthesis applicable to diverse individuals and groups. *In* Theoretical Models of Human Development. Volume 1 of Handbook of Child Psychology. Sixth ed. R.M. Lerner, Vol. Ed., W. Damon & R.M. Lerner, Editors-in-chief.: 829–893. Wiley. Hoboken, NJ.
20. THELEN, E. & L.B. SMITH. 2006. Dynamic systems theories. *In* Theoretical models of human development. Volume 1 of Handbook of Child Psychology. Sixth edition. R.M. Lerner, Vol. Ed., W. Damon & R.M. Lerner, Editors-in-chief.: 258–312. Wiley. Hoboken, NJ.
21. OVERTON, W.F. 2006. Developmental psychology: philosophy, concepts, methodology. *In* Theoretical Models of Human Development. Volume 1 of Handbook of Child Psychology. Sixth edition. R.M. Lerner, Vol. Ed., W. Damon & R.M. Lerner, Editors-in-chief.: 18–88. Wiley. Hoboken, NJ.
22. MASTEN, A.S., K. BURT & J.D. COATSWORTH. 2006. Competence and psychopathology in development. *In* Developmental Psychopathology, Vol 3, Risk, Disorder and Psychopathology. Second edition. D. Cicchetti & D. Cohen, Eds.: 696– 738. Wiley. New York.
23. MASTEN, A.S. & A.H. GEWIRTZ. 2006. Vulnerability and resilience in early child development. *In* Handbook of Early Childhood Development. K. McCartney & D. Phillips, Eds.: 22–43. Blackwell. Malden, MA.
24. MASTEN, A.S. & A. SHAFFER. 2006. How families matter in child development: reflections from research on risk and resilience. *In* Families Count: Effects on Child and Adolescent Development. A. Clarke-Stewart & J. Dunn, Eds. Cambridge University Press. Cambridge.

25. STEINBERG, L., *et al.* 2006. Psychopathology in adolescence: integrating affective neuroscience with the study of context. *In* Developmental psychopathology, Vol. 2: Developmental Neuroscience. Second edition. D. Cicchetti & D. Cohen, Eds.:710–741. Wiley. New York.
26. BRANDTSTÄDTER, J. 2006. Action perspectives on human development. *In* Theoretical Models of Human Development. Volume 1 of Handbook of Child Psychology. Sixth edition. R.M. Lerner, Vol. Ed., W. Damon & R.M. Lerner, Editors-in-chief.: 516–568. Wiley. Hoboken, NJ.
27. LERNER, R.M. 2005. Promoting positive youth development: theoretical and empirical bases. White Paper Prepared for the Workshop on the Science of Adolescent Health and Development, National Research Council/Institute of Medicine. National Academies of Science, Washington, DC, September.
28. LERNER, R.M., *et al.* 2005. Positive youth development, participation in community youth development programs, and community contributions of fifth grade adolescents: Findings from the first wave of the 4-H Study of Positive Youth Development. J. Early Adol. **25:** 17–71.
29. HIRSCH, J. 2004. Uniqueness, diversity, similarity, repeatability, and heritability. *In* Nature and Nurture: The Complex Interplay of Genetic and Environmental Influences on Human Behavior and Development. C. Garcia Coll, E. Bearer & R.M. Lerner, Eds.:127–138. Lawrence Erlbaum Associates. Mahwah, NJ.
30. LERNER, R.M. 1984. On the nature of human plasticity. Cambridge University Press. New York.
31. BENSON, P.L., P.C. SCALES, S.F. HAMILTON & A. SESMA, JR. 2006. Positive youth development: theory, research, and applications. *In* Theoretical Models of Human Development. Volume 1 of Handbook of Child Psychology. Sixth edition. R.M. Lerner, Vol. Ed., W. Damon & R.M. Lerner, Editors-in-chief.: 894–941. Wiley. Hoboken, NJ.
32. THEOKAS, C. & R.M. LERNER. 2006. Observed ecological assets in families, schools, and neighborhoods: conceptualization, measurement and relations with positive and negative developmental outcomes. Appl. Dev. Sci. **10:** 61–74.
33. DAMON, W. 2004. What is positive youth development? Ann. Am. Acad. Pol. Social Sci. **591:** 13–24.
34. ECCLES, J.S. & J.A. GOOTMAN, Eds. 2002. Community Programs to Promote Youth Development/Committee on Community-Level Programs for Youth. National Academy Press, Washington DC.
35. FLOYD, D.T. & L. MCKENNA. 2003. National youth serving organizations in the United States: Contributions to civil society. *In* Handbook of Applied Developmental Science: Promoting Positive Child, Adolescent, and Family Development Through Research, Policies, and Programs: Vol. 3. Promoting Positive Youth and Family Development: Community Systems, Citizenship, and Civil Society. D. Wertlieb, F. Jacobs & R.M. Lerner, Eds.: 11–26. Sage. Thousand Oaks, CA.
36. PITTMAN, K., M. IRBY & T. FERBER. 2001. Unfinished business: further reflections on a decade of promoting youth development. *In* Trends in Youth Development: Visions, Realities and Challenges. P.L. Benson & K.J. Pittman, Eds.:4–50. Kluwer. Norwell, MA.
37. WHEELER, W. 2003. Youth leadership for development: Civic activism as a component of youth development programming and a strategy for strengthening civil society. *In* Handbook of Applied Developmental Science: Vol. 2. Enhancing the

Life Chances of Youth and Families: Contributions of Programs, Policies, and Service Systems. F. Jacobs, D. Wertlieb & R.M. Lerner, Eds.: 491–505. Sage. Thousand Oaks, CA.

38. CUMMINGS, E. 2003. Foreword. *In* Promoting Positive Youth and Family Development: Community Systems, Citizenship, and Civil Society: Vol. 2. Handbook of Applied Developmental Science: Enhancing the Life Changes of Youth and Families: Contributions f Programs, Policies, and Service Systems. F. Jacobs, D. Wertlieb & R.M. Lerner, Eds.: ix–xi. Sage. Thousand Oaks, CA.
39. GORE, A. 2003. Foreword. *In* Developmental Assets and Asset-Building Communities: Implications for Research, Policy, and Practice. R.M. Lerner & P.L. Benson, Eds.: xi–xii. Kluwer. Norwell, MA.
40. ROTH, J.L. & J. BROOKS-GUNN. 2003. What is a youth development program? Identification and defining principles. *In* Handbook of Applied Developmental Science: Vol. 2. Enhancing the Life Chances of Youth and Families: Contributions of Programs, Policies, and Service Systems. F. Jacobs, D. Wertlieb & R.M. Lerner, Eds.:197–223. Sage. Thousand Oaks, CA.
41. ROTH, J.L. & J. BROOKS-GUNN. 2003. What exactly is a youth development program? Answers from research and practice. App. Dev. Sci. **7:** 94–111.
42. HIRSCH, B. 2005. A place to call home: After-school programs for urban youth. Teachers College Press. Washington, DC: Am. Psychol. Assoc. New York.
43. MAHONEY, J., R. LARSON & J. ECCLES, Eds. 2005. Organized activities as contexts of development: extracurricular activities, after-school and community programs. Erlbaum. Hillsdale, NJ.
44. JELICIC, H., D. BOBEK, E. PHELPS, R.M. LERNER & J.V. LERNER. 2007. Using positive youth development to predict contribution and risk behaviors in early adolescence: Findings from the first two waves of the 4-H Study of Positive Youth Development. Int. J. Behav. Dev. In press.
45. ZIMMERMAN, *et al.* 2006. Changes in Positive Youth Development (PYD) Across Early Adolescence: Initial Findings of the First Three Waves of the 4-H Study. Presented at the Biennial Conference of Society for Research on Adolescence. San Francisco, CA, March 24.
46. GESTSDOTTIR, S. & R.M. LERNER. 2007. Intentional self-regulation and positive youth development in early adolescence: findings from the 4-H Study of Positive Youth Development. Dev. Psych. In press.
47. ERIKSON, E.H. 1968. Identity, youth, and crisis. Norton. New York.
48. FREUD, A. 1969. Adolescence as a developmental disturbance. *In* Adolescence. G. Caplan & S. Lebovici Eds.: 5–10. Basic Books. New York.
49. HALL, G.S. 1904. Adolescence: Its Psychology and its Relations to Psychology. Anthropology, Sociology, Sex, Crime, Religion, and Education. Appleton. New York.

Risk, Resilience, and Gene × Environment Interactions in Rhesus Monkeys

STEPHEN J. SUOMI

Laboratory of Comparative Ethology, National Institute of Child Health & Human Development, National Institutes of Health, Bethesda, Maryland, USA

ABSTRACT: Recent research with both humans and rhesus monkeys has provided compelling evidence of gene–environment (GxE) interactions throughout development. For example, a specific polymorphism ("short" allele) in the promoter region of the serotonin transporter (5-HTT) gene is associated with deficits in neurobehavioral functioning during infancy and in poor control of aggression and low serotonin metabolism throughout juvenile and adolescent development in monkeys who were reared with peers but not in monkeys who were reared with their mothers and peers during infancy. In contrast, monkeys possessing the "long" allele of the 5-HTT gene exhibit normal neurobehavioral functioning, control of aggression, and serotonin metabolism regardless of their early social rearing history. One interpretation of these GxE interaction data is that the "long" 5-HTT allele somehow confers resiliency to adverse early attachment relationships on those individuals who carry it ("good genes"). An alternative interpretation of the same data is that secure attachment relationships somehow confer resiliency to individuals who carry alleles that may otherwise increase their risk for adverse developmental outcomes ("maternal buffering"). These two interpretations are not mutually exclusive, but the difference in their respective implications for developing prevention and even intervention strategies is considerable. Moreover, the allelic variation seen in certain genes in rhesus monkeys and humans but apparently not in other primate species may actually contribute to their remarkable adaptability and resilience at the species level.

KEYWORDS: rhesus monkeys; fear; aggression; GxE interactions; species differences

Address for correspondence: Stephen J. Suomi, Ph.D., Laboratory of Comparative Ethology, NICHD, NIH 6705 Rockledge Drive, Suite 8030, Bethesda, MD 20892-7971. Voice: 301-496-9550; fax: 301-496-0630.
e-mail: ss148k@nih.gov

Ann. N.Y. Acad. Sci. 1094: 52–62 (2006). © 2006 New York Academy of Sciences.
doi: 10.1196/annals.1376.006

INTRODUCTION

Why are some individuals more resilient than others? In study after study of the emotional, psychological, and physiological sequelae of trauma and other forms of stress, one basic finding stands out: There are dramatic differences among individuals of all ages and in every culture in the manner in which they respond to stress, be it acute or chronic. On the one hand, even in the face of an overwhelming disaster such as the Pacific tsunami of 2004 or Hurricane Katrina of 2005 many individuals with direct exposure to traumatic events exhibit only minimal immediate effects on their biological, psychological, and emotional functioning and subsequently show scant evidence of any lasting consequences. Many children subjected to the chronic stress of being raised in socially impoverished orphanages have shown remarkable recovery of social, cognitive, and biological functions following adoption into middle- and upper-class families. On the other hand, some individuals consistently respond to even the slightest changes in their physical or social environment with profound emotional, psychological, and physiological distress that often reappears without any obvious subsequent provocation. What are the factors that underlie such dramatic individual differences in response to stress? Are they largely the product of differences in the individuals' genetic heritage, differences in their social and emotional experiences early in life, differences in their current biological and psychological makeup—or some combination of these factors?

Similar questions can be raised about nonhuman primates. This chapter will examine factors contributing to resiliency in rhesus monkeys (*Macaca mulatta*). There are dramatic differences among rhesus monkeys in their behavioral and biological responses to environmental stress throughout development, and numerous studies have identified both genetic and environmental factors that clearly contribute to such individual differences. Recent research has demonstrated that such factors can actually *interact* to shape individual developmental trajectories. The chapter will review some of the relevant findings regarding these gene–environment (GxE) interactions and discuss some implications of those findings from a comparative perspective.

Over the past two decades, my colleagues and I have been studying the development of individual differences in personality or temperament—and the biological substrates that apparently underlie such differences—in the rhesus monkeys we maintain in large social groups at the National Institutes of Health Animal Center (NIHAC) in rural Maryland. During this time we have found that approximately 20% of the monkeys growing up in these naturalistic settings (as well as at two long-term field sites) consistently react to novel, mildly stressful social situations with unusually fearful and anxious-like behavior, accompanied by prolonged hypothalamic-pituitary-adrenal (HPA) axis activation, as indexed by significant and extended elevations of both salivary and plasma cortisol.[1] Another 5–10% of the monkeys growing up in these naturalistic settings are likely to exhibit impulsive and/or inappropriately aggressive patterns of behavioral response under similar circumstances; monkeys in this latter subgroup also show chronic deficits in serotonin metabolism, as indexed by unusually low cerebrospinal fluid (CSF) concentrations of the primary central serotonin metabolite 5-hydroxyindoleacetic acid (5-HIAA).[2]

Development of Individual Differences in Stress Reactivity

Rhesus monkeys growing up in naturalistic settings normally spend virtually all of their first month of life in intimate physical contact with their biological mother, during which time a strong and enduring attachment bond is established between mother and infant. In their second month these infants begin to explore their immediate physical and social environment, using their mother as a "secure base" from which to launch brief exploratory ventures but remaining in physical contact with her at most other times. In the weeks and months that follow the infants spend increasing amounts of time away from their mothers and begin to establish relationships with other members of their social group, most notably with same-aged peers. Throughout the rest of their childhood most juveniles spend several hours each day in active social play with these peers. Virtually every social behavior that will be important for normal adult functioning is developed, practiced, and perfected during the course of peer play, most notably behaviors leading to successful reproduction, as well as the socialization of aggression, which usually first appears in each monkey's behavioral repertoire between 4 and 6 months of age.[3]

Both excessively fearful and excessively aggressive monkeys tend to show significant deviations from this species-normative pattern of social development, beginning very early in life. Fearful infants start leaving their mother to explore their environment at a later age than the rest of their birth cohort, and they continue to exhibit low rates of exploratory behavior in subsequent weeks and months. They also seem reluctant to interact with monkeys other than their mother, and as a result they tend to spend less time playing with peers than others in their birth cohort throughout their childhood years.[4] When these fearful young monkeys become physically separated from their mothers, either in natural settings during the annual breeding season, when females typically leave their social group for short periods to mate with different males, or in the course of laboratory simulations of such maternal separations, they consistently exhibit far greater behavioral distress, accompanied by higher and more prolonged elevations of cortisol, than the rest of their birth cohort.[5] Moreover, such differences in adrenocortical response to separation are predictive of differential responses to other situations later in life. For example, Fahlke and colleagues found that monkey infants who exhibited highly elevated levels of plasma cortisol following brief separations at 6 months of age subsequently consumed significantly more alcohol in a "happy hour" situation when they were 5 years of age than did monkeys whose 6-month cortisol responses were more moderate.[6] Heritability analyses have demonstrated that these individual differences in behavioral and adrenocortical response to separation have a significant genetic component.[7,8]

Overly aggressive infants, especially males, typically display their aggressive tendencies initially in the context of social play with peers. Unlike their fearful counterparts, these youngsters readily respond to play invitations from other monkeys, and they often initiate rough-and-tumble play bouts themselves. However, their rough-and-tumble play bouts with peers often turn out to be *too* rough, escalating into episodes of actual physical aggression with their play partners. Not surprisingly, other monkeys in the social group soon learn to avoid most interactions with these aggressive young males, and as a result they become increasingly isolated socially, even though they are continually in the presence of potential playmates.[9] CSF samples collected from free-ranging juvenile males have revealed a significant negative relationship between the incidence of aggression in the context of play and 5-HIAA concentrations, that is, the most aggressive males tend to have the lowest CSF 5-HIAA concentrations.[10] Laboratory studies have demonstrated that individual differences in CSF 5-HIAA are remarkably stable from infancy to early adulthood in both male and female subjects[11,12] and, as was the case for adrenocortical responses to social separation, they are also highly heritable.[13] Other laboratory studies have demonstrated that like their highly fearful counterparts, impulsively aggressive monkeys consume excessive amounts of alcohol in a "happy hour" situation as adolescents and young adults.[14]

Effects of Differential Social Rearing Environments

The individual differences in behavioral and biological responses to environmental challenges described above were all observed in rhesus monkeys growing up either in naturalistic environments or in captive settings that provided unrestricted access to both their biological mothers and same-aged peers (MP-rearing). However, other rhesus monkeys in our colony at the NIHAC have been reared from birth in the absence of any access to their biological mothers or any other adults but in the continuous presence of 3–4 other like-reared peers after an initial month in our neonatal nursery. After 6 months of such peer-only (PO) rearing, these infants have typically been placed in large social groups containing other same-aged PO-reared monkeys in addition to MP-reared age mates; both the PO- and MP-reared subjects have usually remained in these large social groups until puberty.

PO-reared monkeys rapidly develop strong attachment-like bonds with one another within days of being placed together following their initial month of nursery rearing. However, these "hyperattachments" tend to be essentially nonfunctional, if not outright dysfunctional, largely because a peer is not nearly as good as a mother—even a relatively nonresponsive or punitive mother—in either providing a secure base for exploration or soothing an infant whenever it becomes frightened or otherwise upset.[15] Perhaps as a result, PO-reared infants tend to explore little and play less than their MP-reared counterparts during their first six months. What few play bouts they do experience with one another tend to be rudimentary in nature and short-lived in duration, far less complex than routine play bouts among MP-reared monkeys of comparable age. PO-reared monkeys as a group also exhibit more extreme behavioral and adrenocortical responses to social separation at 6 months of age.[16]

In addition, PO-reared monkeys display many of the same behavioral and serotonergic characteristics that differentiate overly impulsive and aggressive monkeys growing up in naturalistic settings from others in their birth cohort. Perhaps because they are essentially experiencing play deprivation even though they are in the continuous presence of potential playmates, as they grow older they become increasingly aggressive, far more so than most of their MP-reared fellow group members.[17] Importantly, they also consistently exhibit significantly lower CSF 5-HIAA concentrations than MP-reared monkeys from early infancy to early adulthood.[18,19] In addition, as adolescents and young adults they consume more alcohol than MP-reared subjects in a "happy hour" situation.[20] In sum, PO-reared monkeys exhibit many of the same behavioral and biological patterns of response to environmental challenge and social stress that are shown by excessively fearful monkeys and overly impulsive and aggressive monkeys growing up in naturalistic settings. Clearly, at least for rhesus monkeys, early social experiences such as maternal deprivation can have significant and long-lasting effects on behavioral and biological development over and above any contributions to individual differences attributable to heritable factors.

GxE Interactions

In recent years there has been increasing interest in the study of possible GxE interactions, especially in the face of reports such as those of Caspi, Moffitt, and their colleagues, who followed a large sample of young adults prospectively from early childhood onward. Those investigators demonstrated convincingly that allelic variation in the promoter region of the serotonin transporter (5-HTT) gene was associated with significant differences in the number of depressive symptoms observed in these young adults—but *only* if they also had experienced childhood neglect or abuse or were experiencing high levels of concurrent stress.[21] Rhesus monkeys have essentially the same 5-HTT gene and functional polymorphism as do humans.[22] We have recently been able to genotype most monkeys in our colony at the NIHAC, and as a result we have been able to search for possible GxE interactions involving differential early experience (MP- vs. PO-rearing) and allelic variation in the 5-HTT gene.

To date we have found such interactions to be ubiquitous. Monkeys carrying the "short" allele of the 5-HTT gene show delayed early neurobiological development, impaired serotonergic functioning, and excessive aggression, HPA reactivity, and alcohol consumption as they are growing up—*but only if they have been PO-reared.* MP-reared monkeys carrying the "short" 5-HIAA allele exhibit species-normative patterns of early neurobiological development, serotonin metabolism, levels of aggression, and HPA reactivity following separation comparable to those shown by both MP- and PO-reared carrying the "long" 5-HTT allele.[23–26] In addition, MP-reared adolescent and young adult monkeys carrying the "short" 5-HTT allele actually consume *less* alcohol than their MP-reared counterparts carrying the "long" 5-HTT, raising the intriguing possibility that having the functionally less efficient 5-HTT allele may represent a significant risk factor for PO-reared monkeys but may actually be a protective factor for their MP-reared counterparts carrying the same 5-HTT allele.[27] Other studies examining possible GxE interactions involving MP- and PO-reared monkeys carrying functionally different alleles of the MAO-A gene and various measures of aggression have yielded findings paralleling the pattern of GxE interactions involving MAO-A allelic variation and presence/absence of a history of childhood neglect/abuse reported by Caspi and colleagues in the above-mentioned sample of young adults studied prospectively since early childhood.[29,30]

Although it seems apparent that significant GxE interactions involving the 5-HTT gene and differential early experience do occur and are associated with different long-term outcomes for a variety of behavioral and biological measures in both rhesus monkeys and humans, the demonstration of such interactions has been largely statistical to date and hence subject to multiple interpretations. An interpretation initially put forward by Caspi *et al.* for the MAO-A polymorphism is essentially that the more efficient allele "protected" individuals who carried it from possible effects on aggressive behavior stemming early adverse experiences of childhood neglect and/or abuse,[30] that is, a "good" gene offered protection from a "bad" environment. An equally plausible interpretation of a similar pattern of GxE interactions involving the 5-HTT polymorphism and differential early social rearing for a variety of measures of behavioral and biological functioning in rhesus monkeys is essentially that MP-rearing "buffers" individuals carrying the less efficient allele from developing the aberrant patterns exhibited by PO-reared monkeys carrying the same allele,[31] that is, a "good" environment can protect individuals carrying a "bad" gene from deleterious developmental outcomes.

It can be argued that these apparently competing interpretations of the same or similar data sets are not necessarily mutually exclusive, and indeed I believe that different developmental processes representing both interpretations can be taking place in the same individual, even during the same periods of development. Definitive resolution of this potential conflict of interpretation awaits further empirical evidence regarding the actual behavioral and biological process that might underlie such statistical interactions. Some relevant evidence is already beginning to be reported. For example, Meaney, Szyff, and colleagues have demonstrated that differential maternal licking and grooming of rat pups during the second postnatal week can actually alter gene expression in the pups' brains via demethalation processes, with consequences that are not only life-long but actually transmitted to the next generation of offspring.[32] Given such findings, the possibility that specific early social experiences can similarly alter gene expression in primates no longer seems particularly far-fetched. If true, this could have enormous implications for the development of strategies for prevention of adverse outcomes in individuals carrying the less efficient allele of these and other "candidate" genes. At the very least, these recent findings regarding GxE interactions should provide important insights regarding the issue of individual difference in resiliency in the face of experiences with acute and chronic stress in primates, human and nonhuman alike.

A Comparative Perspective

Clearly, there are *both* specific genetic *and* environmental factors that can put individuals at risk for developing adverse responses to environmental stress and challenge, often with long-term consequences. On the other hand, it seems increasingly likely that individual differences in resiliency to such environmental adversity represent the product of complex interactions among multiple genes and characteristics of the physical and social environments within which development takes place. Identifying, characterizing, and understanding the basis for such complex interactions certainly represents a considerable—even daunting—challenge for future research endeavors.

Nevertheless, such endeavors may well be warranted. To put the above-described GxE results from studies of rhesus monkeys and humans into a broader comparative perspective, consider some recent findings regarding the 5-HTT and MAO-A genes carried by other members of the *Macaca* genus. Wendland *et al.*[33] characterized the 5-HTT gene in rhesus monkeys and six other species of macaques. To our considerable surprise, we found that in *none* of these other species was there any allelic variability in the promoter region of the 5-HTT gene. Instead, all of the samples for each species were homozygous for a specific repeat number in that region: Pigtail (*M. nemestrina*), stumptail (*M. arctoides*), Tonkenean (*M. tonkeana)*, and crab-eating (*M. fasicularis*) macaques all were homozygous for the "long" rhesus monkey 5-HTT allele, whereas Barbary macaques (*M. silvanus*) all had an "extra-long" version of this gene and all Tibetan macaques (*M. tibetana*) sampled had an "extra-short" (fewest repeats) 5-HTT promoter region.

Interestingly, there appeared to be a systematic relationship between number of repeats in this region and relative aggressivity at the species level: whereas

Barbary, Tonkenean, stumptail, pigtail, and crab-eating macaques are all generally thought to be considerably less aggressive than rhesus monkeys,[34] a recent field study of Tibetan macaques suggests that this species may be even more aggressive than rhesus monkeys.[35]

But perhaps of potentially greater significance is the finding that *none* of the samples obtained from these other macaque species revealed *any* functional polymorphisms in the 5-HTT gene readily apparent in both humans and rhesus monkeys—nor have any comparable functional 5-HTT polymorphisms been reported for any of the baboon or anthropoid ape species. A similar situation seemingly exists for the MAO-A gene: functional polymorphisms in the promoter region of this gene have been found in humans and rhesus monkeys but to date not in any of the other aforementioned species.[36] What other characteristics might these species' differences in the presence/absence of polymorphisms in these and other genes be related to—what is it about humans and rhesus monkeys that differs from these other primate species?

One characteristic shared by humans and rhesus monkeys—but not these other species—is that they are two of the very few "weed" species of primates.[37] They can live in an extraordinarily wide range of physical range of physical habitats and social environments, and when moved into new settings, more often than not they flourish and actually expand their initial founder populations, unlike all of the other aforementioned species (and most other species of primates).[37] So, to take an admittedly speculative leap, perhaps one of the factors underlying the relative adaptive "success" of both humans and rhesus monkeys derives not from some sort of exquisite genetic specialization but instead from more general genetic *variation*. Consider the truism that there can be no GxE interactions in the absence of any genetic variability. Maybe—just maybe—one of the secrets to the remarkable resiliency shown at the species level by rhesus monkeys and ourselves alike could actually be genetic *diversity*.

SUMMARY

Like humans, rhesus monkeys exhibit striking individual differences in their reactions to environmental stress and challenge. Some rhesus monkeys are excessively fearful in response to changes in their environment throughout development; others are overly impulsive and aggressive. It is possible to identify both genetic and environmental factors that contribute to these different response patterns, but recent evidence suggests that GxE interactions may actually be at least as important in shaping individual developmental trajectories in this species, possibly through mechanisms by which specific aspects of the environment influence the expression of specific genes at specific times during development. Finally, because GxE interactions require genetic variation at the species level in order to take place, the fact that rhesus monkeys—and humans—apparently possess greater allelic variability in certain candidate genes than many other primate species may in fact contribute to their remarkable resilience and adaptive success relative to other primates.

ACKNOWLEDGMENTS

The research summarized in this report was supported by funds from the Division of Intramural Research, National Institute of Child Health & Human Development, National Institutes of Health, DHHS.

REFERENCES

1. SUOMI, S.J. 1991a. Up-tight and laid-back monkeys: individual differences in the response to social challenges. *In* Plasticity of Development. S. Brauth, W. Hall & R. Dooling, Eds.: 27–56. MIT Press. Cambridge, MA.
2. SUOMI, S.J. 2000. A biobehavioral perspective on developmental psychopathology: excessive aggression and serotonergic dysfunction in monkeys. *In* Handbook of Developmental Psychopathology (2nd edition). A.S. Sameroff, M. Lewis & S. Miller, Eds.: 237–256. Plenum. New York.
3. SUOMI, S.J. 1999. Attachment in rhesus monkeys. *In* Handbook of Attachment: Theory, Research, and Clinical Applications. J. Cassidy & P. Shaver, Eds.: 181–197. Guilford. New York, NY.
4. SUOMI, S.J. 1991a. Op. cit.
5. SUOMI, S.J. 1991b. Primate separation models of affective disorders. *In* Neurobiology of Learning, Emotion, and Affect. J. Madden, Ed.: 195–214. Raven. New York.
6. FAHLKE, C, J. *et al.* 2000. Rearing experiences and stress-induced plasma cortisol as risk factors for excessive alcohol consumption in nonhuman primates. Alcoholism: Clin. Exp. Res. **24:** 644–650.
7. SCANLAN, J.S. 1988. Continuity of stress responsivity in infant monkeys (*Macaca* mulatta): state, hormonal, dominance, and genetic status. Ph.D. thesis, University of Wisconsin, Madison, WI.
8. WILLIAMSON, D.E. *et al.* 2003. Heritability of fearful-anxious endophenotypes in infant rhesus macaques: a preliminary report. Biol. Psychiatry **53:** 284–291.
9. SUOMI, S.J. 2000. Op. cit.
10. HIGLEY, J.D. *et al.* 1992. Cerebrospinal fluid moanime metabolite and adrenal correlates of aggression in free-ranging monkeys. Arch. Gen. Psychiatry **49:** 436–444.
11. HIGLEY, J.D., S.J. SUOMI & M. LINOILLA. 1992. A longitudinal assessment of CSF monoamine metabolites and plasma cortisol concentrations in young rhesus monkeys. Biol. Psychiatry **32:** 127–145.
12. HIGLEY, J.D. *et al.* 1996. Stability of interindividual differences in serotonin function and its relationship to severe aggression and competent social behavior in rhesus macaque females. Neuropsychopharmacology **14:** 67–76.

13. HIGLEY, J.D. *et al.* 1993. Paternal and maternal genetic and environmental contributions to CSF monoamine metabolites in thesus monkeys (*Macaca mulatta*). Arch. Gen. Psychiatry **50:** 615–623.
14. HIGLEY, J.D. *et al.* 1991. A new nonhuman primate model of alcohol abuse: effects of early experience, personality, and stress on alcohol consumption. Proc. Natl. Acad. Sci. USA **88:** 7261–7265.
15. SUOMI, S.J. 1999. Op. cit.
16. SUOMI, S.J. 1997. Early determinants of behaviour: evidence from primate studies. Brit. Med. Bull. **53:** 170–184.
17. SUOMI, S.J. 2000. Op. cit.
18. HIGLEY, J.D., S.J. SUOMI & M. LINNOILA. 1992. op. cit.
19. SHANNON, C. *et al.* 2005. Maternal absence and stability of individual differences in CSF 5-HIAA concentrations in rhesus monkey infants. Am. J. Psychiatry **162:** 1658–1666.
20. HIGLEY, J.D. *et al.* 1991. Op. cit.
21. CASPI, A. *et al.* 2003. Influences of life stress on depression: moderation by a polymorphism in the 5-HTT gene. Science **301:** 386–389.
22. LESCH, K.P. *et al.* 1997. The 5-HT transporter gene-linked polymorphic region (5-HTTPR) in evolutionary perspective: alternative biallelic variation in rhesus monkeys. J. Neural Transm. **104:** 1259–1266.
23. CHAMPOUX, M. *et al.* 2002. Serotonin transporter gene polymorphism, differential early rearing, and behavior in rhesus monkey neonates. Mol. Psychiatry **7:** 1058–1063.
24. BENNETT, A.J. *et al.* 2002. Early experience and serotonin transporter gene variation interact to influence primate CNS function. Mol. Psychiatry **7:** 118–122.
25. BARR, C.S. *et al.* 2003. The utility of the non-human primate model for studying gene by environment interactions in behavioral research. Genes Brain Behav. **2:** 336–340.
26. BARR, C.S. *et al.* 2004. Rearing condition and rh5-HTTLPR interact to influence LHPA-axis response to stress in infant macaques. Biol. Psychiatry **55:** 733–738.
27. BENNETT, A.J. *et al.* 1998. Serotonin transporter gene variation, CSF 5-HIAA concentrations, and alcohol-related aggression in rhesus monkeys (*Macaca mulatta*). Am. J. Primatol. **45:** 168–169.
28. NEWMAN, T.K. *et al.* 2005. Monoamine oxidase A gene promoter polymorphism and infant rearing experience interact to influence aggression and injuries in rhesus monkeys. Biol. Psychiatry **57:** 167–172.
29. CASPI, A. *et al.* 2002. Role of genotype in the cycle of violence in maltreated children. Science **297:** 851–854.
30. CASPI, A. *et al.* 2003. Op. cit.
31. SUOMI, S.J. 2005. How gene-environment interactions shape the development of impulsive aggression in rhesus monkeys. *In* Developmental Psychobiology of Aggression. D.M. Stoff & E.J. Sussman, Eds.: 252–268. Cambridge University Press. New York.
32. CHAMPAGNE, F.A. *et al.* 2006. Maternal care regulates methylation of the estrogen receptor alpha 1b promoter and estrogen receptor alpha expression in the medial preoptic area of female offspring. Endocrinology **147:** 2909–2915.
33. WENDLAND, J. *et al.* 2005. Differential functional variability of serotonin transporter and monoamine oxidase A genes in macaque species displaying contrasting levels of aggression-related behavior. Behav. Genet. **36:** 163–172.

34. THIERRY, B. 2000. Covaration of conflict management patterns across macaque species. *In* Natural Conflict Resolution. F. Aureli & F.B.M. de Waal, Eds.: 106–128. University of California Press. Berkeley.
35. BERMAN, C.M., C.S. IONICA, Li. JIN-HUA. 2004. Dominance style among Macaca thibetana on Mt. Hangshan, China. Int. J. Primatol. **25:** 214–227.
36. WENDLAND, J. *et al.* 2005. Structural variation of the monamine oxidase A gene promoter repeat polymorphism in nonhuman primates. Genes Brain Behav. **5:** 40–45.
37. RICHARD, A.F., F.J. GOLDSTEIN & R.E. DEWAR. 1989. Weed macaques: the evolutionary implications of macaque feeding ecology. Int. J. Primatol. **19:** 569–594.

Cumulative, Human Capital, and Psychological Risk in the Context of Early Intervention

Links with IQ at Ages 3, 5, and 8

PAMELA KLEBANOV[a] AND JEANNE BROOKS-GUNN[b]

[a]*Center for Research on Child Wellbeing Princeton University, Princeton, New Jersey, USA*

[b]*National Center for Children and Families, Columbia University, New York City, New York, USA*

ABSTRACT: This article examines the effects of risks for a sample of low birth weight children (2,001 to 2,500 g and family income-to-needs at 250% of the poverty threshold or less; $n = 228$) using data from the Infant Health and Development Program (IHDP, an experiment testing the efficacy of early intervention). Cognitive test scores (IQ) are assessed at 3, 5, and 8 years of age. Links with risks at each age point are examined using three different models—cumulative, human capital, and psychological risks. Similar decrements in IQ scores are found at all ages for the cumulative and human capital models but not for the psychological risk model. Treatment effects are found at 3 years of age (when the intervention ended) for all levels of risk and for all models. Sustained effects of the treatment were found at 5 and 8 years of age for children with moderate levels of human capital risk but were not found for any levels of psychological risk. Implications for early childhood intervention programs are discussed.

KEYWORDS: cumulative risk; low birth weight; early childhood education; IQ

INTRODUCTION

Risks are often broadly defined as biological and environmental conditions that increase the likelihood of negative outcomes. A variety of factors have been investigated, with respect to possible links with child and adolescent health, development, and education. Often, researchers have categorized risk factors

Address for correspondence: Jeanne Brooks-Gunn, National Center for Children and Families, Teachers College, Columbia University, New York City, NY 10027. Voice: 212-678-3369; fax: 212-678-3676. e-mail: brooks-gunn@columbia.edu

Ann. N.Y. Acad. Sci. 1094: 63–82 (2006).
doi: 10.1196/annals.1376.007

as indicative of biological, economic, human capital, demographic, psychological, and parenting risk conditions. Biological factors that often have been considered risks include children's low birth weight, intrauterine growth retardation, early hospitalizations, and low Apgar scores. Economic factors include family income-to-needs ratios, persistent poverty, and assets. Human capital includes parental education, employment, and welfare receipt. Demographic factors include family structure, number of children, and maternal age. Psychological factors include parental mental health, stress, and social support. Parenting factors include knowledge about child rearing, parenting practices (for example, harsh, responsive, detached, or intrusive behaviors), provision of stimulating activities, supervision, and monitoring.[1]

Cumulative risk models originated in the adult literature on morbidity and mortality, with accumulating risks increasing the likelihood of negative outcomes.[2] Research with adults continues on many fronts, including whether individual risks are more important than cumulative risks in predicting outcomes; why low socioeconomic status (SES) and cumulative risks are associated with negative outcomes in adults (SES usually comprises several risk factors in the economic and human capital categories); whether changes in SES or risk alter the likelihood of negative outcomes; whether SES and risk early in life are more or less important in predicting illness in adulthood when compared to SES and risk factors present later in life; and whether relative or absolute indicators of SES and risk are more predictive of negative outcomes.

The work on children has followed a similar trajectory. However, less is known about how risk factors are linked with child and adolescent outcomes than with adult outcomes. In part this is because so much of the adult literature is focused on health; children, by and large, are relatively healthy (although see Case & Paxson, 2000[3]). More work has focused on SES and risk in terms of educational, developmental, and behavioral outcomes (cognitive test scores, achievement, anxiety, juvenile delinquency, depression, and substance use). These lines of work have a 30-year history, although again, many of the questions outlined in the preceding paragraph have not been examined in any detail.

In this article, four issues that are related to the association of risk factors and well-being during childhood are explored using the Infant Health and Development Program (IHDP) data. First, we look at the accumulation of risk factors (nine factors) to see if the number of risk factors is linked to IQ scores similarly at three ages—3, 5, and 8 years. It is expected that similar slopes for more risk and lower IQ scores will be seen at all three ages.[4] Second, we explore associations between two types of risks—human capital and psychological (three of each type)—to see if the two are comparable in predicting lower IQ scores. It is hypothesized that human capital risks will be more important than psychological risks; we expect the primary of human capital risks to be as large at age 8 as at 3 years. This premise is based on the fact that gaps between lower SES and higher SES children (and black and white children) do not diminish when children start school.[5] Third, the IHDP is an experiment testing the efficacy of the provision of intensive early education and parenting services to children in the first three years of their life. Consequently, it is possible to see whether similar treatment effects are seen for children with few, some, or many risk factors. Literature to date is mixed on this premise.[6] We are able to test whether treatment effects at the end of the IHDP intervention (when the children are 3 years of age) are similar or different based on cumulative risk, as well as to see whether sustained effects of the treatment are conditioned on cumulative risk (as the children were seen when they were 5 and 8 years of age, or 2 and 5 years after the intervention ended). It is expected that sustained treatment effects will not be seen for the children with a high number of risks. Fourth, the same question is asked for the human capital and psychological risks. While treatment effects are expected for both models at the time the intervention ended (3 years of age), it is likely that sustained effects will be seen for moderate levels of human capital risk, but not high levels. It is unclear as to how psychological risk will be associated with intervention effects.

The first research question focuses on cumulative risk, testing whether developmental outcomes can better be predicted by combinations of risk factors than by single risk factors. Sameroff and colleagues[7] used the Rochester Longitudinal Study to examine the cognitive and emotional outcomes of children from families in which a large number had mothers with psychopathology. Maternal psychopathology and family SES were individually important correlates of children's outcomes. However, cumulative risk analyses (10 conditions) explained more of the variance in IQ than the individual risks. The 4-year-old children with no risks scored 2 standard deviations higher on IQ tests than children who were considered high risk (8 or more risk factors). More generally, each risk factor was associated with a decrease of 4 IQ points. Subsequent work has examined whether 1 risk factor was "driving" the results. A cluster analysis of risk factors produced five typologies; however, none of the clusters was associated with worse outcomes for children.[8] Few studies have examined the potential cumulative effects of multiple risks experienced by low birth weight children. In a previous analysis of the IHDP data at 3 years of age, we examined 13 risk conditions, paralleling those used in the Rochester Longitudinal Study.[9] The effects of risk were considered separately for poor families (150% or less of the poverty threshold) and nonpoor families. As expected, risk factors were more frequent for poor families than nonpoor families (35% of poor families had 6 or more risks, compared to only 5% of nonpoor families; 2% of poor families had 0 risks, compared to 19% of nonpoor families). Higher risk was associated with lower IQ scores at 3 years of age. Poor and nonpoor children functioned similarly in the presence of high risks. However, a 14-point IQ difference was found when risks were low (0 to 1 risk), as the slope for the nonpoor children was steeper than that for the poor children.

In the previous article, all infants were included. Here, the links between IQ and cumulative risk are examined for one of the two groups of low birth weight (LBW) infants in the IHDP. The IHDP was stratified into two weight groups—those 2,000 g or less at birth and those between 2,001 and 2,500 g at birth. The former is termed the lighter LBW and the latter the heavier LBW group and random assignment was based on this stratification. Since our third and fourth research questions have to do with treatment effects and since sustained treatment effects were only seen in the heavier LBW groups overall, the analyses for all three research questions only include this LBW group.[10] In addition, because our earlier work suggested that the slopes for cumulative risk–IQ links differed for poor and nonpoor 3-year-olds, the current analyses only include lower-income families (when the sample is constrained to the heavier LBW group, the sample size for the higher-income families is not large enough to conduct the risk or risk by treatment comparisons). Not only is family income associated with children's cognitive development[11] but poor families experience more risks than nonpoor families. Consequently, risk is sometimes examined separately for lower- and higher-income families[12] In these analyses, families with income-to-needs ratios up to 250% of the poverty line are included. This decision was based on recent research suggesting that families with less than 250% of the poverty threshold are unlikely to make ends meet. Self-sufficiency has been estimated using basic needs budgeting; families in the bottom two quintiles of the nation's income distribution fall into this category. The poverty threshold in the United States is lower than what is used in other Western nations (who use a relative threshold, often based on 50% of the median income in the country at any point in time). Our poverty threshold falls at less than 32% of the median income.

The second research question considers two separate types of risks—human capital and psychological. These models are presented to examine whether either of these two types of risk is driving any overall cumulative risk–IQ links. It is expected that human capital risk factors will be more highly associated with IQ than psychological resources. The logic is as follows: human capital, in particular parental education, is almost always the strongest family-level predictor of child cognitive and academic test scores; this is true throughout childhood and adolescence.[13] It trumps income, family structure, and maternal age as well as more psychologically oriented constructs, such as maternal mental health and social support.[14] Also, our two other indicators of human capital—maternal employment and welfare receipt—are linked to child cognitive outcomes. Welfare receipt is associated with less optimal cognitive outcomes, with this association holding even when parental education and other demographic characteristics are controlled; even when accounting for income, negative links with welfare receipt are found.[15] Employment of low-income mothers can offset some of these negative links.[16] Also, the large numbers of mothers who received welfare in the past and have entered the workforce in the past decade have been studied; no negative influences of working have been found on preschool children of these low-income mothers.[17] We expect, based on this literature, that children whose mothers have high human capital risk (no work, low education, and welfare receipt) will do appreciably worse than children whose mothers have moderate human capital risk (primarily are working but have low education).

The third research question focuses on the intersection of the accumulation of risk factors and effects of an early childhood intervention. The LBW infants and their families in the IHDP received comprehensive and full-time center-based early childhood education in their second 2 years of life and weekly or bimonthly home visits for their first 3 years of life.[18] When the intervention ended, children who received the treatment had significantly higher cognitive test scores than children in the follow-up group at the end of the intervention (when the children were 3 years of age). The effect of the intervention was larger for the heavier than the lighter LBW children (with the effects for the former being 1 standard deviation or more).[19] The children were followed at 5 and 8 years of age, to look for sustained intervention effects. The heavier LBW children in the treatment group had higher IQ and receptive verbal scores at both ages (ranging from 1/5 to 1/3 of a standard deviation),[20] with the effects being even higher for those children who attended the education centers more than 200 days a year[21] and for those children whose mothers, if they had not been offered the intervention, would not have had their children in center-based child care.[22]

Given the large treatment effects at 3 years of age, it is expected that the number of risk factors will not be associated with treatment; that is, no treatment by risk interaction will be found. However, at 5 and 8 years of age, when the treatment effects are smaller, such an interaction may be found. Our expectation is that sustained treatment effects will be more likely to occur in children whose families have a few or a moderate number of risk factors, rather than having many risk factors (remember that all families are lower income). Our thinking is that in the face of a high accumulation of risk factors, children will be less likely to continue to exhibit positive benefits from the intervention.[23] These analyses differ from those that have been done looking at subgroups based on a specific risk factor (such as being a teenage mother, having less than a high school education, being depressed); some, but not all individual risk factors have been associated with outcomes of early intervention programs.[24]

The fourth research question focuses on treatment by risk interactions for the human capital and psychological risk models. The group with high human capital risk is expected not to show sustained effects of the intervention, while the other two groups (low and moderate risk) are likely to benefit from the intervention into elementary school. In fact, one analysis using the state experiments of welfare reform reports stronger treatment effects (on the mothers and on the use of child care) for mothers who have moderate risk.[25] We expect something similar in the IHDP.

When it comes to examining just the psychological risks, our predictions are on less firm ground. Of the relatively few experimental early childhood interventions that have examined differential treatment effects by psychological risk factors, results are mixed. The Elmira Study of the Nurse Home Visiting

Program[26] found that teenage mothers (who are for the most part, unmarried) were most likely to benefit from the programs. They provided more intellectually stimulating and less restrictive home environments and reported fewer behavior problems in their children. In the Memphis Study, also using the Nurse Home Visiting Program, mothers with lower psychological resources (mental health, personal sense of mastery, and intelligence) benefited more from the intervention than those with higher psychological resources. The children of the former group had fewer health care visits for injuries and ingestions and mothers exhibited more positive interactions with their children.[27] Lyons-Ruth and colleagues,[28] in a nonrandomized study, found a significant treatment by maternal depression interaction for children's cognitive test scores. Children of depressed mothers who received the treatment had significantly higher cognitive scores compared to those who did not receive the treatment. Similarly, Barnard and colleagues[29] found that among mothers who had poor social skills, those who received the treatment had more positive mother–child interaction than the mothers who did not receive treatment (for exceptions, see Ceci and Papierno[30] who found enhanced treatment effects for those families who possess greater psychological resources and Klebanov *et al.* who found no interaction between maternal depressive symptoms and treatment effects on children's IQ). Therefore, we are unable to predict if sustained effects will be more or less likely in children whose mothers have fewer psychological resources.

METHODS

The IHDP is an eight-site randomized clinical trial designed to evaluate the efficacy of a comprehensive early-intervention program for LBW premature infants.[31] Infants weighing 2,500 g or less at birth were screened for eligibility if their postconception age between January 7, 1985, and October 9, 1985, was 37 weeks or less and if they were born in one of the eight participating medical institutions (Arkansas at Little Rock, Einstein, Harvard, Miami, Pennsylvania, Texas at Dallas, Washington, and Yale). A total of 985 infants were randomly assigned either to a medical follow-up only (FUO) or to a comprehensive early childhood intervention (INT) group immediately following neonatal hospital discharge. Because of the higher risk associated with lower birth weights, two-thirds of the infants had birth weights 2,000 g or less, and one-third had birth weights between 2,001 and 2,500 g. Infants in both the INT and FUO groups participated in a pediatric follow-up program of periodic medical, developmental, and familial assessments from 40 weeks conception age (the age at which they would have been born if they had not been premature) to 3 years of age (corrected for premature birth). The intervention program, lasting from hospital discharge until 3 years, consisted of home visits (weekly in the first year, biweekly thereafter), child-care services (a minimum of 4 h per day,

5 days per week, from 1 to 3 years), and parent group meetings (bimonthly, from 1 to 3 years). A coordinated educational curriculum of learning games and activities was used both during home visits and at the center.[32] Home visitors also used a problem-solving curriculum with the parents.[33]

Sample

Of the 1,302 infants who met the enrollment criteria, 274 were excluded because consent was refused and 43 withdrew before entry into their assigned group. The remaining 985 infants constituted the primary analysis group. Of the 637 families who had income-to-needs ratios at ages 1 or 2 years of 250% of the poverty line or less, this study focused upon a subsample of 228 families of heavier birth weight children (2,001–2,500 g). The sample was relatively disadvantaged; almost one-half of the mothers were single parents, had less than a high school education, and had been on welfare. The sample was 57% black, 13% Hispanic, and 29% white.

Measures

Individual Risk Factors

The nine risk factors include human capital, demographic, psychological, and parenting conditions that have been associated with adverse child and parent outcomes in the literature. Whenever possible, risk factors were constructed from measures taken when the child was born (i.e., maternal age and education) or the earliest time the measures were taken (i.e., unemployment data and maternal education were obtained during pregnancy; welfare status, maternal mental health, stressful life events, and father absence were all obtained at 1 and 2 years; social support was obtained at 1 and 3 years; number of children in the household was obtained at 3 years). The risk factors, the criterion used for high risk, and the sample composition of the high-risk groups follow:

1. *Human capital risks* included maternal unemployment (47%), welfare receipt (47%), and less than a high school education (45%).
2. *Psychological risks* included mental health, stressful life events, and low social support. Mothers' mental health was evaluated using the General Health Questionnaire at 12 and 24 months (GHQ).[34] The GHQ is a 12-item scale, which taps depression, somatic symptoms, and anxiety. The overall GHQ score was computed, with higher values signifying more distress (range 0 to 32). High risk was defined as having a score higher than the highest 25% (score of 14 or higher). Mother-reported stressful life events were measured at 12 months. Four items tapped personal illness, illness of others in the family, moves of household members

in and out of the household, and residential moves during the year. High risk was defined as score of 2 or higher (44%). Mothers' social support network was measured by six vignettes asking mothers to report sources of monetary, emotional, and child-care support.[35] An overall score was obtained by summing support across the vignettes (range = 0 to 12), with higher scores indicating greater social support. High risk was defined as a score of less than 7 (26%).

3. *Demographic risks* included teenage motherhood, father absence, and a high number of children in the household. Mothers who were younger than 18 when the child was born were considered high risk (11%). Father absence was determined by whether the husband or father of the child lived in the household when the child was 12 or 24 months old (48% of the households did not have a father in the home). High family density was defined as having four or more children in the household (31%).

Cumulative Risk Factors

The dichotomized nine individual risk factors were summed into a single cumulative risk factor. The distribution of risks for poor, heavier LBW infant indicates 22% experienced 0–1 risks, 34% experienced 2–3 risks, 34% experienced 4–5 risks, and 10% experienced 6 or more risks.

Human Capital Risk Variables

Based on the research by Alderson and colleagues,[36] we also conceptualize risk using three human capital risk variables: Maternal work status during pregnancy, maternal education at the time of the child's birth, and maternal welfare status at 12 or 24 months. Three levels of disadvantage are defined: (1) low—mothers who worked, had a high school degree, and were not on welfare at 12 or 24 months (27%); (2) high—mothers who did not work, had less than a high school degree, and who received welfare at 12 or 24 months (22%); (3) moderate—the rest of the mothers (i.e., had 1 or 2 but not 3 risk factors: 51%)

Psychological Risk Variables

Using 3 of the 9 cumulative risk variables, high life events (2 or more out of 4 events), low social support (less than 7 out of 12 items), and high depressive symptoms (score a 14 or more on a 32-point scale). More than a third (37%) did not have any psychosocial risks; 38% had 1 risk, 25% had 2 or 3 risks.

Cognitive Test Scores

The Stanford–Binet Intelligence Scale Form L-M, third edition[37] provides a measure of cognitive performance at 3 years of age (corrected for premature birth). It is the most widely used intelligence test for this age group.[38] Reliability data are not available for the third edition; however, for the fourth edition it is 0.97.[39] The mean was 86.98 (SD, 14.22). Cognitive functioning at 5 years of age is measured by the Wechsler Preschool and Primary Scale of Intelligence (WPPSI[40]), a test developed for use with children between the ages of 4 and 6.5 years. The reliability of verbal IQ and performance IQ is 0.94 and 0.93, respectively.[41] The mean was 90.98 (SD, 14.68). Cognitive functioning at 8 years of age is measured by the Wechsler Intelligence Scale for Children-III (WISC-III[42]). The mean, was 91.64 (SD, 14.43). These standardized tests are normed so that the mean score is 100 and the standard deviation is 15 for the WPPSI and WISC and the standard deviation of 16 for the Stanford–Binet.

Covariates

Study site, child's sex, race/ethnicity, neonatal health, and mother's immigrant status were included as covariates in all regressions.

RESULTS

Cumulative Risk and IQ Scores

The main effects of the 9 individual risk variables upon the heavier LBW children's cognitive test scores at 3, 5, and 8 years of age are summarized below (results control for the effects of treatment, site, neonatal health status, ethnicity, and gender; complete results available from the authors upon request). Few individual risk factors were significantly associated with children's cognitive test scores. Welfare receipt was associated with about a third of a standard deviation decrease in WPPSI scores at age 5 (4.8 points, $\beta = -0.16$, $P < 0.05$). Less than a high school education was associated with close to a half standard deviation decrease in WISC scores at 8 years of age (7.4 points, $\beta = -0.26$, $P < 0.001$).

Next, the cumulative effects of 9 risk factors are examined. Similar to previous work, because of sample size limitations,[43] the 9 risk factors are collapsed into the following categories: 0 to 1 risks, 2 to 3 risks, 4 to 5 risks, and 6 or more risks. The main effect of cumulative risks was significant for cognitive test scores at 3, 5, and 8 years of age (Fs > 3.38, Ps < 0.02). Greater risks were associated with worse cognitive scores. As shown in FIGURE 1, there is a significant association between risks and children's IQ scores at 3, 5, and 8 years of age. Children with few or no risks scored 3/4 to almost a full standard

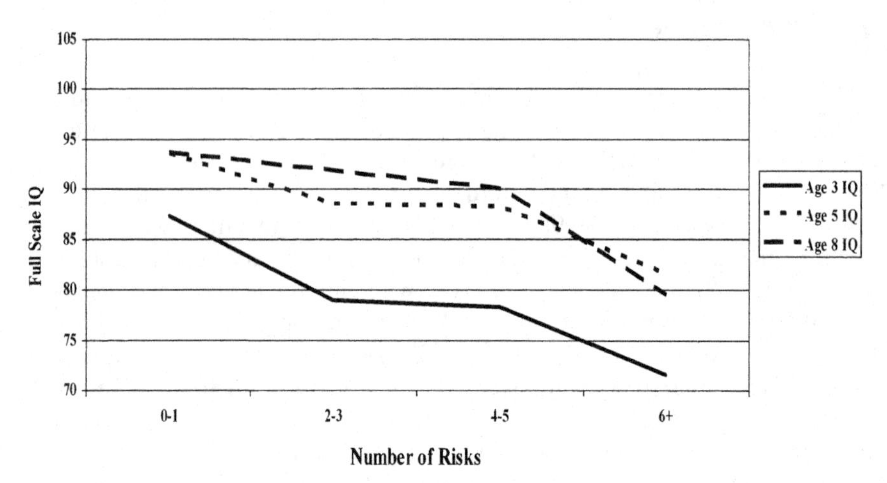

FIGURE 1. Cumulative risk and IQ over time: IHDP heavier LBW group ($n = 228$).

deviation higher on IQ tests than children who were considered high risk (6 or more risk factors). The negative effect of having 2 to 3 risks, compared to having little or no risks, was greater for 3-year-old children than for 5- or 8-year-old children.

Human Capital and Psychological Risks and IQ Scores

Next, the effects of two qualitatively different sets of risk factors upon heavier LBW children's IQ scores are examined. Two types of analyses are conducted. The first examines the cumulative risk of human capital risks and psychosocial risks separately. The second examines the cumulative risk for both in same regression. The proportion of variance in children's cognitive test score accounted for by each set of risks is compared to determine which set of risks is more explanatory of children's cognitive development.

A significant association was found between greater human capital disadvantage and heavier LBW children's IQ scores at 3, 5, and 8 years of age (Fs > 4.04, Ps < 0.05; FIG. 2). Children who had low human capital risks scored from more than 1/2 to more than 3/4 of a standard deviation higher on IQ tests than children who were in the high human capital risk group. The decrement in test scores was greater between low and moderate human capital risk groups at 3 and 5, and 8 years of age, compared to the decrement between moderate and high human capital risk groups. In contrast, to the findings for human capital risks, psychosocial risks were not associated with decrements in children's IQ scores at 3 through 8 years of age (Fs <1, Ps > 0.69; FIG. 2). However, the decrements in IQ scores appeared somewhat greater from 0 to 1 risk than from 1 to 2 or greater risks for 8 years of age (although the F-test was ns). When

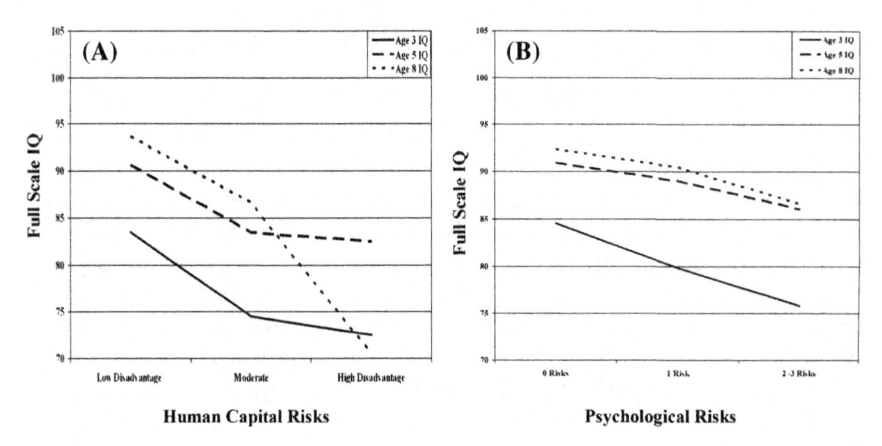

FIGURE 2. Human capital and psychological risks and IQ over time: IHDP: heavier LBW group ($n = 228$).

the effects of both human capital and psychosocial risks are examined in the same regression model, we find overwhelming support for the importance of human capital risks.

As presented in TABLE 1, the adjusted R-squares for the three regression models presented are as follows: At 3 years of age, it is 0.46 for human capital risks, 0.39 for psychological risks, and 0.49 for both. At 8 years of age, the comparable R-squares are 0.26, 0.20, 0.26. Human capital risks are negatively associated with IQ scores from 3, 5, and 8 years of age ($\beta = -0.21$, -0.20, and -0.19, respectively, $Ps < 0.01$). With the exception of a marginally significant negative effect of psychosocial risks upon IQ at 3 years of age ($\beta = -0.10$, $P < 0.08$), psychosocial risks are not associated with cognitive test scores (β at age 5 and 8 = -0.03 and -0.08, $Ps > 0.26$). In the regressions with both risk categories included, human capital risks account for more than 80% of the variance explained by both.

TABLE 1. Adjusted R-squares from three regression models of cognitive test scores on psychosocial risks, human capital risks, and combined risk

Dependent variable:	Age 3 Stanford binet	Age 5 WPPSI total	Age 8 WISC total
Regression model			
Psychosocial risks	0.39	0.22	0.20
Human capital risks	0.46	0.29	0.26
Psychosocial and human capital risks	0.49	0.27	0.26

NOTE: Control variables include: 7 site dummy variables, ethnicity, gender, neonatal health, mother's immigant status, dummy variables for missing data.

Cumulative Risk and Treatment Effects

As reported in previous articles, the effect of the intervention was highly significant for children's IQ scores at 3, 5, and 8 years of age. These effects were also found when controlling for the cumulative effects of the 9 risk variables (Fs > 4.26, Ps < 0.05). Interactions between treatment and the cumulative risk categories were not significant (Fs < 1.67, Ps > 0.18). The differences between treatment and follow-up groups for cognitive test scores at 3 years were significant for each level of risk (about a 1 to 1 and 1/3 of a standard deviation treatment benefit; FIG. 3). The difference between treatment and follow-up groups exists only for 8-year-olds who experience few or no risks (1/2 of a standard deviation) and for children who experience 6 risks or more (3/5 of a standard deviation; FIG. 3).

Human Capital and Psychological Risks and Treatment Effects

The effect of treatment was significant at each level of risk for the 3-year-olds (FIG. 4). By 5 and 8 years of age, however, a significant treatment by human capital risk interactions was found with the treatment effect only being seen for the moderate human capital risk group ($F = 2.98$, $P < 0.05$; FIG. 4). In contrast, none of the interactions were significant for psychological risk factors (results not shown but available upon request).

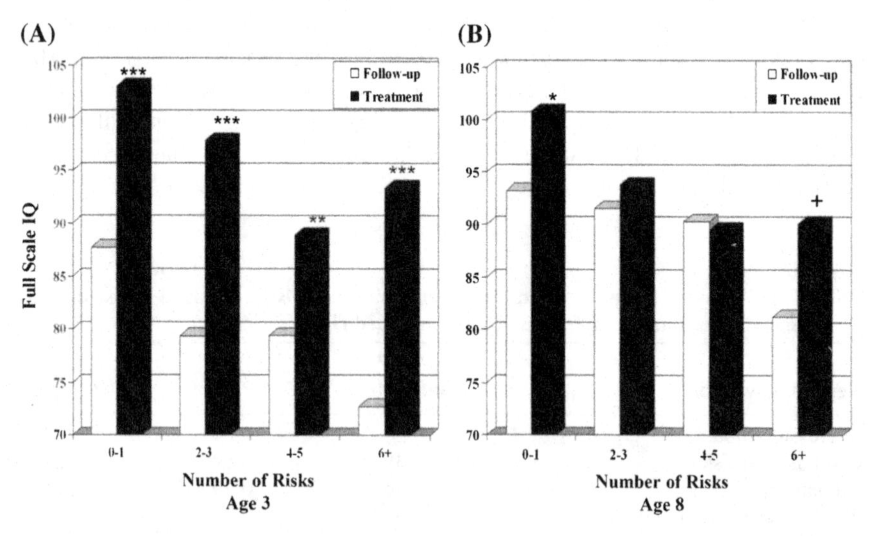

FIGURE 3. Cumulative risk × treatment IHDP: IQ at ages 3 and 8 for heavier LBW group ($n = 228$).

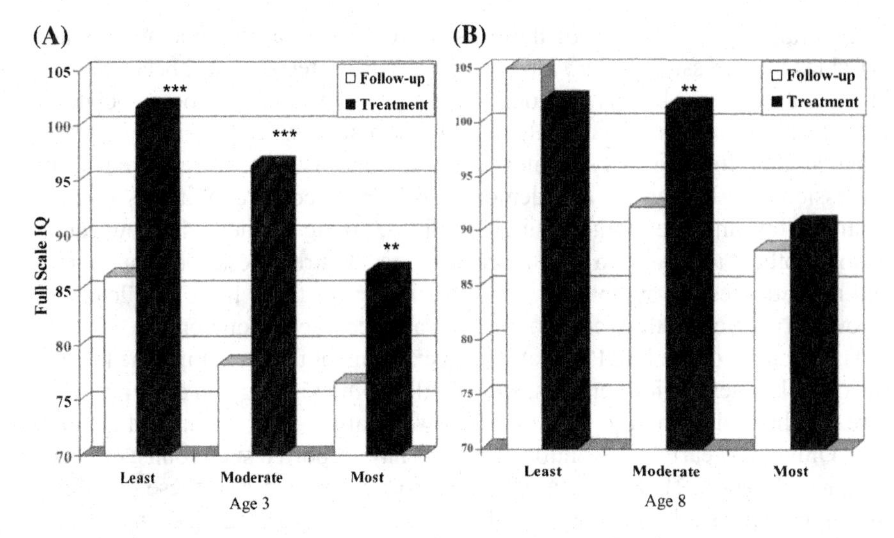

FIGURE 4. Human capital risk × treatment for IQ at ages 3 and 8 IHDP: heavier LBW group ($n = 228$).

DISCUSSION

In brief, cumulative risk is negatively associated with IQ scores in low-income, heavier LBW infants, similar to findings with normal birth weight infants. These negative slopes are seen at 3, 5, and 8 years of age in the sample reported here, with the slopes being quite similar. Our sample is comprised of only low-income families, unlike earlier studies that included middle- and high-income families as well. Our results, then, cannot be attributed to income (given that low-income families have more risk factors than middle- and high-income families).

Of particular interest is the relative contribution to risk–IQ links of human capital and psychological risk factors. It is clear that in this sample, human capital risks are much more strongly associated with IQ declines, than are psychological risks. Parental education, workforce experience, and avoidance of welfare all are probably associated with the home environment and parenting.[44] More educated parents talk more to their children, use less harsh discipline techniques, spend more time teaching their children, and provide more stimulating environments, all of which contribute to higher cognitive test scores.[45] These effects hold true even when controlling for income.[46] While the evidence is more limited for links between home environment and welfare receipt, the same pattern is seen.[47] Employment for low-income mothers also seems to be beneficial for children,[48] especially if work raises income above the poverty line (Morris, Gennetian, Duncan, 2005).[49] It may come as a surprise that the psychological risks, however, were not linked with IQ scores.

In general, the correlations of these risks are lower than for human capital variables in regressions where individual risks are entered, as has been shown in these analyses. Also, psychological risks are more likely to be associated with behavior problems than with cognitive test scores.[50] Also, in many previous studies looking at psychological risk, controls were not entered into regressions for human capital, demographic, and income conditions. If, for example, low-income mothers, single mothers, young mothers, and low education mothers are likely to have more emotional distress, less social support, and more depressive symptoms[51] not accounting for these links may lead to an overestimation of their contribution to variance in child outcomes.

The strength of the IHDP is that it is an experiment that examines the benefits of early intervention services, specifically home visiting and center-based care. At the end of the program, benefits were large—over a standard deviation. Only a few early intervention programs have reported such robust effects (see, Koraly *et al.*, 1998 and Barnett, 1995 for reviews).[52] And these benefits were seen across all risk groups analyzed here. However, sustained benefits, which were more modest, were not seen across all risk groups. Of particular interest is the finding for human capital. The group with moderate, not low or high risk, exhibited large IQ effects at 5 and 8 years, or 2 and 5 years after the intervention ended. The families in the moderate group had 1 or 2, but not 3, of the following risks—low education, unemployment, and/or welfare receipt. Children from families with all 3 risks did not continue their earlier gains. Similarly, those with no human capital risks do not either. Why might this be the case? In an earlier analysis where several different clusters of children were identified, using their IQ scores at ages 1, 2, and 3 years of age, a group of children who had relatively high IQ scores at all three ages were identified.[53] When the characteristics of this group were examined, it turned out that of mothers with low education at the birth of the child, virtually all in the high-stable IQ group had received the intervention. In another analysis, when looking at 3-year IQ for three education groups and two ethnic groups, positive effects were seen for black and white mothers who had a high school education or less, but not for white mothers with more than a high school education.[54] However, in regressions entering maternal education as an interaction term (with other such terms also included), no maternal education by treatment group effect was seen at 3 years of age,[55] the earlier findings either took into account IQ scores at 3 age points or maternal education by ethnicity by treatment interactions). Also, at 5 years of age, no maternal education by treatment interaction was reported.[56] We build on these analyses, in that maternal education alone did not condition the treatment effect at 5 or 8 years of age. However, when considered in combination with welfare receipt and unemployment, low education does matter. If all 3 risk factors are present, it may be that families are too overwhelmed to continue to benefit from the early intervention. Very high risk families may not have the ability to manage their lives well, get their children into good schools, provide their children stimulating environments, or deliver consistent care giving. Perhaps these ingredients (or at least one of them) are necessary for sustained effects[57] on the possible importance of elementary school quality in predicting success of early intervention programs. These results parallel those of Alderson and colleagues[58] where welfare families most likely to benefit from income supplements or special services who had moderate, not high human capital risk. The content and intensity of services needed to help families who have been labeled "hard to employ" might need to be quite different from what is offered in most programs.

At the same time, the low-risk families may not have benefited because they had the wherewithal to organize their own, their family, and their children's school experiences. In fact, the original welfare reform act of 1996 had provisions for a subgroup of the welfare population that was expected to have difficulty entering the workforce (thereby exceeding the term limits set forth by the act). The question has always been how large this group might be. The low-risk findings parallel, in part, the findings that mothers with more than a high school education were less likely to benefit from the program at 3 years of age than those with less education.

ACKNOWLEDGMENTS

We wish to thank all of those who funded the Infant Health and Development Program, most notably the Robert Wood Johnson Foundation, the Pew Charitable Trusts, NICHD, and the Maternal and Child Health Bureau of the Department of Health and Human Services. We also are grateful for the contribution of our collaborators and site directors—Marie McCormick, Cecelia McCarton, David Scott, Judith Bernbaum, Charles Bauer, Kurt Bennett, Patrick Casey, and Mark Swanson.

REFERENCES

1. Brooks-Gunn, J. & L. Markman. 2005. The contribution of parenting to ethnic and racial gaps in school readiness. Future Children **15**(1)**:** 139–168; Garmezy, N. M. Rutter, 1983. Stress, coping and development in children. New York, NY: Mcgraw-Hill; Sameroff, A. J. & Chandler, M. J. 1975. Reproductive risk and the continuum of caretaking casualty. *In* Review of child development research, Vol. 4. F. D. Horowitz, M. Hetherington, S. Scarr-Salapatek & G. Siegel, Eds.: 187–244. Chicago; University of Chicago; Sameroff, A. J., R. Seifer, R. Barocas, *et al.* (1987). Intelligence quotient scores of 4-year-old children: Social environmental risk factors. Pediatrics **79:** 343–350.
2. Adler, N.E., W.T. Boyce, M.A. Chesney, *et al.* 1993. Socioeconomic inequalities in health. No easy solution. JAMA **269:** 3140–3145.
3. Case, A. & C. Paxson. 2000. Mothers and others: who invests in children's health? Nat. Bur. Eco. Res. Retrieved from http://www.nber.org/papers/w7691

4. SAMEROFF, A.J. 2007. Psychosocial constraints on the development of resilience. Ann. N. Y. Acad. Sci. This volume.
5. BROOKS-GUNN, J., G. DUNCAN & P. REBELLO. 1999. Are socioeconomic gradients for children similar to those for adults? Achievement and health in the United States. *In* Developmental health and the wealth of nations: social, biological and educational dynamics. D. Keating & C. Hertzman, Eds.: 94–124. Guilford. New York; ROUSE, C., J. BROOKS-GUNN & S. MCLANAHAN. 2005. Introducing the issue, 'School readiness: closing racial and ethnic gaps.' The Future of Children, **15:** 1, 5–14; DUNCAN, G.J., & J. BROOKS-GUNN, 1997. Income effects across the lifespan: integration and interpretation. *In* G.J. Duncan & J. Brooks-Gunn (Eds).: Consequences of growing up poor (pp.596–610). New York, NY: Russell Sage; JENCKS, C. & M. PHILLIPS, 1998. The black white test score gap. Washington, DC: Brookings Institution Press; KLEBANOV, P.K., J., BROOKS-GUNN, C., MCCARTON, & M.C. MCCORMICK. 1998. the contribution of neighborhood and family income to developmental test scores over the first three years of life. Child Development, **69:** 1420–1436; PHILLIPS, M., J. BROOKS-GUNN, G.J. DUNCAN, P.K. KLEBANOV & C. Jencks. 1998. Family background, parenting practices, and the black-white test score gap. *In* The Black-White test score gap C. Jencks & M. Phillips, Eds.: 103–145. Washington, D.C: Brookings Institute; SMITH, J. R., J. BROOKS-GUNN & P.K. KLEBANOV. 1997. The consequences of living in poverty for young children's cognitive and verbal ability and early school achievement. *In* Consequences of growing up poor G.J. Duncan & J. Brooks-Gunn Eds.: 132–189. New York, NY: Russell Sage.
6. BROOKS-GUNN, J., J. WALDFOGEL & W. HAN. 2002. Maternal employment and child outcomes in the first three years of life: The NICHD study of early childcare. child development **73:** 1052–1072; LIAW, F. R. & J. BROOKS-GUNN. 1993. Patterns of low birth weight children's cognitive development and their determinants. Dev. Psychol. **29:** 1024–1035; LOVE, J. M., E. E. KISKER, C. M. ROSS, et al. 2002). Making a difference in the lives of infants and toddlers and their families: the impacts of Early Head Start. Washington, DC: U.S. Department of Health and Human Services; OLDS, D. L., C. R. JR. HENDERSON, H. S. KITZMAN, et al. 1999. Prenatal and infancy home visitation by nurses: recent findings. The Future of Children **9** 44–65.
7. SAMEROFF, A.J., R. SEIFER, A. BALDWIN. & C. BALDWIN. 1993. Stability of intelligence from preschool to adolescence: the influence of social and family risk factors. Child Dev. **64:** 80–97.
8. SAMEROFF, A.J. 2006. Biopsychosocial influences on the development of resilience. This issue.
9. LIAW, F. & J. BROOKS-GUNN. 1994. Cumulative familial risks and low birth weight children's cognitive and behavioral development. J. Clin. Child Psychol. **23:** 360–372.
10. MCCARTON, C., J. BROOKS-GUNN, I. WALLACE, *et al.* 1997. Results at 8 years of intervention for low birth weight premature infants: the infant health development program. J. Am. Med. Assoc. **227:** 126–132.
11. BROOKS-GUNN, J. & G.J. DUNCAN. 1997. The effects of poverty on children Future Children **7:** 55–71; DUNCAN, G. J., J. BROOKS-GUNN & P. K. KLEBANOV. 1994. Economic deprivation and early-childhood development. Child Development. **65:** 296–318; SMITH, J. R., J. BROOKS-GUNN & P. K. KLEBANOV. 1997.

12. LIAW, F.R. & J. BROOKS-GUNN. 1993: MCLOYD, V.C. 1990. The impact of economic hardship on black families and children: psychological distress, parenting, and socioemotional development. Child Development. **61:** 311–346; MCLOYD, V.C. 1998. Socioeconomic disadvantage and child development. Am. Psychol. **53:** 185–204.
13. DUNCAN, G.J. & J. BROOKS-GUNN. 1997; MAYER, S. 1997. *What money can't buy: The effect of parental income on children's outcomes.* Cambridge, MA: Harvard University Press.
14. KLEBANOV, P.K., J. BROOKS-GUNN & M.C. MCCORMICK. 2001. Maternal coping strategies and emotional distress: results of an early intervention program for low birth weight young children. Dev. Psychol. **37:** 654–667.
15. BAYDAR, N., J. BROOKS-GUNN & F.F. FURSTENBERG, JR. 1993. Early warning signs of functional illiteracy: predictors in childhood and cence. Child Dev. **64:** 815–829: BROOKS-GUNN, J., G. GUO & F. F. JR. FURSTENBERG. 1993. Who drops out of and who continues beyond high school?: A 20-year follow-up of black urban youth. *Journal of Research on Adolescence,* **3**: 271–294: GUO, G., J. BROOKS-GUNN & K.M. HARRIS. 1996 Parent's labor-force attachment and grade retention among urban Black children. *Sociology of Education,* 217–236: HAVEMAN, R. & B. WOLFE 1994. *Succeeding Generations: on the effects of investments in children.* New York: Russell Sage Foundation: SMITH, J. R., J. BROOKS-GUNN, D. KOHEN & C. MCCARTON. 2001. Transitions on and off AFDC: implications for parenting and children's cognitive development. Child Dev. **72:** 1512–1533.
16. SMITH, J.R., J. BROOKS-GUNN, P. KLEBANOV & K. LEE. 2000. Welfare and work: complementary strategies for low-income mothers? J. Marriage Fam. **62:** 808–821.
17. CHASE-LANSDALE, P.L., R.A. MOFFITT, B.J. LOHMAN, *et al.* 2003. Science **299:** 1548–1552.
18. GROSS, R., D. SPIKER & HAYNES, Eds.: 1997. Helping low birthweight, premature babies: the Infant Health and Development Program. Stanford University Press. Stanford, CA.
19. THE INFANT HEALTH AND DEVELOPMENT PROGRAM STAFF. 1990. Enhancing the outcomes of low birthweight, premature, infants: a multisite, randomized trial. JAMA.
20. BROOKS-GUNN, J., C. MCCARTON,P. CASEY, *et al.* 1994. Early intervention in low birth weight, premature infants: results through age 5 years from the infant health and development program. **272:** 1257– 1262; MCCARTON, C., J. BROOKS-GUNN, I. WALLACE, *et al.* 1997. Results at 8 years of intervention for low birth weight premature infants: the infant health development program. J. Am. Med. Ass. **227:** 126–132.
21. HILL, J., J. WALDFOGEL. & J. BROOKS-GUNN. 2002. Assessing the differential impacts of high-quality child care: a new approach for exploiting post-treatment variables. J. Pol. Anal. Manag. **21:** 601–627.
22. HILL, J., J. BROOKS-GUNN & J. WALDFOGEL. 2003. Sustained effects of high participation in an early intervention for low-birth-weight premature infants. Dev. Psychol. **39:** 730–744.
23. LIAW, F.R. & J. BROOKS-GUNN. 1993.
24. BROOKS-GUNN, J., R.T. GROSS, H.C. KRAEMER. 1992. Enhancing the cognitive outcomes of low-birth-weight, premature infants: for whom is the intervention

most effective? Pediatrics **89:** 1209–1215; LIAW, F. R. & J. BROOKS-GUNN. 1993; LOVE, J. M. 2002: LOVE, G.M., E. KISKER, C. ROSS, *et al.* 2005. The effectiveness of early head start for 3-year old children and their parents: lesson for policy and programs. Dev. Psychol. **41:** 885–901; OLDS, *et al.* (1999).

25. ALDERSON, D.P., L. DOWSETT, C.J. IMES & A.E. HUSTON. Economic, child care and child outcome effects of employment-based programs by prior levels of family disadvantage. Manuscript submitted for publication.
26. OLDS, *et al.* 1999.
27. IBID.
28. LYONS-RUTH, K., D.B. CONNELL, H.U. GRUNEBAUM & S. BOTEIN. 1990. Infants at social risk: maternal depression and family support services as mediators of infant development and security of attachment. Child Dev. **61:** 85–98.
29. BARNARD, K.E., D. MAGYARY, G. SUMNER, *et al.* 1988. Prevention of parenting alterations for women with low social support. Psychiatry **51:** 248–253; BOOTH, C.L., S. K. MITCHELL K.E. BARNARD & S.J. SPIEKER. 1989. Development of maternal social skills in multiproblem families: effects on mother-child relationship. Dev. Psychol. **25:** 403–412.
30. CECI, S.J. & P.B. PAPIERNO. 2005. The rhetoric and reality of gap closing: when the "have nots" gain but the "haves" gain even more. Am. Psychol. **60:** 149–160: Klebanov *et al.* 2001.
31. BAYDAR. *et al.* 1993; BROOKS-GUNN *et al.* 1993; Duncan *et al.* 1994; BROOKS-GUNN, J., R. T., GROSS, H. C., KRAEMER, D., SPIKER, & S. Shapiro. 1992. Enhancing the cognitive outcomes of low-birth-weight, premature infants: for whom is the intervention most effective? Pediatrics **89** (8): 1209–1215; GROSS, R., D. SPIKER & HAYNES (Eds).: 1997. Helping low birthweight, premature babies: the infant health and development program. Stanford, CA: Stanford University Press; GROSS *et al.* 1997; LIAW *et al.* 1993.
32. RAMEY, C.T., D.M. BRYANT, B.H. WASIK, *et al.* 1992. The Infant Health and Development Program for low birthweight, premature infants: program elements, family participation and child intelligence. Pediatrics **3:** 454–465; SPARLING, J.J. & I. LEWIS. 1984. *Partners for learning.* Lewisville, NC; KAPLAN, SPARLING, J.J., I. LEWIS, C.T. RAMEY, *et al.* 1991. Partners: a curriculum to help premature low birthweight infants get off to a good start. Topics in Early Childhood Special Education, **11:** 36–55.
33. WASIK, B.H. 1984. Coping with parenting through effective problem solving: a handbook for professionals. Unpublished manuscript. (Chapel Hill; Frank Porter Graham Child Development Center, University of North Carolina at Chapel Hill.): WASIK, B.H., D.B. BRYANT, J.J. SPARLING & C.T. RAMEY. 1997. Maternal problem solving. *In* Helping Low Birthweight, Premature Babies: The Infant Health and Development Program. R.T. Gross, D. Spiker & C.W. Haynes, Eds.: 276–289. Stanford University Press: Stanford.
34. GOLDBERG, D. 1978. Manual of the general health questionnaire. NFER.London.
35. COHEN, J.B. & R.S. LAZARUS. 1977. Social support questionnaire. University of California, Berkeley; MCCORMICK, M. C. & BROOKS-GUNN, J. 1989. Health care for children and adolescents. *In* H. Freeman & S. Levine Eds.: Handbook of Medical Sociology (pp. 347–380). Englewood Cliffs, NJ: Prentice Hall.
36. ALDERSON, *et al.* (Submitted for Publication).
37. TERMAN, L.M. & M.A. MERRILL. 1973. *Stanford-binet intelligence scale: Manual for the third revision, form L-M*. Houghton Mifflin.Boston.

38. ANASTASI, A. 1988. *Psychological testing.* Sixth edition. Macmillan. New York:BARNARD K. E., D. MAGYARY, G. SUMNER, *et al.* 1988. Prevention of parenting alterations for women with low social support. Psychiatry. **51:** 248–253; SATTLER, J.M. 1992. *Assessment of children's intelligence and special abilities.* Boston: Allyn & Bacon.
39. THORNDIKE, R.L., E.P. HAGEN & J.M. SATTLER. 1986. Guide for administering and scoring the Stanford-Binet Intelligence Scale. 4th ed. Riverside. Chicago.
40. WECHSLER, D. 1967. Wechsler Preschool and Primary Scale of Intelligence. Psychological Corp. San Antonio, TX.
41. SATTLER. 1992.
42. WECHSLER, D. 1991. WISC-III: Wechsler Intelligence Scale for Children- 3 edition Manual. Psychological Corporation.San Antonio, TX.
43. LIAW, *et al.* 1994.
44. BRADLEY, R.H. 2004. Chaos, culture, and covariance structures: a dynamic systems view of children's experiences at home. *In* Handbook of Parenting. M.H. Bornstein (Ed.), Vol. 4: Science and Practice. 243–258. Mahwah, NJ. Lawrence Erlbaum Associates; BRADLEY 2001, CORWYN, R.H., R.F., BURCHINAL, M. MCADOO, P.H., & GARCIA COLL, C. 2001. The home environments of children in the United States Part II: relations with behavioral development through age thirteen. Child Dev. **72:** 1868–1886.
45. BORNSTEIN, M.H. 2002 Handbook of Parenting: children and Parenting. Mahwah, N.J. Lawrence Erlbaum Associates BROOKS-GUNN & MARKMAN. (2005); GERSHOFF, E. T. 2002. Corporal punishment by parents and associated child behaviors and experiences: a meta-analytic and theoretical review. Psychol. Bull. **128:** 539–579; HART, B. & T. RISLEY. 1999. *The Social World of Children Learning to Talk.* Baltimore: Paul Brookes Publishing; YEUNG, J., M. LINVER & J. BROOKS-GUNN 2002. How money matters for young children's development: parental investment and family processes. Child Dev. **73:** 1861–1879.
46. BROOKS-GUNN & DUNCAN. 1997: LINVER, M., J. BROOKS-GUNN & D. KOHEN. 2002. Family processes as pathways from income to young children's development. Dev. Psychol. **38:** 719–734; SMITH, *et al.* 1997.
47. SMITH, *et al.* (2000, 2001).
48. CHASE-LANSDALE, *et al.* 2003; JACKSON, A., J. BROOKS-GUNN, C. HUANG & M. GLASSMAN. 2000. Single mothers in low-wage jobs: Financial strain, parenting, and preschoolers' outcomes. Child Dev. **71:** 1409–1423; ZASLOW, M., K. MOORE, J.L. BROOKS, *et al.* 2002. Experimental studies of welfare reform and children. The Future of Children, **12:**(1) 78–95.
49. DUNCAN & BROOKS-GUNN. 1997: MORRIS, P.A. 2002. The effects of welfare reform policies on children. *Society for Research in Child Development Social Policy Report*, XVI(1).S; MORRIS, P.A., L.A. GENNETIAN & G. DUNCAN. 2005. Effects of welfare and employment policies on young children: new findings on policy experiments conducted in the early 1990s. Society for Research in Child Development Social Policy Report, XIX(II).
50. YEUNG, *et al.* 2002.
51. ADLER, *et al.* 1993: Mclloyd. 1990, 1998.
52. KORALY, L.A., P.W. GREENWOOD, S.S. EVERINGHAM, *et al.* 1998. Investing in our children: what we know and don't know about cost and benefit of early childhood interventions. Santa Monica, CA; RAND & W.S. BARNETT, 1995. Long-term effects of early childhood programs and on cognitive school outcomes. The Future of Children, **5:** 25–50.

53. LIAW & BROOKS-GUNN. 1993.
54. BROOKS-GUNN, *et al.* 1992.
55. BROOKS-GUNN, *et al.* 1993: IHDP. 1990.
56. BROOKS-GUNN, 1994.
57. LEE, V.E., S. LOEB & S. LUBECK. 1998. Contextual effects of prekindergarten classrooms for disadvantaged children on cognitive development: the case of chapter 1. Child Dev. **69**: 479–44.
58. ALDERSON, *et al.* (Submitted for Publication)

The Inherent Stress of Normal Daily Life and Social Interaction Leads to the Development of Coping and Resilience, and Variation in Resilience in Infants and Young Children

Comments on the Papers of Suomi and Klebanov & Brooks-Gunn

ED TRONICK

Child Development Unit, Children's Hospital Boston, Harvard Medical School, Boston, Massachusetts, USA

ABSTRACT: The hypothesis is advanced that behavioral and physiologic resilience develops in part from infants' and young children's experience coping with the inherent normal stress of daily life and social interaction. Data on the stress of normal social interactions and perturbated interactions from the Face-to-Face Still-Face Paradigm (FFSF) are presented for young infants. These findings, including behavioral, heart rate and vagal tone, and electrodermal reactivity demonstrate the stress inherent in normal interaction and how coping with normal stress develops infants' coping with more intense environmental and social stressors.

KEYWORDS: infants; Face-to-Face Still-Face Paradigm; FFSF; microtemporal communicative processes; mutual regulation model; MRM; resilience; stress; electrodermal; vagal tone

Michael Rutter[1] has defined resilience as individual variation in the relative resistance to environmental risk experiences. Though many factors affect the development of resilience, I want to advance the hypothesis that behavioral and physiologic resilience develops in part from infants' and young children's experience coping with the inherent normal stress of daily life and social interaction. This hypothesis, which we call the normal stress resilience hypothesis, is framed by a dynamic systems perspective on development of behavior and

Address for correspondence: Ed Tronick, Child Development Unit, Children's Hospital Boston, 1295 Boylston Street, Suite 320, Boston, MA 02215. Voice: 617-355-6948; fax: 617-730-0074.
e-mail: ed.tronick@childrens.harvard.edu

Ann. N.Y. Acad. Sci. 1094: 83–104 (2006). © 2006 New York Academy of Sciences.
doi: 10.1196/annals.1376.008

the brain and the processes that regulate development, in particular the interactive communicative engagements between infants/children and caretakers that regulate stressful experiences. In this article I will present a dynamic systems perspective on development, the mutual regulation model (MRM) of the child-caregiver communicative exchanges, and recent behavioral and physiologic data from my laboratory on the nature of the interactive process. The normal stress resilience hypothesis begins with the idea from a dynamic systems perspective and supported by empirical evidence that stress inevitably and ubiquitously travels with normal developmental change and paradoxically stress also travels with the interactive regulatory processes that regulate the stress of developmental change.[2,3] Second, based on developmental theory and empirical evidence of behavioral and brain plasticity it argues that as a consequence of coping with normal developmental and regulatory stresses children develop both new coping capacities and increase the effectiveness of their capacities for resisting normal and even more intense nonnormal (traumatic) levels of stress. Furthermore, that individual variation in children's relative resistance to stress—their resilience—is in part determined by the unique experience of success or failure of each child in coping with normal stressors.[4]

An analogy for this normal stress resilience hypothesis is training for a marathon. Runners do not run marathon distances to train for a marathon. They run a specific amount each day and week and increase the distance over the course of weeks and days. However, it is not until they actually run the marathon that they run the full distance. The earlier training leads to the development of the capacity to extend themselves to the full distance. The daily training in a sense developed their coping capacities such that they had the resilience to go the full distance. Of course, without the training had they tried to go the full—traumatic—distance they would have failed.

COMPLEXITY AND DISSIPATION IN OPEN SYSTEMS

Prigogine and Stengers[5] state that a primary principle governing the activities of open biological systems is that they must acquire energy from the environment to maintain and increase their coherence and complexity, their distance from entropy. The energy must have a particular form to be useful (i.e., what Sander[6] calls fittedness for the organism). For example, though the food that prey eat has plenty of energy, if predators eat it, they cannot utilize the energy—it has no metabolic fittedness, no "meaning" for the animal. Complex systems are systems that have a hierarchical organization operating at multiple size and temporal scales and they are information-rich with local contextual interactions. Complex systems exhibit emergent properties at different levels that are neither fixed nor chaotic. Self-organizing processes generate these emergent properties and lead to an increase in the complexity of the system, but there are always limits on a system's maximum complexity. Mature and healthy open biological systems are in a dynamic state of organization that approaches these limits, such that the mature organism attempts to garner energy to maintain and optimize its level of coherence and complexity. However, in mature systems emergence of new properties is limited and variation in the relative complexity among individuals is primarily related to the success or failure in gaining fitted energy. Furthermore, for mature organisms, self-organized maintenance of complexity becomes increasingly energetically demanding and when there is a failure to achieve sufficient amounts of energy the system begins to dissipate and lose complexity. In the extreme there is shift to a less complex state or phase. Baltes *et al.*,[7] for example, argue that aging is a losing fight against the dissipation of complexity within an already achieved state of organization and an inevitable shifting into a lower state of organization, such as death.

In contrast to the mature system, the developing organism is in a time limited period in which the second law of thermodynamics is locally violated. For a developing organism the developmental process is aimed at increasing and optimizing complexity. This aim has high energetic demands because the organism must garner sufficient energy to maintain its level of complexity and to make state and phase shifts to higher levels of complexity and coherence. Successful developing systems manifest emergent properties as well as directionality, that is, movement toward optimization of complexity and coherence. However, making stage and phase shifts are unpredictable and the shifts are potentially dissipative. Dissipation is possible because of how a complex system is organized and changes. The organism exists as a coherent assemblage of many interacting elements with both constitutive and integrative levels. At the point when a system is about to shift into a new emergent phase, it is close to a chaotic edge and the transition is inherently unstable. Failure to make the shift is dissipative; that is there is loss of complexity and increase in entropy.

In a typically developing system in a typical environment failure is unlikely, yet even in systems that are successfully increasing their complexity there is the necessity of disorganizing the extant state and assembling a new state. The disorganization of the extant state during a transforming transition is always associated with a loss of complexity and coherence. Thus there is a paradox of the emergence of the new: it is at one and the same time fulfilling the first principle of increasing complexity and at the same time threatening dissipation. The system is both optimizing and imperfecting itself and the outcome is unpredictable until it coalesces. As we shall see, these changes at both the macrolevel of development and the microregulatory level are stressful.[3]

Humans have developed an exceptional (though hardly unique) way to garner more energy from the environment and avoid dissipation by forming a dyadic regulatory system. The MRM attempts to describe the operation of this dyadic system.[8] In the MRM there is a working together of two individuals such that they form an integrated dyadic system for acquiring energy. Though a dyadic system of course has limits, it is able to garner more resources and become more complex than either individual would be able to garner or to achieve on their own. As a component in a dyadic system each individual can appropriate energy to itself and consequently increase its own complexity. For the infant and young child, the disorganization that comes with increasing complexity and associated dissipation is dyadically regulated by the microtemporal interplay of the infant/child's self-organizing capacities and external organizing input provided by an adult (caretaker) system. The interplay of internal and external organizing capacities is regulated by a bidirectional communicative system that can be conceptualized as interchange of signals and receptors, but for humans both the child and adult simultaneously and sequentially play both roles. This simultaneous and sequential shifting of roles makes the workings of this dyadic system astonishingly complicated. When the interplay or coordination of signaling and reception is adequate the infant/child and adult/caretaker form a more complex dyadic system made up of two major component systems from which each appropriates fitted energy and as a consequence gains in complexity. But even when successful the process is stressful because there is a loss of complexity as the old organization is dissembled and because of the unpredictability of the outcome. Of course the stress is even greater when the system is unsuccessful and complexity is lost.

DEVELOPMENT AND ITS REGULATION

Development is one source of stress because it does not proceed smoothly but is characterized by periods of disorganization in one domain to new more coherent forms of organization within that domain (e.g., changes in motor systems for mobility; see Refs. 9 and 10, in particular chapters by Plooij and Trevarthen). Periods of disorganization are an inherent characteristic of developing self-organizing systems. They can be thought of as the "avalanches" of Bak's[11] sand pile model from which new organization emerges from self-organizing processes at the edge of chaos. Adding to the complexity, the disorganization of one system disorganizes other systems. For example, the infant who is beginning to change from crawling to walking not only becomes disorganized motorically, but other systems such as sleep/activity cycling, emotions and mood, and even perception become disorganized as well (see FIG. 1). As with temperature regulation, a portion of the task of regulating this disorganization falls to the internal self-organizing resources of the infant. However, the infant's resources are inadequate to the task and must be supplemented by external regulation. Without external caretaker provisioned regulatory resources development would be derailed. Under normal circumstances the formation of a dyadic regulatory system, a combination of internal and external processes, is adequate to meet the regulatory demands and development moves forward. However, when the dyadic system fails, when internal and external resources are inadequate, development may be seriously disrupted. Disorganization increases and coherence and complexity are lost. Note however, a critical feature of the model is that disorganization is part of the normal process. It is

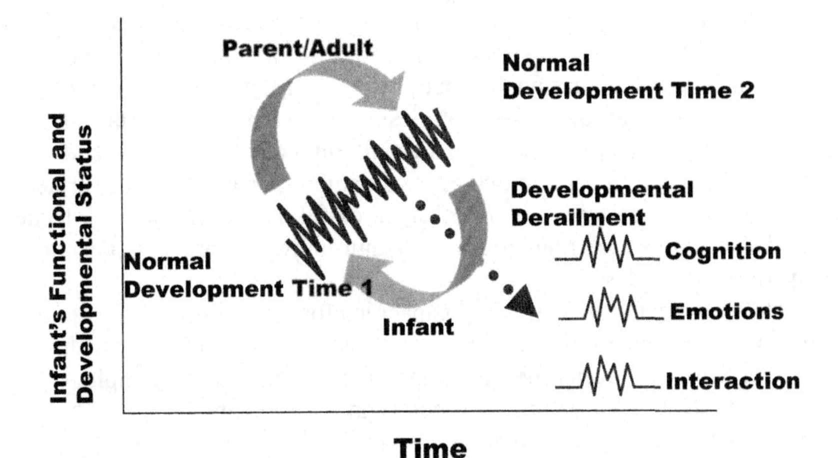

FIGURE 1. Normal development involves a disorganization from Time 1 to Time 2 and this disorganization will disorganize other functions.

necessary for the emergence of something new and for an increase of complexity and coherence—disorganization is the wellspring of change and the new. But again, change is costly.

DYADIC REGULATION: THE WORKINGS OF THE MICROTEMPORAL REGULATORY PROCESS

What is the structure of the microtemporal communicative processes, which in the accumulation of moment-by-moment interchanges, regulates development and leads to the growth of complexity. The development of walking takes months but it is worked on during millions of moment-by-moment exchanges. To understand mutual regulation I want to start with an example far from macrodevelopmental processes as well as the issue of resilience—infant temperature regulation. I choose this example because it illustrates the dyadic regulatory process for a psychobiological state that is most typically seen solely as a self-organized process.

Temperature regulation is a process governed by a simple rule: maintain homeothermic status but it leads to complex system behavior.[12] Fulfilling the rule is complicated and this regulatory system is hierarchically organized with a multitude of subsystems from metabolic processes to behavioral systems. It is a system that operates to maintain equilibrium, and though it changes with development (e.g., the loss of brown fat) and is influenced by environmental factors (e.g., the increase in capillary networks in the hand in cold environments), its change and development is limited compared to other psychobiological systems (e.g., respiratory systems, motor systems, or coping systems). Infants have self-organizing capacities to upregulate a below normal temperature, such as increasing their activity level, preferentially metabolizing high energy brown fat, or moving into less energetic behavioral states (e.g., sleep). But these self-organized capacities are limited and immature, and will eventually fail, an especially quick event for infants with their high surface-to-volume ratio. Such failure is obviously stressful. However, though Claude Bernard saw temperature regulation as a within-individual process, it is not. It is a dyadic process.

Infants' self-organized regulatory capacities for operating on temperature control are supplemented by external regulatory input by caregivers that is specifically fitted to overcome the infant's limitations.[13] For example, caregivers place infants against their own chests and share their body heat with their infants, which in turn reduces their infants' surface heat loss. This dyadic regulatory process itself is guided by communicative signals from the infant. These communicative signals convey the state of the infant to a receptive caregiver. When done successfully the input provided by the adult is fitted (meaningful) to the infant's temperature regulatory system and the system becomes dyadic and more coherently organized than the infant would be on his/her own.

A major consequence for the developing organism of the formation of a dyadic system, is that the capacity/effectiveness of its self-organized regulatory capacities actually will increase, such that later in development the infant will be able to self-regulate temperature without as much external regulatory scaffolding. One reason for the increase is because the energetic demands on the infant are reduced and the saved energy can be channeled into the growth of regulatory capacity. This increase in the self-organizing capacity of the individual by its participation in a dyadic regulatory system is not unlike Vygotsky's[14] concept of the zone of proximal development. By contrast, were the formation of a dyadic system to fail, the infant would lose control of his temperature, and his homeostatic state would dissipate. When the failure is chronic the infant's self-regulatory capacities might maintain themselves at a cost to other systems but there would be no energy for growth of regulatory capacity. The system would lose complexity and coherence and eventually move to a less complex state of organization. Keeping this dyadic model of temperature in mind, let us examine the process of development and the microtemporal dyadic communicative system that regulates it.

The perspective is based on the MRM and empirical work examining the organization of the regulatory process.[8,15,16] The MRM stipulates that caregivers/mothers and infants/children are linked subsystems of a dyadic system and each component, infant and caregiver/mother, regulate disorganization and its costs by a bidirectional process of behavioral and expressive signaling and receiving. However, the communicative process between the developing human and the adult is inherently imperfect, unstable, and unpredictable. The infant signals to the caregiver may vary one moment to another. The caregiver's reception of them and of course the caregiver's input to the infant also varies. Moreover, the infant signals that worked one time may not work the next time, and the same is true for the caregiver's response. Thus the mutual regulatory process is "messy" and energetically costly. Nonetheless, over time it is likely that the activities that work more often will become more and more a part of the workings of the dyadic regulatory process, the process will become less costly, and energy will be freed up for growing self-organized regulatory processes and increasing self-system complexity.

THE FACE-TO-FACE STILL-FACE PARADIGM: A SOCIAL STRESSOR ON BEHAVIOR AND PHYSIOLOGY

To study the dyadic microregulatory process, I developed the Face-to-Face Still-Face Paradigm (FFSF).[17] The FFSF confronts the young infant with three interactive contexts: (i) an episode of "normal" face-to-face social interaction with a caregiver (typically the mother) during which the caregiver is asked to play with the infant, followed by (ii) a SF episode, during which the caregiver is instructed to keep an unresponsive poker face and not smile, touch, or talk to the baby, followed by (iii) a reunion episode during which the caregiver and infant resume face-to-face social interaction. Each episode typically lasts 2 min. The paradigm has primarily been used with infants ranging in age from 2 to 15 months, with a mean age of 5.2 months,[18] but a modified form has also been used with 30-month-olds and even with adults.

The FFSF paradigm demonstrates the costliness of the stress of an experimental disruption of the mutual regulatory process, and as I will show it serves as a model for the stress inherent in normal interactions. The FFSF exposes infants to a unique social-emotional stressor (maternal SF) that differs from inanimate stressors as well as typical forms of social interaction and elicits well-documented emotional reactions and stress in infants. Over the past 25 years, hundreds of infants have been videotaped in FFSF paradigm.[17] The FFSF has proven to be a fruitful methodological tool for evaluating young infants' ability to cope with an interactive perturbation and an emotional stressor.[17–23]

Infants typically respond to the SF with what Adamson and Frick have labeled the "still-face effect"[18] (FIG. 2). In study after study, infants respond with a signature decrease in positive affect and an increase in negative affect and gaze aversion.[20,23,24] In studies using microanalytic signal scoring systems, infants have additionally been shown to react to the SF with an increase in visual scanning, pick-me-up gestures, distancing behavior such as twisting and turning in their seat, and autonomic stress indicators such as spitting up.[23–27] The "still-face effect" is seen with infants and children over a wide age range. Gender differences have been found in young infants' reactions to the FFSF. For instance, in a study from our lab,[27] 6-month-old male infants had more difficulty than female infants in maintaining affective regulation during the FFSF.

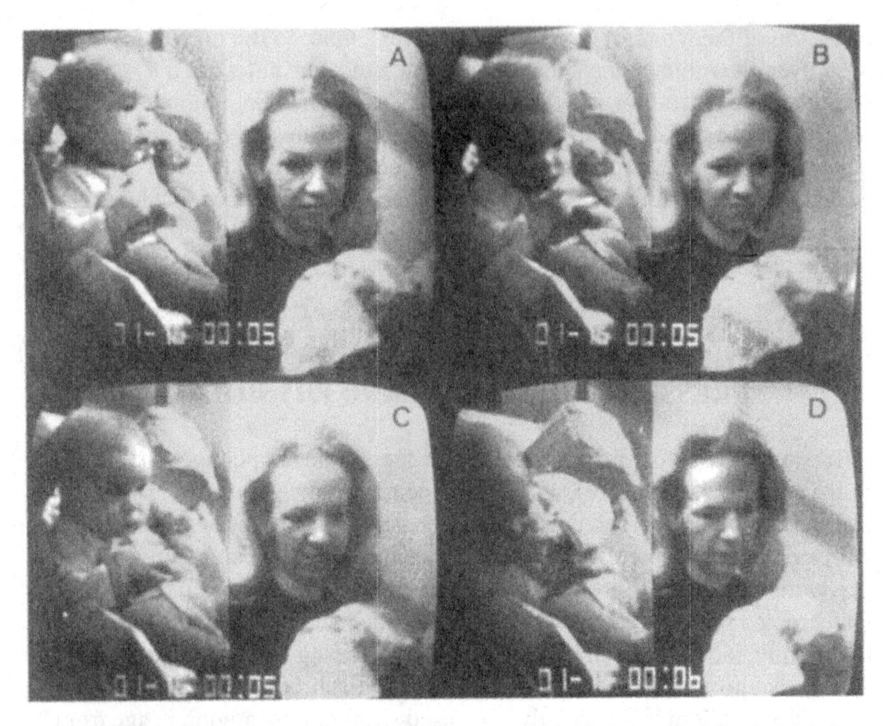

FIGURE 2. The sequence from A–D illustrates the still-face effect. In A the infant looks at the still-faced mother. He turns away in B but glances at her in C. In D he loses postural control and self-comforts.

Infants' neurophysiologic reactions also index the stressfulness of the FFSF. Whereas heart rate reflects degree of physiological arousal, respiratory sinus arrhythmia (RSA) reflects neural regulation of the heart via the vagal nerve, and is sometimes measured in terms of vagal tone (VT), an index of cardiac activity related to respiratory function mediated by the parasympathetic nervous system.[28] Changes in RSA reflect a functional relation between the central nervous system and the heart as mediated by the vagus[29,30] and are thought to serve an important regulatory function in human social engagement.[30,31] The regulation of vagal control of the heart is associated with the ability to engage and disengage with people and objects in one's environment. High RSA measured at rest reflects a baseline of neural integrity and a readiness to respond to social engagement or the environment. Prior research[32–35] has shown that higher RSA measured at rest is related to less negative behavior and less difficult temperament in infants and preschoolers.[32,35,36] Moreover, a decrease in RSA is thought to reflect an individual's active coping in reaction to stressors or an increase in attention to (or engagement with) the environment. For instance, greater suppression of RSA during challenging situations is related to better state regulation, greater self-soothing, more attentional control, and greater capacity for social engagement.[32] In contrast, a deficit in the ability to suppress RSA in challenging contexts may be related to a lack of behavioral and emotional control.[37,38] In general, the research is consistent with a view that RSA is an index of the manner in which an individual actively engages with the environment and regulates emotion and behavior in the face of environmental challenge.[30,39–41]

Only a few studies have evaluated changes in infants' RSA during the FFSF. In a prior study in my lab using the FFSF with 6-month-olds,[23] infants' VT dropped significantly during the SF episode compared to the first play episode, and recovered to baseline levels in the reunion episode. Also, in my laboratory, Jacob Ham has recently replicated these findings of a suppression of VT to the stress of the SF.[89] Similar findings were reported in a study evaluating stranger–infant interaction using a modified version of the FFSF.[42] Using a modified version of the FFSF paradigm, Haley and Stansbury[43] found an increase in infants' heart rate during each SF episode (VT was not evaluated). In a study of 3-month-olds, Moore and Calkins, and Moore *et al.*[28,44] investigated changes in infants' VT, heart rate, and behavioral reactivity during the FFSF and found that infants exhibited decreased VT and increased heart rate and negative affect during the SF episode, indicating physiological regulation of distress. Of note, individual differences in VT reactivity were also observed. Infants who did not suppress VT in the SF evidenced less positive affect, higher reactivity, and lower VT during the play and reunion episodes with their mothers.

In an innovative and unique as aspect of his study, Ham successfully utilized skin conductance with infants as a measure of the activation of the sympathetic nervous system to the FFSF paradigm. This measure had long been thought not to be usable with infants. Ham developed sensors for use with infants that could be bound to the soles of their feet eliminating much of the movement artifact and with modern computer technology and programming was able to get clean and stimulus responsive measures. The development of this technique is an important contribution because it provides a pure measure of sympathetic nervous system control and another window into the functioning of the infant nervous system. Ham found that skin conductance increased from the first play episode to the SF episode and that it further increased in the reunion play episode. These findings substantiate the arousing and stressful effect of the SF as well as the cost of recovering from it in the subsequent normal play episode. These findings parallel behavioral findings indicating that infants' arousal (e.g., levels of negative affect) are higher in the reunion episode than in the first play episode.

In another methodologic advance, Ham was also able to simultaneously record VT and skin conductance from the mothers during the FFSF episodes. As was the case for the infants, the mothers' reactions demonstrated the stressful nature of the SF. Furthermore, in results similar to the relations found between the behavioral signals of infants and mothers during the FFSF, there were relations between infant and maternal physiologic reactions. For example, there were significant positive relations between infant and mother skin conductance, positive relations between infant heart rate and maternal skin conductance, and infant VT and maternal heart rate. These results are suggestive of mutual regulation of physiology by infants and mothers not unlike the relations seen in their behavior or the relations seen in animal studies.

The reactivity of the hypothalamic-pituitary-axis (HPA) as measured by the level of glucocorticoids also has been examined using the FFSF paradigm.[43,45] Similar to the view based on animal work,[46–48] HPA activity in humans is viewed as a measure of the stress response as well as a regulator of emotional and social behavior. For example, Gunnar *et al.*,[49,50] utilized pre- and post-salivary cortisol reactions as a measure of infant stress and found that stressful events such as inoculations lead to an elevation in infants' cortisol levels. Though the relation between cortisol response and stress is now viewed as more complicated than originally thought, peak cortisol response is still seen as an indicator of physiologic reactivity.[51] In a recent review of the relation between acute stress and cortisol reactivity in adults and older children, Dickerson and Kemeny[52] conclude that perceived uncontrollable social threat to the self are strongly predictive of cortisol reactivity. Although this interpretation is based on the adult and older child literature, it theoretically could be applied to infants confronting the SF, which is an uncontrollable and possibly threatening event.

Several recent studies have examined infants' cortisol reactivity during the FFSF. Ramsey and Lewis[45,53] found a significant but modest increase in cortisol level in 6-month-old infants following exposure to the SF. However, they found no significant association between peak cortisol response and response dampening or behavioral reactivity. In a second study, Lewis and Ramsey[45] found that peak cortisol response was related to infants' expressions of sadness but not anger. Haley and Stansbury[43] evaluated 5- to 6-month-olds' behavior, heart rate, and cortisol reactivity during a modified FFSF in which infants were exposed to two SF and two reunion episodes to increase the stress level and likelihood of a cortisol response. Infants exhibited a significant increase in heart rate and cortisol response. The different measures of reactivity were not highly correlated although higher baseline cortisol was positively correlated with more infant negative affect during the SF. Others have also reported a lack of tight coupling among behavioral and physiologic reactivity measures during infancy.[45,54,55] Moreover, the level of cortisol change reported in these studies was relatively modest, especially in comparison to the cortisol changes observed in the animal literature, which show an inverted U-shaped relation between cortisol and memory.[56,57] In sum, the SF demonstrates that breaking the mutual regulatory process is a powerful psychobiologic stressor and that the infant has self-organized capacities for coping with it.

THE EFFECTS OF REPARATION ON DEVELOPMENT

The SF is an experimental paradigm and though it may be thought of "unnatural," a lack of regulatory reception-signaling between mother and child often occurs (e.g., a lack of response to the infant when the adult is driving in a car, talking on a phone, or being out of proximity to the child) suggesting that the infant is often exposed to stressful experience. More importantly, the FFSF paradigm actually serves as a model for *normal* interactions and the stress that accompanies them. The FFSF paradigm has an experimentally induced miscoordination or mismatch in the interaction of the mother/adult and infant (i.e., the infant attempting to interact and the mother "refusing") and their reestablishment of coordination in the reunion play. The mismatch and match of the FFSF has a time course of minutes but in our research on normal face-to-face and play interactions we have found a pattern of matching and mismatching of behavior, affect, and communicative expressions at the microtemporal level (tenths of a second) of the mutual regulatory process. These mismatches are inherent to the interaction because of: (i) the speed at which signals are emitted, (1–4 times per second); (ii) the demands on infants' and adults' receptor apparatus to detect and decode the signals; (iii) the response time demands, again on the order of tenths of a second; (iv) the occurrence of miscues; (v) the likelihood of missed signals given their rate of occurrence; and (vi) the mismatching of intentions between the interactants and changes in their intentions as affected by their ongoing interactive state.[58–62] In addition, add to these reasons the fact that the child has limited and immature regulatory, behavioral, and attentional capacities and the likelihood of mismatches and miscoordinations become quite high. In our studies, we have found that periods of mismatching make up as much as 70% or 80% of the interaction[63].

Importantly, using the SF as a model, the microtemporal mismatches are microstressors and are associated with negative affect (Fig. 3). By contrast, matching states are associated with positive affect, though at high intensity they too can be stressful. The level of stress associated with mismatches is of course small compared to the stress induced by the SF and it is also of shorter duration. However, these mismatches and microstressors occur frequently, on the order of 4–10 times per minute. The interaction moves from matching to mismatching states and back again; that is, from positive affective nonstressful microstates to negative affective microstressful states at a very high rate. I have labeled the change from a mismatching to a matching state a repair because it leads to a change of negative to positive affect and a reduction in stress.[64] A metaphor is to think of dancing with lots of miscoordinations such as stepping on toes, but the dancers are wearing socks and they quickly get off each others' feet. The interaction is stressful, but in successful interactions the stress from mismatches, miscommunications, and misattunements is quickly repaired and over time matches again become miscoordinated and stressful, and again they are re-repaired. Critically, the process of mismatch and stress, reparation, and the reduction of stress literally occurs thousands of times in the course of a day and millions of times over the course of the year such that as the microeffects of matches, mismatches, and reparation accumulate they have profound effects.

THE INDUCTION OF RESILIENCE AND INDIVIDUAL DIFFERENCES

How does the experience in normal interactions of matching and mismatching and reparation lead to resilience? And how is individual variation in resilience induced? The normal interactive stress hypothesis is that the reparation of interactive mismatches and associated stress has a powerful inducing effect on resilience (capacity to regulate or resist stress), and that the reparation process helps shape individual differences in resilience.[65] In interactions characterized by normal rates of reparation, the infant learns which communicative strategies are effective in producing reparation and consequently effective in reducing stress. The infant also learns new self-organized ways of coping that are effective in reducing that stress, for example, averting gaze from a stressor or engaging in self-comforting behaviors. With the experiential accumulation of successful reparations, and the attendant transformation of negative affect and stress into positive affect, the infant establishes a robust positive affective core (Emde 1983).[8] A positive affective core biases experience by increasing the likelihood that an event is experienced as positive rather than as negative and stressful; in other words, an optimistic, implicit attitude about events. Importantly, the infant also learns that he or she has control over social interactions. Specifically, the infant develops a

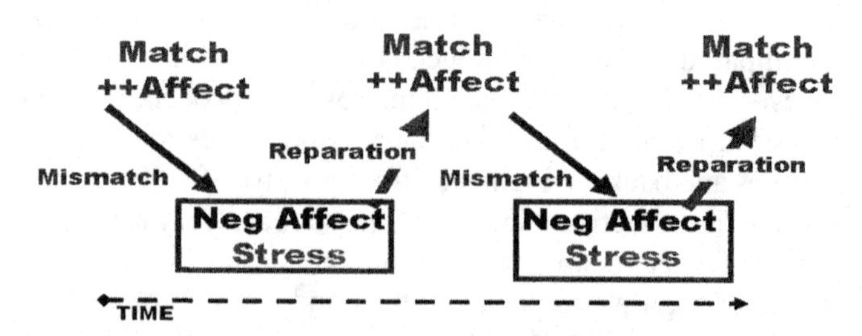

FIGURE 3. Normal interactions are characterized by periods of matching in which both partners (infant and adult) do the same behaviors and have the same intentions and periods of mismatching in which they do different behaviors and have different intentions. Matches are accompanied by positive affect and mismatches by stress and negative affect. Moving from a mismatch to a matching state is a reparation and reparations have positive developmental effects whereas failures of reparation have negative consequences.

representation of himself or herself as effective, and of his or her interactions as positive and reparable. He or she also learns that the caretaker is a reliable and trustworthy regulatory partner. These representations are crucial for the development of a sense of self that has coherence, continuity, and agency and for the development of stable and secure relationships, all of which add to resilience (Tronick, 1980; Tronick, Cohn & Shea, 1986). Thus a child who has a normal range of interactive experience develops robust resources and resilience for confronting stressors and effectively coping with them. By contrast, we know that infant animals and humans who have confronted overwhelming stress early in development fail to develop normally. And while we refer to these situations with a single word such as deprivation, the effect actually emerges from millions of reiterated moments in which reparation fails to resolve the stress.

Research supports the hypothesis that individual differences in resilience in part emerge from different experiences with stress and reparation at the microtemporal level. Research has demonstrated short- and long-term stability in infants' reactions to the SF. Tronick and Gianino [63] found significant stability across a 10-day period in infant signaling, attention, and self-comforting at 6 months of age. Recently, Tronick *et al.*[66] found short-term stability in 6-month-old infants' behavior between the administrations of the FFSF 2 weeks apart. The proportion of time infants spent averting from the mother, looking at objects, socially attending to the mother, and playing with the mother were significantly correlated over time. Moore *et al.*[44] evaluated stability and change in infants' negative and positive affect and gaze away from mother in response to the FFSF at 2, 4, and 6 months. Although there was no stability in infant positive affect, there were stable individual differences in negative affect from 4 to 6 months and in gazing away from 2 to 4 months and from 4 to 6 months. Similarly, Shapiro *et al.*[67] evaluated stability and change in the FFSF from 3 to 6 months. They found cross-time stability in infants' expression of interest and joy and in prepointing behaviors. In addition, Rosenblum and Muzik[68] recently reported stability in infants' positive and negative affective responses during the SF from 7 to 15 months of age.

Neurophysiologic measures have been found to be stable and related to interactive experiences. In typically developing children, measures of VT exhibit small-to-moderate levels of stability across contexts and over time during infancy and early childhood.[34,40,42,69–75] Individual differences in VT have been reported, which are associated with observations of infants' negative behavior during challenging tasks, although the correlations between infants' physiological and behavioral responses are typically not high.[70,76,77] In a study of 3-month-olds, Moore and Calkins, and Moore *et al.*[28,44] investigated changes in infants' VT, heart rate, and behavioral reactivity during the FFSF. They found individual differences in VT reactivity. Infants who did not suppress VT in the SF evidenced less positive affect, higher reactivity, and lower VT during the play and reunion episodes with their mothers. Calkins and Keane[77] found that children who displayed a pattern of stable and high VT suppression during challenging tasks from 2 to 4 years of age were less emotionally negative, and had fewer behavior problems and better social skills than other children. Investigators have also observed that children exhibit decreased VT during attention-demanding activities indexing individual differences in how an individual actively engages with the environment and regulates emotion and behavior in the face of environmental challenge.[30,39–41] Gunnar *et al.*[71] found that newborns' VT measures were related to their distress to limitations (frustration) at 6 months of age, as assessed via maternal report. In a study examining the relation between VT and later compliance in 5-, 10-, and 18-month-old infants, Stifter *et al.*[75,78] found that the younger infants' VT was related to their later noncompliance at 18 months. In a second study using a modified stranger-infant FFSF procedure with 5- to 6-month-olds,[42] infants' VT and behavioral responses were correlated across different episodes of the FFSF.

There are also individual differences in cortisol reactivity. Ramsay and Lewis[53] collected saliva samples from 33 infants at 2, 4, 6, and 18 months of age before, immediately before and 20 min after routine inoculations. When infants were divided into low-, moderate-, and high-reactor groups, significant correlations were found, indicating that infants within groups retained their relative rank-ordering in reactivity from 6 to 18 months of age. Nachmias and colleagues,[79] observed 18-month-olds in two moderately stressful procedures administered 1 week apart. Significant cross-age correlations were found between the baseline levels and the peak responses. Goldberg *et al.*[80] examined the stability of cortisol reactivity 1 week apart in 12- to 18-month-old infants. The stressors used were Ainsworth's Strange Situation and a "coping" task in which three novel events were presented to the infant (e.g., a noisy clown). Baseline levels of cortisol were collected at home, and in the lab cortisol was assessed repeatedly (20–40 min) after exposure to the stressors. Significant stability was found for the cortisol measures made within each stressful context. In a study of low-income preschoolers,[81] multiple measures of cortisol made on the same day were significantly correlated. Taken together, these findings indicate that infants' cortisol response to stressors shows moderate short-term stability.

These findings of stability in infants' behavioral and physiologic reaction to the SF and other stressors help us to understand the findings on the development of infants of depressed mothers and how a lack of reparation affects resilience.[82] Infants of depressed mothers experience fewer interactive reparations and can be under chronic stress. These infants develop self-organized patterns of coping that include looking away during interactions and higher levels of self-comforting to help reduce stress, but the cost is evident in higher levels of negative affect and less engagement with the inanimate environment. Their negative mood and disengagement compromise their interactions with others and their cognitive capacities with the consequence of compromising their development and making them less resilient. Furthermore, we have found that infant sons of depressed mothers are more stressed by their interactions with their mothers than are infant daughters.[83] These findings make sense given our studies showing that infant boys of clinically normal mothers are more stressed by the SF than are infant girls. Thus the coping of all infants is affected by the chronic moment-by-moment stress of their interactions with their depressed mothers and a lack of reparation, with the boys being more stressed because they have less ability in general to self-regulate stress compared to girls. We believe that this inability to self-regulate continues to compromise boys' as contrasted to girls' experience with reparation, resulting in more disorganized behavior and coping by boys throughout development.

There is a well-established relation between infants' early experience and their coping and resilience to challenges. Much of this literature is about the quality of infants' and young children's attachment relationship. The attachment relation, secure, ambivalent, avoidant, or disorganized, can be viewed as indicating the ways in which young children cope with stress, in particular the stress of separation from their primary caregiver (i.e., mother). The secure child, for example, has multiple strategies for dealing with stress whereas the disorganized child is overwhelmed by stress. In clinically normative studies, infants' reactions to the SF as well as to the normal FF interactions are predictive of infants' security of attachment. The infants' reactions to the SF are thought to index infants' accumulated experience with their mothers. For example, infants who repeatedly solicit their mothers' attention during the SF and are positive during the normal interaction have learned to trust their mothers and to expect positive interactions with her. Supporting this interpretation in a recent study Fuertes found that the quality of the mothers' reactions to their infants during play as well as the infants' reactions to the SF were predictive of infants' attachment security.[93]

There is also a large literature demonstrating the relation between early maternal sensitivity in caretaking and infants' coping with separation from the mother. Indeed it is widely accepted that sensitive caretaking is a primary factor affecting the quality of an infant's attachment to their mother. Importantly, recent research by Beebe and her colleagues,[84] and by Belsky,[85] demonstrates that sensitivity in the midrange is most predictive of infant secure attachments. Midrange sensitivity is characterized by a pattern of mismatching and reparation back to matching. In contrast, high and low sensitivity index a lack of reparation albeit in different ways: low sensitivity reflects a lack of reparation of long duration mismatches and high sensitivity reflects vigilance, too long lived matching with little opportunity for reparation. Infants' experience of midrange sensitivity develops ways of coping with the stress of separation, whereas infants experiencing low sensitivity are constantly overwhelmed by stress and fail to develop ways of coping, and the high sensitivity infants do not confront a sufficient amount of stress to develop their own resources, but end up relying on parental regulation to cope with stress. Thus normal interactive experience with mismatching, reparation, and stress have a strong relation to individual variation in the quality of infants' capacity for coping with stress and their resilience in the face of stress. Of course, when the infant is resilient, the mother has a better chance to find the midrange because it is wider, than the mother of a vulnerable infant whose midrange is narrow forcing the mother into one extreme or the other.

CONCLUSIONS

The MRM and the normal interactive stress hypothesis argue that normal and typical experience with reparation, matching, and mismatching has a profound effect on the development of coping and individual differences in resilience in the face of stress. The effects are not only behavioral but also neurophysiologic as indicated by the research on the sympathetic, parasympathetic, and HPA systems. These systems are not tightly linked, which allows for adaptive flexibility in the face of stress (e.g., gaze aversion is a fast and less costly way of coping with stress than is sympathetic nervous system activation) but all of these systems are affected by moment-to-moment events and experience. Though the literature is far too great to be summarized here, this normal interactive stress hypothesis also is strongly supported by the animal research on the effects of stress on development of brain and behavior.[57,86–88] I believe that taking a normal interactive stress perspective on many animal experiments that manipulate the environment (e.g., avoidance conditioning, handling, environmental impoverishment, or enrichment) can give us a better understanding of how stress has its long-term effects. Like the SF many of the manipulations used in animal work serve to highlight the stress that is inherent, normal, and typical in the animal's environment. The SF in humans highlights the match-mismatch-reparation process of normal interactions. Rats that are handled more by humans develop coping capacities, not because handling by humans is special but because the normal contact they have with other conspecifics, which is mimicked by human handling, is the way they normally develop coping and resilience. When the dominance hierarchy of a monkey troop is manipulated, individual animals have to cope with the change, but it has its effects not because it is a dramatic manipulation, but because the manipulation mimics the daily moment-by-moment experience of animals coping with dominance, and that experience is one way in which they develop coping and resilience.

By contrast to normal stress manipulations, manipulations that are traumatic, ones that exceed the individual's capacity for coping, highlight the limits of the system. Such traumatic experiences do not lead to resilience. However, individuals vary in what is or is experienced as traumatic based on their experience with levels of stress that they have been able to cope with. The adage that what does not kill you will make you stronger likely is not true. Rather, more likely is the hypothesis that a whole lot of small well-coped-with stressors make you more resilient.

Fortunately, everyday life provides plenty of small stressors. The mature organism has to cope with the stresses of garnering specifically fitted energy to maintain their current level of complexity and coherence. Finding and acquiring resources is one source of stress. In normal environments the stress is not overwhelming. In the developing young human even more energy has to be obtained to permit growth. Development itself is messy and unpredictable and a source of stress. In normal development the stress is not overwhelming and to meet these demands, humans have evolved a highly effective dyadic (and larger) mutually regulated system for garnering energy for both maintenance and growth and for coping with stress. It is a system that is more effective in garnering resources than individuals can gain on their own and for regulating stressors individuals would not be able to regulate on their own. Paradoxically, the interactive system in and of itself is inherently stressful but normally is not overwhelming. As a consequence of coping with these normal stressors all individuals' develop and grow their coping capacities and their unique experience with stressors makes for differences in resilience.

REFERENCES

1. RUTTER, M. 2006. Genes and Behavior. Blackwell. Malden, MA.
2. TRONICK, E.Z. 2003. Infant moods and the chronicity of depressive symptoms: the co-creation of unique ways of being together for good or ill. Paper 1: the normal process of development and the formation of moods. Zeitschrift für Psychosomatische Medizin und Psychotherapie **4:** 408–425.
3. TRONICK, E.Z. 2005. Why is connection with others so critical? Dyadic meaning making, messiness, and complexity-governed selective processes which co-create and expand indviduals' states of consciousness: the assembling of states of consciousness and experiential impelling certitude from the messiness of age-possible meanings of emotions, actions and symbols. *In* Emotional Development. J. Nadel & D. Muir, Eds.: 293–315. Oxford University Press. New York.
4. TRONICK, E.Z. 2003. Of course all relationships are unique: how co-creative processes generate unique mother-infant and patient-therapist relationships and change other relationships. Psychol. Inq. **23:** 473–491.
5. STENGERS, I. & I. PRIGOGINE. 1997. The End of Certainty. Simon & Schuster. New York.
6. SANDER, L. 1995. Thinking about developmental process: wholeness, specificity, and the organization of conscious experiencing. Paper presented at the Division 39 meeting of the American Psychological Association. Santa Monica, CA.
7. BALTES, P., U. LINDENBERGER & M. STAUDINGER (Ed.). 1998. Life-Span Theory in Developmental Psychology (Vol. 1). John Wiley & Sons. New York.
8. GIANINO, A. & E.Z. TRONICK. 1988. The mutual regulation model: the infant's self and interactive regulation, coping, and defensive capacities. *In* Stress and Coping. T. Field, P. McCabe & N. Schneiderman, Eds.: 47–68. Erlbaum. Hillsdale, NJ.

9. BRAZELTON, T.B. 1992. Touchpoints: Your Child's Emotional and Behavioral Development. Addison-Wesley. Reading, MA.
10. HEIMANN, M. 2003. Regression Periods in Human Infancy. Lawrence Erlbaum Associates. London.
11. BAK, P. 1996. How Nature Works. Srpinger-Verlag. New York.
12. FREEMAN, W.J. 2000. How Brains Make Up Their Mind. Columbia University Press. New York.
13. HOFER, M.A. 1984. Relationships as regulators: a psychobiologic perspective on bereavement. Psychosom. Med. **46:** 183–197.
14. VYGOTSKY, L.S. 1967. Play and its role in the mental development of the child. Soviet Psychol. **5:** 6–18.
15. BEEBE, B. & F. LACHMANN. 1998. Co-constructing inner and relational process: self and mutual regulation in infant research and adult treatment. Psychoanal. Psychol. **15:** 1–37.
16. BEEGHLY, M. & E.Z. TRONICK. 1994. Effects of prenatal exposure to cocaine in early infancy: toxic effects on the process of mutual regulation. Infant Ment. Health J. **15:** 158–175.
17. TRONICK, E.Z., H. ALS, L. ADAMSON, *et al.* 1978. The infant's response to entrapment between contradictory messages in face-to-face interaction. J. Am. Acad. Child Adolesc. Psychiatry **17:** 1–13.
18. ADAMSON, L. & J. FRICK. 2003. The Still-Face: a history of a shared experimental paradigm. Infancy **4:** 451–473.
19. COLE, P.M., S.E. MARTIN & T.A. DENNIS. 2004. Emotion regulation as a scientific construct: methodological challenges and directions for child development research. Child Dev. **75:** 317–333.
20. STACK, D.M. & D.W. MUIR. 1990. Tactile stimulation as a component of social interchange: new interpretations for the still-face effect. Br. J. Dev. Psychol. **8:** 131–145.
21. TRONICK, E.Z. 1989. Emotions and emotional communication in infants. Am. Psychol. **44:** 112–119.
22. TRONICK, E.Z. 2001. Emotional connections and dyadic consciousness in infant-mother and patient-therapist interactions. Psychoanal. Dialogues **11:** 187–194.
23. WEINBERG, M.K. & E.Z. TRONICK. 1996. Infant affective reactions to the resumption of maternal interaction after the still-face. Child Dev. **67:** 905–914.
24. TODA, S. & A. FOGEL. 1993. Infant response to the still-face situation at 3 and 6 months. Dev. Psychol. **29:** 532–538.
25. KOGAN, N. & A.S. CARTER. 1996. Mother-infant reengagement following the still-face: the role of maternal emotional availability in infant affect regulation. Infant Behav. Dev. **19:** 359–370.
26. ROSENBLUM, K.L., S. MCDONOUGH, M. MUZIK, *et al.* 2002. Maternal representations of the infant: associations with infant response to the still-face. Child Dev. **73:** 999–1015.
27. WEINBERG, M.K., E.Z. TRONICK, J.F. COHN & K.L. OLSON. 1999. Gender differences in emotional expressivity and self-regulation during early infancy. Dev. Psychol. **35:** 175–188.
28. MOORE, G.A. & S.D. CALKINS. 2004. Infants' vagal regulation in the still-face paradigm is related to dyadic coordination of mother-infant interaction. Dev. Psychol. **40:** 1068–1080.
29. BERNTSON, G.G., S. HART & M. SARTER. 1997. The cardiovascular startle response: anxiety and the benzodiazepine receptor complex. Psychophysiology **34:** 348–357.

30. PORGES, S.W. 1995. Cardiac vagal tone: a physiological index of stress. Neurosc. Biobehav. Rev. **19:** 225–233.
31. PORGES, S.W. 2001. The polyvagal theory: phylogenetic substrates of a social nervous system. Int. J. Psychophysiol. **42:** 123–146.
32. CALKINS, S.D. 1997. Cardiac vagal tone indices of temperamental reactivity and behavioral regulation in young children. Dev. Psychobiol. **31:** 125–135.
33. DONZELLA, B., M.R. GUNNAR, W.K. KRUEGER & J. ALWIN. 2000. Cortisol and vagal tone responses to competitive challenge in preschoolers: associations with temperament. Dev. Psychobiol. **37:** 209–220.
34. DOUSSARD-ROOSEVELT, J., L. MONTGOMERY & S. PORGES. 2003. Short-term stability of physiological measures in kindergarten children: respiratory sinus arrhythmia, heart period, and cortisol. Dev. Psychobiol. **43:** 230–242.
35. PORGES, S.W., J.A. DOUSSARD-ROOSEVELT, A.L. PORTALES & P.E. SUESS. 1994. Cardiac vagal tone: stability and relation to difficultness in infants and 3-year-olds. Dev. Psychobiol. **27:** 289–300.
36. HUFFMAN, L.C., Y.E. BRYAN, R. DEL CARMEN, *et al.* 1998. Infant temperament and cardiac vagal tone: assessments at twelve weeks of age. Child Dev. **69:** 624–635.
37. DEGANGI, G., J. DIPIETRO, S.W. PORGES & S. GREENSPAN. 1991. Psychophysiological characteristics of the regulatory disorded infant. Infant Behav. Dev. **14:** 37–50.
38. PORGES, S.W., J.A. DOUSSARD-ROOSEVELT, A.L. PORTALES & S.I. GREENSPAN. 1996. Infant regulation of the vagal "brake" predicts child behavior problems: a psychobiological model of social behavior. Dev. Psychobiol. **29:** 697–712.
39. PORGES, S.W. 2003. The polyvagal theory: phylogenetic contributions to social behavior. Physiol. Behav. **79:** 503–513.
40. BORNSTEIN, M.H. & P.E. SUESS. 2000. Child and mother cardiac vagal tone: continuity, stability, and concordance across the first 5 years. Dev. Psychol. **36:** 54–65.
41. RICHARDS, J.E. 1987. Infant visual sustained attention and respiratory sinus arrhythmia. Child Dev. **58:** 488–496.
42. BAZHENOVA, O.V., O. PLONSKAIA & S.W. PORGES. 2001. Vagal reactivity and affective adjustment in infants during interaction challenges. Child Dev. **72:** 1314–1326.
43. HALEY, D.W. & K. STANSBURY. 2003. Infant stress and parent responsiveness: regulation of physiology and behavior during Still-Face and reunion. Child Dev. **74:** 1534–1546.
44. MOORE, G.A., J.F. COHN & S.B. CAMPBELL. 2001. Infant affective responses to mother's still face at 6 months differentially predict externalizing and internalizing behaviors at 18 months. Dev. Psychol. **37:** 706–714.
45. LEWIS, M. & D. RAMSAY. 2005. Infant emotional and cortisol responses to goal blockage. Child Dev. **76:** 518–530.
46. DE QUERVAIN, D.J., B. ROOZENDAAL & J.L. MCGAUGH. 1998. Stress and glucocorticoids impair retrieval of long-term spatial memory. Nature **394:** 787–790.
47. LUPIEN, S.J., A. FIOCCO, N. WAN, *et al.* 2005. Stress hormones and human memory function across the lifespan. Psychoneuroendocrinology **30:** 225–242.
48. MCEWEN, B.S. & R.M. SAPOLSKY. 1995. Stress and cognitive function. Curr. Opin. Neurobiol. **5:** 205–216.
49. STANSBURY, K. & M.R. GUNNAR. 1994. Adrenocortical activity and emotion regulation. *In* The Development of Emotion Regulation: Biological and Behavioral Considerations, 59 edition. N.A. Fox, Ed.: 108–134. Monographs of the Society for Research in Child Devleopment. Blackwell Publishing. Malden, MA.

50. WHITE, B.P., M.R. GUNNAR, M.C. LARSON, *et al.* 2000. Behavioral and physiological responsivity, sleep, and patterns of daily cortisol production in infants with and without colic. Child Dev. **71:** 862–877.
51. GODLBERG, S., R. LEVITAN, E. LEUNG, *et al.* 2003. Cortisol concentrations in 12- to 18-month-old infants: stability over time, location and stressor. Biol. Psychiatry **54:** 719–726.
52. DICKERSON, S.S. & M.E. KEMENY. 2004. Acute stressors and cortisol responses: a theoretical integration and synthesis of laboratory research. Psychol. Bull. **130:** 355–391.
53. RAMSAY, D. & M. LEWIS. 2003. Reactivity and regulation in cortisol and behavioral responses to stress. Child Dev. **74:** 456–464.
54. BUSS, K.A., J.R.M. SCHUMACHER, I. DOLSKI, *et al.* 2003. Right frontal brain activity, cortisol, and withdrawal behavior in 6-month-old infants. Behav. Neurosc. **117:** 11–20.
55. GUNNAR, M.R., S. MANGELSDORF, M. LARSON & L. HERTSGAARD. 1989. Attachment, temperament, and adrenocortical activity in infancy: a study of psychoendocrine regulation. Dev. Psychol. **25:** 355–363.
56. MCGAUGH, J.L. 2004. The amygdala modulates the consolidation of memories of emotionally arousing experiences. Ann. Rev. Neurosc. **27:** 1–28.
57. ROOZENDAAL, B., G.L. QUIRARTE & J.L. MCGAUGH. 1997. Stress-activated hormonal systems and the regulation of memory storage. *In* Psychobiology of Posttraumatic Stress Disorder. Eds.: A.C. McFarlane & R. Yehuda: 247–258. New York Academy of Sciences. New York.
58. COHN, J.F. & M. ELMORE. 1988. Effect of contingent changes in mothers' affective expression on the organization of behavior in 3-month-old infants. Infant Behav. Dev. **11:** 493–505.
59. COHN, J. & E. TRONICK. 1987. Mother-infant face-to-face interaction: the sequence of dyadic states at three, six, and nine months. Devel. Psych. **23:** 68–77.
60. COHN, J.F. & E. TRONICK. 1988. Mother-infant face-to-face interaction: influence is bidirectional and unrelated to periodic cycles in either partner's behavior. Dev. Psychol. **24:** 386–392.
61. COHN, J.F. & E.Z. TRONICK. 1987. Mother-infant face-to-face interaction: the sequence of dyadic states at 3, 6, and 9 months. Dev. Psychol. **23:** 68–77.
62. TRONICK, E., J. COHN & E. SHEA. 1986. The transfer of affect between mothers and infants. *In* Affective Development in Infancy. Eds.: 11–25. T.B. Brazelton & M.W. Yogman, Ablex Publishing Corp. Norwood, NJ.
63. TRONICK, E.Z. & A. GIANINO. 1986. Interactive mismatch and repair: challenges to the coping infant. Zero to Three: Bulletin of the National Center for Clinical Infant Programs **6:** 1–6.
64. TRONICK, E.Z. & J.F. COHN. 1989. Infant-mother face-to-face interaction: age and gender differences in coordination and the occurrence of miscoordination. Child Dev. **60:** 85–92.
65. TRONICK, E.Z. & M.K. WEINBERG. 1997. Depressed mothers and infants: failure to form dyadic states of consciousness. *In* Postpartum Depression and Child Development. L. Murray & P.J. Cooper, Eds.: 54–81. Guilford Press. New York.
66. TRONICK, E.Z., M.K. WEINBERG, M. BEEGHLY & K.L. OLSON. 2003. Short-term stability and change in infant, maternal, and mutual regulatory behavior during the face-to-face still-face paradigm. Presented at the biennial meetings of the International Conference on Infant Studies. Chicago, IL.

67. SHAPIRO, B., J. FAGEN, J. PRIGOT, *et al.* 1998. Infants' emotional and regulatory behaviors in response to violations of expectancies. Infant Behav. Dev. **21:** 299–313.
68. ROSENBLUM, K.L. & M. MUZIK. 2004. Mothers' representations of their infants and infant still face response: individual differences from 7- to 15-months. International Conference on Infant Studies. Chicago.
69. DOUSSARD-ROOSEVELT, J.A., B.D. MCCLENNY & S.W. PORGES. 2001. Neonatal cardiac vagal tone and school-age developmental outcome in very low birth weight infants. Dev. Psychobiol. **38:** 56–66.
70. EL-SHEIKH, M. 2005. Stability of respiratory sinus arrhythmia in children and young adolescents: a longitudinal examination. Dev. Psychobiol. **46:** 66–74.
71. GUNNAR, M.R., F.L. PORTER, C.M. WOLF, *et al.* 1995. Neonatal stress reactivity: predictions to later emotional temperament. Child Dev. **66:** 1–13.
72. PORGES, S.W. 1992. Vagal tone: a physiological marker of stress vulnerability. Pediatrics **90:** 498–504.
73. PORGES, S.W., J.A. DOUSSARD-ROOSEVELT, C.A. STIFTER, *et al.* 1999. Sleep state and vagal regulation of heart period patterns in the human newborn: an extension of the polyvagal theory. Psychophysiology **36:** 14–21.
74. STIFTER, C.A. & N.A. FOX. 1990. Infant reactivity. Physiological correlates of newborn and 5-month temperament. Develop. Psych. **26**(4)**:** 582–588.
75. STIFTER, C.A., N.A. FOX & S.W. PORGES. 1989. Facial expressivity and vagal tone in 5- and 10-month-old infants. Infant Behav. Dev. **12:** 127–138.
76. CALKINS, S., S.E. DEDMON, K.L. GILL, *et al.* 2002. Frustration in infancy: implications for emotion regulation, physiological processes, and temperament. Infancy **3:** 175–197.
77. CALKINS, S. & S. KEANE. 2004. Cardiac vagal regulation across the preschool period: stability, continuity, and implications for childhood adjustment. Dev. Psychobiol. **45:** 101–112.
78. STIFTER, C.A. & A. JAIN. 1996. Psychophysiological correlates of infant temperament: stability of behavior and autonomic patterning from 5 to 18 months. Dev. Psychobiol. **29:** 379–391.
79. NACHMIAS, M., M. GUNNAR, S. MANGELSDORF, *et al.* 1996. Behavioral inhibition and stress reactivity: the moderating role of attachment security. Child Dev. **67:** 508–522.
80. GOLDBERG, S., R. LEVITAN, J.B. EMANS, *et al.* 2003. Cortisol concentrations in 12- and 18-month-old infants: stability over time, location and stressor. Biol. Psychiatry **54:** 719–726.
81. BLAIR, C., D. GRANGER & R.P. RAZZA. 2005. Cortisol reactivity is positively related to executive function in preschool children attending Head Start. Child Dev. **76:** 554–567.
82. TRONICK, E.Z. & T. FIELD. 1987. Maternal Depression and Infant Disturbance. Jossey-Bass. San Francisco, CA.
83. WEINBERG, M.K., E.Z. TRONICK, J.F. COHN & K.L. OLSON. 1999. Gender differences in emotional expressivity and self-regulation during early infancy. Devel. Psych. **35:** 175–188.
84. JAFFE, J., B. BEEBE, S. FELDSTEIN, C.L. CROWN & M.D. JASNOW. 2001. Rhythms of Dialogue in Infancy. Blackwell Publishing. Malden, MA.
85. BELSKY, J. 1999. Interactional and contextual determinants of attachment security. *In* Handbook of Attachment. Theory, Research, and Clinical Applications. J. Cassidy & P.R. Shaver, Eds.: 249–264. The Guilford Press. New York.

86. LUPIEN, S.J. & B.S. MCEWEN. 1997. The acute effects of corticosteroids on cognition: integration of animal and human model studies. Brain Res. Rev. **24:** 1–27.
87. MCGAUGH, J.L. 2000. Memory: a century of consolidation. Science **287**: 248–251.
88. SMYTHE, J.W., C.M. MCCORMICK & M.J. MEANEY. 1996. Median eminence corticotrophin-releasing hormone content following prenatal stress and neonatal handling. Brain Res. Bull. **40:** 195–199.
89. HAM, J. & E. TRONICK. 2006. Infant resilience to the stress of the still-face. Ann. N. Y. Acad. Sci. This volume.
90. EMDE, R.N. (1983, March). The *affective core*. Paper presented at the Second World Congress of Infant Psychiatry, Cannes, France.
91. TRONICK, E. 1980. The primary of social skills in infancy. *In* Exceptional infant, Vol. 4: Psychosocial risks in infant-environment transactions. D.B. Sawin, Hawkins R.C., L.O. Walker, J.H. Penticuff, Eds.: 144–158. Bruner/Mazel. New York.
92. TRONICK, E., J. COHN & E. SHEA. 1986. The transfer of affect between mothers and infants. *In* Affective development in infancy. Norwood. T.B. Brazelton, M.W. Yogman, Eds.: 11–25. NJ: Ablex Publishing Corporation.
93. FUERTES, M., *et al.* More maternal sensitivity shopes attachment. Ann. N. Y. Acad. Sci. This volume.

Conceptual Issues in Studies of Resilience

Past, Present, and Future Research

SUNIYA S. LUTHAR,[a] JEANETTE A. SAWYER,[a]
AND PAMELA J. BROWN[b]

[a] *Teachers College, Columbia University, New York, New York, USA*

[b] *Yale University School of Medicine, New Haven, Connecticut, USA*

ABSTRACT: We begin this article by considering the following critical conceptual issues in research on resilience: (1) distinctions between protective, promotive, and vulnerability factors; (2) the need to unpack underlying processes; (3) the benefits of within-group experimental designs; and (4) the advantages and potential pitfalls of an overwhelming scientific focus on biological and genetic factors (to the relative exclusion of familial and contextual ones). The next section of the article is focused on guidelines for the selection of vulnerability and protective processes in future research. From a basic science standpoint, it is useful and appropriate to investigate all types of processes that might significantly affect adjustment among at-risk individuals. If the research is fundamentally applied in nature, however, it would be most expedient to focus on risk modifiers that have high potential to alter individuals' overall life circumstances. The final section of this article considers conceptual differences between contemporary resilience research on children versus adults. Issues include differences in the types and breadth of outcomes (e.g., the tendencies to focus on others' ratings of competence among children and on self-reports of well-being among adults respectively).

KEYWORDS: resilience; protective processes; risk modifiers; interventions

INTRODUCTION

The value of empirical data on childhood resilience rests upon our conceptual understanding of the issues central to this research. It is therefore essential for scholars engaging in the study of resilience to critically appraise ongoing dialogues on the themes salient to this body of work. This article touches

Address for correspondence: Dr. Suniya S. Luthar, Teachers College, Columbia University, 525 West 120th Street, Box 133, New York, NY 10027. Voice: 212-678-3798; fax: 212-678-3483.
e-mail: Sl504@columbia.edu

Ann. N.Y. Acad. Sci. 1094: 105–115 (2006).
doi: 10.1196/annals.1376.009

briefly on six such themes. The first three are issues that have been discussed for years in the literature, but there are still some points of confusion; these have to do with what we mean by labels of protective and vulnerability factors, the need to unpack underlying processes or mechanisms, and the usefulness of interaction effects (as opposed to using within-group studies). The other three issues have not been discussed quite as much in the past; these pertain to the focus on biological and genetic indices, research priorities in our future work, and differences between resilience research on children versus adults. In discussing all these issues, a common underlying consideration is how we, in science, can best intervene to help vulnerable children and families: a theme that undergirds much (if not most of) contemporary research on resilience.

DISTINCTIONS BETWEEN PROTECTIVE, PROMOTIVE, AND VULNERABILITY FACTORS

The central objective of resilience researchers is to identify vulnerability and protective factors that might modify the negative effects of adverse life circumstances, and having accomplished this, to identify mechanisms or processes that might underlie associations found.[1–4] In the literature on resilience, discussions on the notions of vulnerability and protection have reflected considerable confusion around definition, measurement, and interpretation of statistical findings. Clarification of the meaning of terms "protective factors" and "vulnerability factors" is therefore vital for further research.[5]

The term "protective factor," referring to something that modifies the effects of risk in a positive direction, clearly has positive connotations, referring to something that is helpful or beneficial. What is less clear is whether this is also the inverse of "vulnerability factor," with the two terms reflecting two sides of the same coin, as it were. Until recently, many suggested that this is the case—as high IQ is protective, low IQ connotes vulnerability. However, this is not necessarily true for all variables, and caution must be exercised in choosing between labels.

We illustrate the need for care in this regard with a data-based example. In a study of children of mothers with major mental illness,[6] we found positive links between maternal warmth and child competence. This might suggest, logically, that mothers' warmth served as a protective or promotive factor. However, when the distributions of children's scores were examined, this is not what was revealed. On the measure of competence used in this study, T scores of 50 reflect the population average so that scores of 60 or more—at one standard deviation above the average—would imply excellence and those of 40 or less would connote significant vulnerability. In our own at-risk sample, children with high maternal warmth were close to national averages (with T scores of about 52); they did not reflect "superior" competence. On the other hand, those with low closeness fared quite poorly, clearly in the clinically significant range (with mean competence T scores of about 36). In this case, therefore, high closeness was not particularly promotive—rather, low maternal closeness connoted significant vulnerability. In future research, therefore, it would be useful for researchers to examine such distributions of scores to determine the "polarity," as it were, of apparently bipolar variables, to see whether most of the effects occur at the positive end, the negative end, or in fact, equally at both.

THE NEED TO UNPACK UNDERLYING PROCESSES

The need to unpack processes is critical not only with reference to risk modifiers but also the risk indices themselves. With regard to risk modifiers (or protective and vulnerability factors), this issue has been written about frequently in the past with questions, such as, "What is it, exactly, about family support that might promote resilience: A sense of security? High self-esteem? Feelings of control?" Less often discussed is the need to unpack processes that underlie the risk indices themselves. We know well that risk factors tend to coalesce or coexist.[7,8] Research has shown us, for example, that maternal drug abuse tends to co-occur with diagnoses of depression or anxiety, and also with major life stressors. A critical question to be addressed is the following: If one considered all of these risks together, which ones would prevail in actually representing high risk? The answer to this question is not necessarily intuitive. Recent evidence suggests that maternal depression actually seems to connote more risks for children than does maternal substance abuse in itself.[9] Unpacking the relative impact of different processes linked with a global risk factor, therefore, is critical in understanding antecedents of vulnerability and resilience.

Findings such as these can have major policy implications. To continue with the preceding example, drug-abusing mothers tend to be seen as having willfully jeopardized their children's well-being and are subject to punitive measures, such as revocation of parental rights.[10] In comparison, mothers with depression are often seen as victims of genetic predisposition or life circumstances. As we weigh such disparities in attitudes, it is worthwhile to consider that the evidence suggests that maternal drug dependence is not necessarily more inimical for children than is maternal depression. Like depression, it is a psychiatric condition that emerges from multiple vulnerabilities, and like depression, it can show considerable improvement with therapeutic attention.

ASSUMPTIONS REGARDING "HIGH" AND "LOW" RISK

These findings on maternal drug abuse lead to another broader issue warranting careful attention in our research, and this pertains to commonplace assumptions about what a risk condition is, or is not. Again, presumptions in this regard are not necessarily based on reality, as is evident from findings on children at the socio-economic status (SES) extremes.[11]

Whereas youth in urban poverty are commonly and appropriately thought of as being at high risk, recent evidence shows that those at the other end of the socioeconomic extreme can reflect as much disturbance or more. In a comparative study based on data gathered about a decade ago, affluent, suburban youth reported significantly higher levels of cigarette, alcohol, and marijuana use as compared to their counterparts in serious poverty.[12] Suburban youth also reported higher levels of substance use when compared with national normative samples. More recent data collected from another suburban community[11,13] and from a private high school in a large city,[14] replicated these findings; again, use levels were higher among these affluent youth as compared to norms.

Elevated problems were also seen on other adjustment indices, both internalizing and externalizing in nature. Affluent girls in particular have been found to show elevated levels of depression and anxiety symptoms[11,15] and both boys and girls show striking elevations in rule-breaking behaviors. In national normative samples, about 7% of youth have T scores of 65 on rule breaking,[16] and in our suburban and urban affluent samples, rates were two to three times as high.

Collectively, these data indicate the need for researchers to be careful about assuming that particular demographic groups are necessarily at "low" risk. There is no question that children living in chronic poverty face significant risks to their well-being. This does not imply, however, that their counterparts in affluence experience salutary life circumstances, or for that matter, even stress-free ones.

INTERACTION EFFECTS VERSUS WITHIN-GROUP ANALYSES

A third critical conceptual issue has to do with the role of statistical interaction effects in resilience research. As frequently noted, interaction effects are conceptually very intriguing.[17] On the other hand, searching for them can sometimes be counterproductive.[18] We illustrate this with a hypothetical example from a study on youth in poverty. The focus here is on various family predictors with the hypothesis that stringent limit setting will be a critical "protective factor." This is, in fact, borne out by simple correlations in this study, with high limit setting linked with responsible, prosocial behaviors. In multivariate regressions, moreover, this effect remained significant even with the inclusion of several other family-level variables.

If the researchers then wished to document interaction effects—showing benefits of stringent limit-setting among low-income youth but not others—they would include a comparison group of middle class youth. Multivariate regressions would then be conducted based on the entire sample, with initial controls for several variables (e.g., age, gender, ethnicity of the child), and then main effects (e.g., limit-setting along with other family dimensions), followed by interaction terms: SES by limit setting, and in interaction with other family variables.

Whereas limit setting showed positive simple correlations with competence among low-income children, it was negatively correlated with competence among middle-income youth (for whom stringency can imply harshness[5]). With all the children considered together in the regressions, then, these effects would serve to work against each other, rendering the main effect for limit-setting weak or statistically nonsignificant. Furthermore, the multiple interaction terms included in the equation would use several degrees of freedom so that the block as a whole also could become nonsignificant. Thus, the pursuit of interaction effects might essentially have obscured the fact that stringent limit setting was, in fact, potentially beneficial for youth in urban poverty.

The point underlying this illustration goes well beyond whether or not researchers should focus on interaction effects; we are arguing for more *within-group analyses* with discrete groups of people at risk. When researchers work with particular at-risk children, they seek to illuminate what makes a difference for *these* youth—not whether these factors affect sundry other comparison groups. Reverting to the previous example, then, the critical question is not whether limit setting "matters more" for poor youth than for their more affluent counterparts, but rather, "Given the different forces salient in the lives of low-income teens, which particular ones prevail in compensating for their adversities?" Fortunately, the value of within-group studies is being increasingly acknowledged.[19–24] Developmental scholars endorse shifts in designs from comparative approaches that document group differences, to within-group analyses illuminating the particularly critical processes for youth from given subcultural backgrounds. Such studies are often the strategy of choice when seeking to learn about intervention priorities in subgroups of the population about whom we currently understand little.[5]

FOCUS ON BIOLOGICAL AND GENETIC FACTORS: CONSIDERATIONS FROM AN APPLIED PERSPECTIVE

For decades, resilience research was focused entirely on psychological or behavioral variables; and we are now well into a new era with concerted attention to biology and genetics as well.[25,26] In a seminal overview paper, Curtis and Cicchetti[27] explained the importance of diverse biological processes ranging from neuroendocrinology to capacities for emotion regulation. With regard to genetic influences, Rutter, Caspi, Kim-Cohen, Moffitt, and their colleagues have written extensively on genetic factors potentially involved in resilience.[4,28,29] Recent studies have identified gene–environment interactions—wherein both genes and child-specific environmental influences contribute to behavioral resilience—as well as specific gene markers that contribute to protection or vulnerability in the face of childhood adversities.[30,31]

From an intervention perspective, there are several obvious advantages of these lines of inquiry. Most obviously, we are making great scientific strides as we learn about the biological aspects of the human body that impose constraints, or confidence intervals, within which environments can be helpful. Another benefit is that in demonstrating the power of environmental inputs, biological evidence tends to be particularly compelling. If intervention researchers could demonstrate that good early interventions result in increased brain mass and enriched neural networks, this tends to be more powerful evidence, to the minds of many, than simply reports of improvements in children's observed or self-reported adjustment. Similarly, attempts to prevent adolescent substance use might be bolstered if families and youth are made aware of the neurodevelopmental risks involved, especially the high plasticity and hence vulnerability of the developing brain during adolescence.

At the same time, researchers operating from an intervention perspective need to be careful about moving hastily to an overwhelming focus on genes and biology. This cautiousness is warranted for at least two reasons. First, as exciting as discoveries of gene markers are, we are limited in how much we can change these. Second, we have limited funds for research to promote resilience (unfortunately, increasingly limited funds for health-related research altogether). And the reality is that as we devote more to studying biology and genes, we have that much less toward developing creative interventions to alter factors that we already *know very well* can make an enormous difference—not just factors like poverty and community violence, but also maltreatment in homes, lack of services for families, and so on.

If a fundamental goal is to promote the psychosocial well-being of vulnerable children and families, therefore, we believe that it is critical to ensure balance in our scientific priorities. Discovering biological risk and gene markers constitutes groundbreaking science. At the same time, much is still to be learned about using research-based interventions that attenuate potent and well-known environmental risks affecting the lives of thousands of today's children.

GUIDELINES FOR THE SELECTION OF VULNERABILITY AND PROTECTIVE PROCESSES IN FUTURE RESEARCH

In considering future research on resilience, we consider, next, how we might most productively focus our future inquiry on psychosocial vulnerability and protective factors. There are so many candidate constructs from which to choose, all potentially alleviating or exacerbating risk. Weighing this issue again, from an applied or interventions perspective, we present a set of four criteria that might be helpful.[5]

First, given a particular at-risk condition, there must be concerted attention to factors that are *salient in that particular life context,* those that affect a relatively large number of people in that group. Second, we should prioritize attention to indices that are relatively *malleable*—risk modifiers amenable to change via external interventions or "modifiable modifiers." Third, focus should be afforded to indices that tend to be relatively *enduring* in a child's life, or those that continue to exert their (positive or negative) effects for some length of time. Finally, it is critical to attend to indices that are *generative* of other assets; those that set into motion "cascades"[2] wherein they catalyze other protective processes.

Reviews of more than 50 years of research on childhood resilience[5,32] show that across different risks—ranging from parental divorce and bereavement to maltreatment and community violence—close, supportive family relationships clearly meet all four criteria. These relationships are obviously salient and proximal in children's lives; they can be changed via interventions; parents are present in children's lives for almost two decades or longer; and good parent–child relationships can generate other assets, such as feelings of confidence, security, and self-efficacy.

At the same time, there is still a great deal more to be learned about parents, families, relationships, and resilience. Most importantly, we have very little research on what *makes for* good parenting.[5] In child development studies, parenting dimensions are almost always predictor variables and almost never outcomes, so that we know little about how it is that parents facing formidable challenges are still able to function reasonably well. Thus, in future research it must be a priority to understand how parents, particularly mothers who are usually primary caregivers, are able to do well despite considerable odds (e.g., chronic poverty along with serious psychiatric problems).

We also need more research on the specific demands of parents in particular risk contexts, and on how to optimally harness the resources available from adults other than parents. As an illustration relevant to the first point, parental monitoring and supervision are critical in violence-prone, inner-city settings whereas in upper-class suburbia, guarding against crushing achievement pressures can be crucial.[10] With regard to the recommended increased focus on nonparent adults, this is important because the reality is that even with our best efforts, we will not be able to reach some parents at high risk. Juxtaposed with this unfortunate reality, however, is a more comforting one (a truism put forth decades ago by pioneers in resilience[33–35])—what is critical is a strong, enduring relationship with *at least one caring adult*; this may or may not be a biological parent. For vulnerable children in contemporary society, there are in fact many adults who could potentially fulfill this function—not only informal mentors, but also teachers at school, often cited as having turned people's lives around.[5] Stated differently, we know without question that good relationships are fundamental to children's resilient adaptation. We need, now, to work harder on developing interventions that harness the relationship resources existing in children's lives, toward systematically fostering strong, supportive relationships in the lives of vulnerable youth.

CONCEPTUAL DIFFERENCES BETWEEN RESILIENCE RESEARCH ON CHILDREN VERSUS ADULTS

The last set of issues we will address concerns conceptual differences between contemporary research on resilience in children versus resilience in adults. A particularly intriguing difference pertains to the types of outcomes typically considered. In work with children, researchers usually consider behavioral competence, or the degree to which they meet society's expectations in stage salient tasks.[30] Assessments are based on reports from their teachers, their classmates, and their parents, about whether they are getting good grades, getting on with peers, and are generally well behaved. In the adult literature, conversely, the focus is on how the person herself or himself feels. Prominent are indices, such as subjective well-being, happiness, self-reported absence of distress, and so on.

The two approaches to assessing well-being—based on others' versus self-reports—have apparently been largely exclusive to children and adults, respectively. Few if any studies on resilience among adults have defined "doing well" in terms of others' ratings of them, gauging whether they functioned as good spouses, parents, bosses, or mentors. In parallel, researchers do not ask children about their subjective well-being. Feelings of depression or anxiety are commonly measured, but for some reason, assessments of happiness have not been considered relevant for our children. In future studies on resilience, therefore, researchers working with adults and children would each do well to borrow a little from each others' methodologies as they consider different strategies to define and explore resilient adaptation.

SUMMARY

To summarize the different themes touched upon within this article: First, as we uncover statistical "main effect" findings, labels of "protective" factors versus "vulnerability" factors should not be chosen arbitrarily. Examining the distribution of scores vis-à-vis norms can be critical in illuminating whether the construct connotes exceptional well-being at one end, or exceptional dysfunction at the other. Second, the need to unpack underlying processes is important not only with regard to risk modifiers, but with risk indices themselves. Effects of particular parent mental illness, for example, can operate through many conduits, and disentangling which of these is the most prominent is critical to guide interventions. Third, when the goal is to inform interventions for a given at-risk group, within-group designs are optimal; these help us understand which of several major influences are most potent in affecting children's lives. Fourth, increased attention to biology and genes is invaluable, illuminating critical aspects of the human body that can compromise well-being. At the same time, we must ensure balance in our research priorities; there is still much to be learned about context-specific environmental risks, and about how we can effectively mitigate the many risks already well known to have profound ill effects.

If researchers seek to guide interventions, it would be prudent to prioritize somewhat, in choosing "risk modifiers" for our studies. Especially useful would be a focus on factors known to be *salient* in that risk context, that are *malleable* or amenable to interventions, that are *enduring*, affecting children for relatively long periods, and that are *generative* of other assets. Strong relationships with adults meet all these criteria; at the same time, we need much more research on antecedents of good parenting—within different risk contexts—and how to optimally use other adults, such as mentors or teachers, to promote resilience. Finally, researchers working with children and adults could usefully learn from each others' methodologies. In particular, it would be useful to define adults' resilience in terms of others' views of how well they are doing and not just their own feelings of well-being, as it would help to look at what makes for children's subjective feelings of happiness.

The field of resilience research has grown momentously over the last several decades, and with further integration of diverse approaches to science, research in the years ahead will be invaluable in helping the children and families with whom we work. This research can inform interventions that help at-risk individuals to function adaptively, and to feel some sense of personal well-being, despite the many and considerable adversities with which they contend.

ACKNOWLEDGMENT

The preparation of the manuscript was funded in part by grants from the National Institutes of Health (RO1-DA10726, RO1-DA11498, and R01-DA14385), the William T. Grant Foundation.

REFERENCES

1. LUTHAR, S.S. & D. CICCHETTI. 2000. The construct of resilience: implications for interventions and social policies. Dev. Psychopathol. **12:** 857–885.
2. MASTEN, A. 2001. Ordinary magic: resilience processes in development. Am. Psychol. **56:** 227–238.
3. RUTTER, M. 2000. Resilience reconsidered: conceptual considerations, empirical findings, and policy implications. *In* Handbook of Early Childhood Intervention (Second ed). J.P. Shonkoff & S.J. Meisels, Eds.: 651–682. Cambridge. New York.
4. RUTTER, M. 2003. Genetic influences on risk and protection: implications for understanding resilience. *In* Resilience and vulnerability: Adaptation in the context of childhood adversities S.S. Luthar, Ed.: 489–509. Cambridge. New York.

5. LUTHAR, S.S. 2006. Resilience in development: A synthesis of research across five decades. In Developmental Psychopathology: Risk, disorder, and adaptation D. Cicchetti & D.J. Cohen, Eds.: 740–795. Wiley. New York.
6. LUTHAR, S. & C. SEXTON. Maternal drug abuse versus maternal depression: Vulnerability and resilience among school-age and adolescent offspring. Dev. Psychopathol. In press.
7. RUTTER, M. 1987. Psychosocial resilience and protective mechanisms. Am. J. Orthopsychiat. **57:** 316–331.
8. SAMEROFF, A., L. J. GUTMAN & S.C. PECK. 2003. Adaptation among youth facing multiple risks: prospective research findings. *In* Resilience and Vulnerability: Adaptation in the Context of Childhood Adversities, S.S. Luthar, Ed.: 364–391. Cambridge. New York.
9. LUTHAR, S.S. & C.C. SEXTON. In press. Maternal drug abuse versus maternal depression: Vulnerability and resilience among school-age and adolescent offspring. Dev. Psychopathol.
10. LUTHAR, S.S., K. D'AVANZO & S. HITES. 2003. Parental substance abuse: risks and resilience. *In* Resilience and Vulnerability. Adaptation in the Context of Childhood Adversities. S.S. Luthar, Ed.: 104–129. Cambridge. New York.
11. LUTHAR, S.S. 2003. The culture of affluence: psychological costs of material wealth. Child Dev. **74:** 1581–1593.
12. LUTHAR, S.S. & K. D'AVANZO. 1999. Contextual factors in substance use: a study of suburban and inner-city adolescents. Dev. Psychopathol. **11:** 845–867.
13. LUTHAR, S.S. & A. GOLDSTEIN. 2006. Substance use and related behaviors among suburban late adolescents: the importance of perceived parent containment. Manuscript submitted for publication.
14. LUTHAR, S.S. & L. TEEL. 2006. High socioeconomic status youth in cities versus suburbia: a comparison of vulnerabilities and resources. Manuscript in preparation.
15. LUTHAR, S.S., S. MUST & R.P. PRINCE. 2006. Challenges in feminine development: Body image and relationship issues among suburban sixteen-year-olds. Manuscript submitted for publication.
16. ACHENBACH, T.M. & L.A. RESCORLA. 2001. Manual for the ASEBA School-Age Forms and Profiles. University of Vermont, Research Center for Children, Youth, & Families. Burlington, VT.
17. LUTHAR, S.S., D. CICCHETTI & B. BECKER. 2000a. The construct of resilience: a critical evaluation and guidelines for future work. Child Dev. **71:** 543–562.
18. LUTHAR, S.S. & A. GOLDSTEIN. 2004. Children's exposure to community violence: implications for understanding risk and resilience. J. Clin. Child Adolesc. Psychol. **33:** 499–505.
19. GARCIA COLL, C., G. LAMBERTY, R. JENKINS, *et al.* 1996. An integrative model for the study of developmental competencies in minority children. Child Dev. **67:** 1891–1914.
20. GARCIA COLL, C., A. AKERMAN & D. CICCHETTI. 2000. Cultural influences on developmental processes and outcomes: implications for the study of development and psychopathology. Dev. Psychopathol. **12:** 333–356.
21. HOBFOLL, S.E., C. RITTER, J. LAVIN, *et al.* 1995. Depression prevalence and incidence among inner-city pregnant and postpartum women. J. Consult. Clin. Psychol. **63:** 445–453.
22. LUTHAR, S.S. 1999. Poverty and Children's Adjustment. Sage. Thousand Oaks, CA.

23. Tucker, C.M. & K.C. Herman. 2002. Using culturally sensitive theories and research to meet the academic needs of low-income African American children. Am. Psychol. **57:** 762–773.
24. Smetana, J.G., N. Campione-Barr & A. Metzger. 2006. Adolescent development in interpersonal and societal contexts. Ann. Rev. Psychol. **57:** 255–284.
25. Cicchetti, D. 2003. Foreword. *In* Resilience and Vulnerability: Adaptation in the Context of Childhood Adversities. S.S. Luthar, Ed.: xix–xxvii. Cambridge. New York.
26. Rutter, M. 2002. The interplay of nature, nurture, and developmental influences: the challenge ahead for mental health. Arch. Gen. Psychiatry **59:** 996–1000.
27. Curtis, W.J. & D. Cicchetti. 2003. Moving research on resilience into the 21st century: theoretical and methodological considerations in examining the biological contributors to resilience. Dev. Psychopathol. **15:** 773–810.
28. Caspi, A., K. Sugden, T.E. Moffitt, *et al.* Influence of life stress on depression: moderation by a polymorphism in the 5-HTT gene. Science **301:** 386–389.
29. Kim-Cohen, J., T.E. Moffitt, A. Caspi & A. Taylor. 2004. Genetic and environmental processes in young children's resilience and vulnerability to socioeconomic deprivation. Child Dev. **75:** 651–668.
30. Moffitt, T.E. 2005. The new look of behavioral genetics in developmental psychopathology: gene–environment interplay in antisocial behaviors. Psychol. Bull. **131:** 533–554.
31. Moffitt, T.E., A. Caspi & M. Rutter. 2005. Strategy for investigating interactions between measured genes and measured environments. Arch. Gen. Psychiatry **62:** 473–481.
32. Luthar, S.S. & L.B. Zelazo. 2003. Research on resilience: an integrative review. *In* Resilience and Vulnerability: Adaptation in the Context of Childhood Adversities S.S. Luthar, Ed.: 510–549. Cambridge. New York.
33. Garmezy, N. 1974. The study of competence in children at risk for severe psychopathology. *In* The child in his family: children at psychiatric risk: III. E.J. Anthony & C. Koupernik, Eds.: 547. Wiley. New York.
34. Rutter, M.1979. Protective factors in children's responses to stress and disadvantage. *In* Primary Prevention in Psychopathology: Vol. 3. Social Competence in Children. M.W. Kent & J.E. Rolf, Eds.: 49–74. Hanover, University Press of New England. NH.
35. Werner, E.E. & R. Smith. 1977. Kauai's Children Come of Age. University of Hawaii Press. Honolulu.

Psychosocial Constraints on the Development of Resilience

ARNOLD J. SAMEROFF AND KATHERINE L. ROSENBLUM

Center for Human Growth and Development, University of Michigan, Ann Arbor, Michigan, USA

ABSTRACT: Although resilience is usually thought to reside in individuals, developmental research is increasingly demonstrating that characteristics of the social context may be better predictors of resilience. When the relative contribution of early resilience and environmental challenges to later child mental health and academic achievement were compared in a longitudinal study from birth to adolescence, indicators of child resilience, such as the behavioral and emotional self-regulation characteristic of good mental health, and the cognitive self-regulation characteristic of high intelligence contributed to later competence. However, the effects of such individual resilience did not overcome the effects of high environmental challenge, such as poor parenting, antisocial peers, low-resource communities, and economic hardship. The effects of single environmental challenges become very large when accumulated into multiple risk scores even affecting the development of offspring in the next generation.

KEYWORDS: resilience; adaptation; risk; mental health; intelligence; longitudinal studies

DEFINING RESILIENCE

Resilience connotes positive adaptation by individuals despite severe adversity. However, there has been sharp criticism concerning the construct of resilience and the methods used by resilience researchers.[1] One of the main criticisms concerns the absence of a unifying conceptual framework that encompasses its integration across disciplines and specialized areas. A scientific basis for intervention research necessitates precise terminology to build upon earlier classifications and to ensure its continued vitality. A consistent and systematic framework is essential to facilitate the work of researchers and practitioners who pursue work in this area, to integrate findings across diverse

Address for correspondence: Arnold J. Sameroff, Center for Human Growth and Development, University of Michigan, 300 N. Ingalls Ann Arbor, MI 48105. Voice: 734-764-2443; fax: 734-936-9288.
e-mail: sameroff@umich.edu

Ann. N.Y. Acad. Sci. 1094: 116–124 (2006).
doi: 10.1196/annals.1376.010

fields, as well as provide guidance for the identification and implementation of age-appropriate, optimal targets for preventive interventions.[2]

Although resilience is usually conceptualized as adaptive response to extraordinary challenge, it is not clear how it differs from adaptive responses to ordinary challenge except in some surprising ways. Extraordinary challenges can be separated into general and personal categories. In the general category are stressors that affect everyone in a community, such as war or earthquakes. Personal stressors are those specific to a particular family or individual, such as death or divorce.

What then are ordinary challenges? Essentially it is the stuff of life, the ordinary developmental stressors that individuals experience as they grow up. These again can be divided into general stressors, such as the educational systems and personal ones, such as coping with siblings. When children go to school, each curriculum is constructed as a series of challenges where as soon as the student overcomes one, such as learning to add, they are confronted with another, such as subtraction. In the family children must adapt to the requirements of others and the changes in relationships, for example, as their increasing autonomy skills are restricted by parental concerns with safety.

Is there evidence for a relation between responses to ordinary challenges and responses to extraordinary ones? The field of developmental psychopathology provides many examples where this seems to be the case. For several disorders that were thought to have a unique course, for example, acute schizophrenia, postpartum depression, and posttraumatic stress disorder, there is evidence that the amount of individual competence during the premorbid condition was highly predictive of the postmorbid resilience.[3–5]

OPERATIONALIZATION OF RESILIENCE

Although a prescriptive definition of resilience may not be forthcoming, many of its ingredients have been identified including resourcefulness, intelligence, and mental health. Resourcefulness is almost a synonym for resilience with its ingredients of the ability to solve problems, to bounce back, and to learn from mistakes. The definition of intelligence has been broadening to include such elements as effective adaptation to the environment, learning from experience, and overcoming obstacles by taking thought.[6]

Modern conceptions of mental health include everyday adaptations to varying situations, which is the opposite of mental illness, which is the lack of everyday adaptation. Mental illness is the opposite of resilience in that behavior does not change with the situation. There is poor regulation of affect, behavior, and cognition. Healthy individuals may become saddened by the death of a relative but then move on, whereas depressives are saddened in all situations. Healthy children are hyperactive on the playground, but hyperactive children cannot regulate their behavior when they return to the classroom. Healthy individuals can attend to many different things but can focus down when it is a requirement of the task, but children with attention problems cannot adapt to the special situation. All these problems in self-regulation are evidence of a lack of resilience.

OPERATIONALIZATION OF CHALLENGE

Because resilience is defined as response to challenge, our next concern is to identify those factors that challenge individuals. Over the past three decades, studies of resilience have focused on individual variation in response to risky conditions, such as stressful life events,[7] exposure to community violence,[8] maltreatment,[9] poverty,[10] divorce,[11] and maternal mental illness.[12] These studies have brought sharper attention to the social factors that influence stress resistance in children and adolescents.

Challenges are the equivalents of risk factors, defined as variables that increase the incidence of nonoptimal development. A representative set of such risk factors can be found in our longitudinal studies of families from the time target children were born until they were 30 years of age. From the data available in our study we chose a set of 10 social–environmental variables.[13] We then tested whether poor preschool cognitive and social–emotional resilience, defined here as competence, was related to the risk factors associated with low socioeconomic circumstances. The 10 environmental risk variables were: (1) a history of maternal mental illness, (2) high maternal anxiety, (3) parental perspectives that reflected rigidity in the attitudes, beliefs, and values that mothers had in regard to their child's development, (4) few positive maternal interactions with the child observed during infancy, (5) head of household in unskilled occupations, (6) minimal maternal education, (7) disadvantaged minority status, (8) single parenthood, (9) stressful life events, and (10) large family size. Each of these risk factors has a large literature documenting their potential for deleterious developmental effects, but there are many others not included in our list. Each of our 10 variables turned out to be a risk factor for preschool competence.

Because risk factors tend to cluster in the same individuals, many investigators soon realized that focusing on a single risk factor or challenge does not address the reality of most children's lives.[14] As a way of improving predictive power, Rutter[15] argued that it was not any particular risk factor but the number of risk factors in a child's background that led to psychiatric disorder. When we used this strategy in our study and created a multiple risk score that was the total number of risks for each individual family, major differences were found on mental health and intelligence measures between those children with few risks and those with many. On the intelligence test children with no environmental risks scored more than 30 points higher than children with 8 or 9 risk factors.[13] No preschoolers in the zero-risk group had IQs below 85, 26%

of those in the high-risk group did. On average, each risk factor reduced the child's IQ score by 4 points. Four-year-olds in the high-risk group (5 or more risk factors) were 12.3 times as likely to be rated as having clinical mental health symptoms.

CONTINUITY OF ENVIRONMENTAL CHALLENGE

We completed new assessments of the sample when the children were 13 and 18 years of age.[16] Because of the potent effects of our multiple risk index at 4 years, we calculated new multiple environmental risk scores for each family based on their situation 9 and 14 years later. To our surprise there were very few families that showed major shifts in the number of risk factors across the intervening periods.

The typical statistic reported in longitudinal research is the correlation between early and later performance of the children. We too found such correlations. Intelligence at 4 years correlated 0.72 with intelligence at 13 years and 0.67 from 13 to 18 years. The usual interpretation of such numbers is that there is a continuity of competence or incompetence in the child. Such a conclusion cannot be challenged if the only assessments in the study are of the children. In our study we examined and were able to correlate environmental challenges across time as well as child ones. We found a high correlation of 0.77 for environmental risk scores between 4 and 13 years and 0.80 between 13 and 18 years. These were greater than the continuities for the child measures. Whatever the child's ability for showing resilience and achieving higher levels of competence, it was severely undermined by the continuing number of environmental challenges. Whatever the capabilities provided to the child by individual factors, the environment seemed to limit further opportunities for development. Those children who had been living in high-risk environments at 4 years of age were still living in them at 13 and 18 years of age.

The 13- and 18-year high-risk contexts were producing the same negative effects on competence as the earlier 4-year ones had done. FIGURE 1 shows the relation between the IQ of these children and risk levels at the three assessments. The curves overlap substantially with similar ranges of outcomes at each age. We found the same relationship between the number of risk factors and the child's intellectual competence at each age; those children from families with no risk factors scored more than 30 points higher on intelligence tests than those with the most risk factors and had significantly better mental health.

CAN INDIVIDUAL RESILIENCE OVERCOME SOCIAL CHALLENGE?

We have demonstrated that the accumulation of environmental challenge has negative effects on a child's competence through adolescence. But what

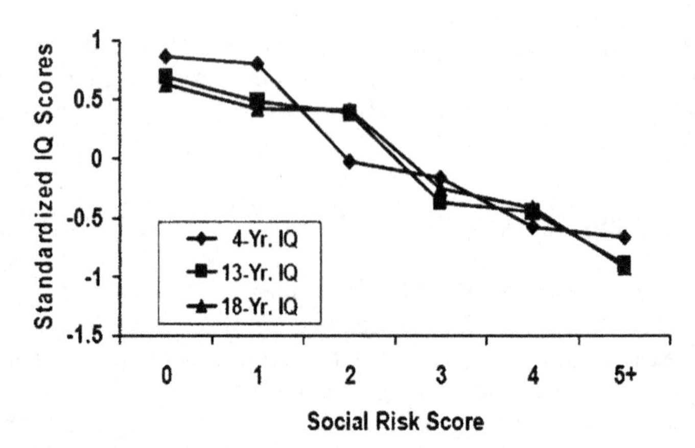

FIGURE 1. Relation of contemporary cumulative social risk score to standardized IQ scores at 4, 13, and 18 years of age.

about resilience? Would those children with higher levels of competence be better at overcoming social risk factors? Our study provided an opportunity to answer this question because we had measures of competence and challenge from infancy through adolescence. We could see how infant competence affected preschool competence, and then how preschool competence affected high school competence.

We started by testing whether infant competence could overcome challenges. For each infant we created a resilience or "multiple competence" score that included 12 factors from the data collected during the first year of life. Competence/resilience was defined as better scores on newborn medical and behavioral tests, temperament assessments, and developmental scales. We then divided the sample into groups of high and low resilient infants and examined as outcomes their 4-year IQ and social–emotional functioning scores to determine if these personal characteristics could overcome the negative effects of social adversity. We found no relation between infant competence and 4-year IQ or mental health problems.[17] The single predictor of 4-year mental health and IQ was the multiple environmental risk score. Competent infants did no better than incompetent ones.

Infant developmental scales may be weak predictors because they assess different developmental functions than are captured by later cognitive and personality assessments. As many have argued, infant developmental scales do not incorporate aspects of mental functioning that are central to later IQ tests. Perhaps, if we move up the age scale we would find that the mental health and intelligence of these children at 4 years of age, when more cognitive functions are incorporated into IQ tests and greater social–emotional competence is possible, may be protective for later competence during adolescence.

We divided the 4-year-olds into high and low mental health groups and high and low IQ groups in two analyses. We then compared these groups on how they did at 18 years on their mental health and measures of school achievement. Competent preschoolers did better on average than less competent ones but when we controlled for environmental risk, the differences between children with high and low levels of early competence paled when compared to the differences in performance between children in high- and low-risk social environments. We found that high competent children in high-risk environments did worse than low competent children in low-risk environments.

If 4-year competence is still too ephemeral to resist the negative consequences of adverse social circumstance, would competent 13-year-olds fare better at 18 years? We divided the 13-year-olds into high and low mental health groups and high and low intelligence groups, and examined their 18-year behavior. Again, in each case, 13-year-old youth with better mental health and intelligence did better within the same social risk conditions, but groups of children with high levels of competence living in conditions of high environmental risk did worse than low competent children in low-risk environments.[18]

DEVELOPMENTAL TRAJECTORIES

We have reported the effects of risk across two ages at a time, however, interactive processes between risk and protective factors often rely on chains of connections over time rather than on a multiplicative effect at any single time point. Understanding the factors that influence children's academic trajectories over many time points may help explain why some high-risk youth either catch up or fall further behind their more advantaged peers as they progress through school.

In our study we examined school records and obtained grades and attendance records for the participants from first to twelfth grade. We used hierarchical linear modeling (HLM) to examine the trajectories of the children throughout their school careers.[19] We could then determine how the growth curves were influenced by their 4-year multirisk scores. We could also determine the degree to which their early mental health and intelligence interacted with environmental risk to see if there was evidence of resilience in predicting school grades from first to twelfth grades.

These analyses confirmed our less sophisticated prior analyses: early risk had an adverse effect on academic trajectories during the entire period children were in school from the first to twelfth grades. For children in higher-risk families, having a higher IQ score was not a protective factor. There were no differences between the growth curves (see FIG. 2). But for children in low-risk families, higher IQ was a promotive factor and resulted in a higher grade point trajectory. But consistent with earlier analyses, low resilient 4-year-olds

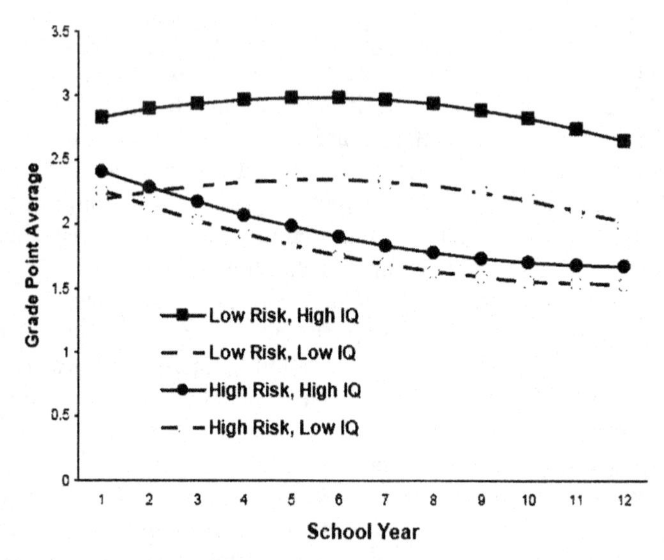

FIGURE 2. Effects of 4-year high and low cumulative social risk score and high and low 4-year verbal intelligence on trajectory of school grades (GPA) from first to twelfth grades (high is one standard deviation above the mean and low is one standard deviation below the mean).

in low-risk conditions consistently had higher GPAs than the high resilient children in high-risk conditions.

When we extend these analyses in time we find continuing predictive power of early risk factors on individual competence. The individuals in our study were contacted when they were 30-year-olds and their mental health assessed using the DSM-IV-R global assessment of functioning (GAF) scores. Using regressions analyses we found that we could explain fully 30% of the variance

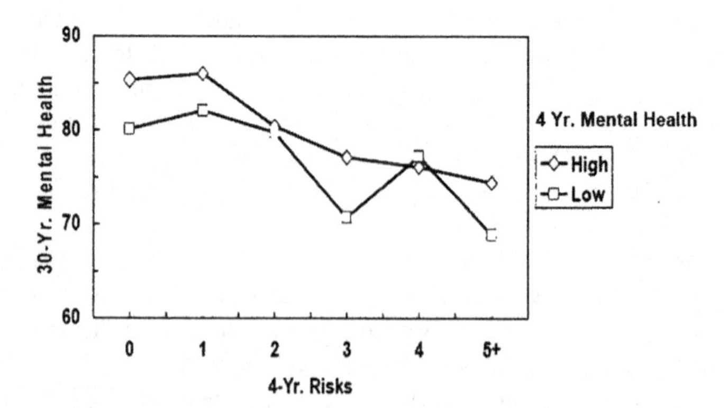

FIGURE 3. Relation of cumulative social risk score at 4 years of age to GAF at 30 years of age for 4-year high and low mental health groups.

in their GAF scores over a span of 26 years. More to our point, the 4-year mental health measure of resilience only added 5% to the variance explained by the 4-year social risk score. FIGURE 3 shows the 30-year GAF mental health scores for groups of high and low 4-year mental health groups as a function of number of 4-year risk scores. Here is another example where high-mental health 4-year-old children in high-risk conditions have worse 30-year mental health than low-mental health 4-year-old children in low-risk conditions.

SUMMARY OF FINDINGS

A focus on resilience as an individual characteristic does not explain more than a small proportion of variance in behavioral development. To truly appreciate the effects of childhood resilience requires attention to the broad constellation of social risk factors that challenge individuals and their families.[20] The concern with preventing developmental failures has often clouded the fact that the majority of children in every social class and ethnic group are not failures. They get jobs, have successful social relationships, and raise a new generation of children. Masten[20] concludes that the most surprising result of risk studies is the ordinariness of resilience and that it is both common and arises from the normative functions of human adaptational systems. In our analyses we have found that individual characteristics of mental health and higher intelligence contribute to developmental competence. However, the effects of such individual resiliencies do not overcome the effects of high environmental risk. In our analyses we consistently found that groups of high resilient children in high-risk environments had lower later mental health and cognitive competence than groups of low resilient children in low-risk environments.

REFERENCES

1. LUTHAR, S.S., D. CICCHETTI, & B. BECKER. 2000. The construct of resilience: a critical evaluation and guidelines for future work. Child Dev. **71:** 543–562.
2. SAMEROFF, A. & L.M. GUTMAN. 2003. Contributions of risk research to the design of successful interventions. *In* Intervention with Children and Adolescents: An Interdisciplinary Perspective. P. Allen-Meares & M.W. Fraser, Eds. New York: Pearson, Allyn & Bacon.
3. GARMEZY, N. & E. RODNICK1959. Premorbid adjustment and performance in schizophrenia: implications for interpreting heterogeneity in schizophrenia. J. Nerv. Ment. Dis. **129:** 450–466.
4. O'HARA, M.W. & A.M. SWAIN. 1996. Rates and risk of postpartum depression-A meta-analysis. Int. Rev. Psychiatry **8:** 37–54.
5. BRESLAU, N., E.L. PETERSON, L.M. POISSON, *et al.* Estimating post-traumatic stress disorder in the community: lifetime perspective and the impact of typical traumatic events. Psychol. Med. **34:** 889.

6. NEISSER, U., G. BOODOO, T.J. BOUCHARD, *et al.* 1996. Intelligence: knowns and unknowns. Am. Psychol. **51:** 77–101.
7. GARMEZY, N., A.S. MASTEN & A. TELLEGAN. 1984. The study of stress and competence in children: a building block of developmental psychopathology. Child Dev. **55:** 97–111.
8. WHITE, K., S. BRUCE, A. FARRELL & W. KLIEWER. 1988. Impact of exposure to community violence on anxiety: a longitudinal study of family social support as a protective factor for urban children. J. Child Family Stud. **7:** 187–203.
9. CICCHETTI, D., S.L. TOTH & A. MAUGHAN. 2000. An ecological-transactional model of child maltreatment. *In* Developmental Psychopathology. Vol 2. D. Cicchetti & D.J. Cohen, Eds.: 689–722. Wiley. New York.
10. MCLOYD, V.C. 1997. Children in poverty: development, public policy, and practice. *In* Child Psychology in Practice. W. Damon, I.E. Siegel & K.A. Renninger, Eds.: 135–208 Handbook of child psychology Fifth edition. Wiley. New York.
11. HETHERINGTON, E.M. 2005. The influence of conflict, marital problem solving, and parenting on children's adjustment in nondivorced, divorced, and remarried families. *In* J. Families Count: Effects on Child and Adolescent Development. A. Clarke-Stewart & J. Dunn. Ed.: Cambridge University Press. Cambridge, UK.
12. SAMEROFF, A.J., R. SEIFER & M. ZAX. 1982. Early development of children at risk for emotional disorder. Monogr. Soc. Res. Child Dev. **47**(7)**:** 1–82.
13. SAMEROFF, A.J., R. SEIFER, B. BAROCAS, M. ZAX & S. GREENSPAN. 1987. IQ scores of 4-year-old children: social–environmental risk factors. Pediatrics **79:** 343–350.
14. MASTEN, A.S. & J.D. COATSWORTH. 1998. The development of competence in favorable and unfavorable environments: lessons from research on successful children. Am. Psychol. **53:** 205–220.
15. RUTTER, M. 1979. Protective factors in children's responses to stress and disadvantage. *In* Primary Prevention of Psychopathology (Vol. 3): Social Competence in Children. M.W. Kent & J.E. Rolf, Eds.: University Press of New England. Hanover, NH.
16. SAMEROFF, A.J., R. SEIFER, A. BALDWIN & C. BALDWIN. 1993. Stability of intelligence from preschool to adolescence: the influence of social and family risk factors. Child Dev. **64:** 80–97.
17. SAMEROFF, A.J. & B.H. FIESE. 2000. Transactional regulation: The developmental ecology of early intervention. *In* Handbook of early childhood intervention. J.P. Shonkoff & S.J. Meisels, Eds.: 135–159. Cambridge University Press. New York.
18. SAMEROFF, A.J., W.T. BARTKO, A. BALDWIN, *et al.* 1998. Family and social influences on the development of child competence. *In* Families, risk, and competence. M. Lewis & C. Feiring, Eds.: Lawrence Erlbaum Associates. Mahwah, NJ.
19. GUTMAN, L.M., A.J. SAMEROFF & R. COLE. 2003. Academic growth curve trajectories from first to twelfth grades: effects of multiple social risk and preschool child factors. Dev. Psychol. **39:** 777–790.
20. MASTEN, A.S. 2001. Ordinary magic: resilience processes in development. Am. Psychol. **56:** 227–238.

Adolescents' Resilience as a Self-Regulatory Process

Promising Themes for Linking Intervention with Developmental Science

THOMAS J. DISHION AND ARIN CONNELL

University of Oregon, Child and Family Center, University of Oregon, Eugene, Oregon, USA

ABSTRACT: **This chapter focuses on the concept of self-regulation as a measure of resilience in children and adolescents. Developmental psychology and neuroscience are converging on the role of attention control as a central ability underlying self-regulation. We collected measures of adolescent attention control from parents and youth, and a measure of self-regulation from teachers. The measures of effortful attention correlated highly with teacher ratings of self-regulation. The composite measure of self-regulation (youth, parent, teacher report) was found to moderate the impact of peer deviance on adolescent antisocial behavior, as well as stress on adolescent depression. These findings suggest that self-regulation is a promising index of adolescent resilience. The construct of self-regulation also provides an excellent target for strategies aimed to improve child and adolescent adjustment in problematic environments and stressful circumstances.**

KEYWORDS: **adolescence; resilience; self-regulation; antisocial behavior; depression**

INTRODUCTION

The gap is closing between current intervention strategies for children and adolescents and developmental research on resilience. Early studies of resilient children seemed to reveal a trait that renders them invulnerable to harsh, extreme, and impoverished child-rearing circumstances, although the nature of this internal trait was unclear.[1] Research identified protective factors that facilitated the likelihood that children raised in harsh circumstances would be resilient with respect to long-term adjustment. Protective factors invariably

Address for correspondence: Thomas J. Dishion, Child and Family Center, University of Oregon, 377 Straub Hall, Eugene, Oregon 97401. Voice: 541-346-5561; fax: 541-346-4858.
e-mail: tomd@uoregon.edu

Ann. N.Y. Acad. Sci. 1094: 125–138 (2006).
doi: 10.1196/annals.1376.012

consisted of positive adult relationships (e.g., with teachers, relatives). Even experiences such as military service could serve as opportunity-enhancing processes that provide a countervailing force to problematic early experiences.[1]

Researchers have also made efforts to consider the complexity of resiliency in children, after having noted that some children may fare positively in terms of one outcome and less well in terms of others.[2] Thus, although some children who have experienced difficult environments do well, it is clear they do not necessarily do well on all outcomes. It is therefore necessary to more closely examine the link between experience, protective factors, patterns of resilience, and outcomes. In this sense, recent research on resilience proposes that we examine specific child competencies[3,4] and childhood resilience as a *process*.[5]

The construct of self-regulation is clearly fundamental to children's development of competence and therefore, to resilience in the context of growing up in disadvantaged environments.[6] Measures of self-regulation and coping have been found to be critical for understanding why some children do well and others do not in the context of divorce, for example.[7] Compas and colleagues also suggested that in adolescence, awareness of and coping with one's psychological state serves as a resiliency factor for a variety of adverse experiences such as serious illness, loss, and family dysfunction.[8] Identifying a key construct such as self-regulation that promotes children's positive adaptation to adverse circumstances provides a clue about how psychosocial interventions can successfully support children in adverse circumstances. Indeed, self-regulation could be seen as the common denominator target of all psychotherapeutic interventions that focus on the individual. Although psychotherapy interventions may differ in terms of which components of self-regulation are emphasized, invariably it is either explicitly or implicitly assumed that the client's positive adaptation will result from his or her successful application of therapeutic experiences to life in the real world.

Research on self-regulation, therefore, can enhance our understanding of the developmental dynamic underlying resilience in children and help us design realistic interventions that promote positive adjustment in children raised in adverse circumstances.

The analysis of self-regulation in children, however, is an emerging area of study that considers complex mechanisms ranging from domain-specific variation to neurological mechanisms underlying the regulation of attention and emotion. With respect to domain-specific variation, the degree of self-regulation in children and adolescents may vary as a function of specific context and activities. Some children may be highly regulated in complex social interactions with peers yet less regulated in quiet classrooms that demand high levels of intellectual activity. Despite the complexity of both the context and the neurological input into self-regulatory strategies, the field is converging on a basic process that may be common to a variety of circumstances in which self-regulation leads to positive outcomes. This process is referred to as *effortful attentional control*.[9]

Effortful attentional control is linked to specific mechanisms within the cerebral systems that account for specific patterns of self-regulation. Functional imaging studies of the human brain suggest that the anterior cingulate cortex is often activated in the context of tasks involving inhibition.[10] Management of one's attention may be the foundation of the ability to self-regulate under a variety of circumstances. Posner and colleagues have been instrumental in identifying the attention systems that are relevant to these micro behavioral shifts: alerting, orienting, and executive control. Although alerting and orienting are certainly relevant to self-regulation, it appears that the ability to have executive control of attention under conditions of perceptual conflict is the key to effortful attentional control. Cognitive tasks that involve executive control consistently activate the prefrontal cingulate cortex, and this ability emerges most likely around the time that children begin to walk.[11,12] Although individual differences in the degree of effortful attentional control prevail, the empirical literature suggests that such differences emerge in part as a function of temperamental genetic predispositions as well as of learning experiences that begin early and persist through childhood and adolescence.[12] Important developmental research, indeed, suggests that effortful attentional control is embedded in family environments that promote self-regulation and that individual differences predict other aspects of social and emotional adjustment.[13]

Although the basic mechanisms of effortful attentional control underlying self-regulation have often been assessed using neurocognitive tasks that involve responding at the millisecond level, it has also been shown that self-regulatory behaviors can be reliably assessed using specific ratings and reports from parents of offspring in early childhood and from youth and parents in adolescence. The temperament questionnaire referred to as the Child Behavior Questionnaire provides an effortful attentional control scale that links to neurocognitive tasks in early childhood and converges with youth report in adolescence.[14] This chapter discusses the extent to which an attention control measure of self-regulation in adolescence can serve as a resiliency factor with respect to two potentially disruptive experiences that can affect adolescent outcomes:

(i) Exposure to deviant peers and its influence on problem behaviors. We will summarize a longitudinal study examining the potential of a composite measure of self-regulation to buffer the effect of exposure to deviant behavior among peers with respect to future problem behavior.[15]

(ii) Exposure to stress and its influence on depression. We will summarize a longitudinal study examining the potential of the same composite measure of self-regulation to buffer the effect of extreme stress on the progression of internalizing symptoms among adolescents.[16]

Researchers have certainly found that coping and self-regulation directly affect long-term child and adolescent outcomes. Much of the current thinking, however, maintains that factors such as self-regulation define a resiliency process that reduces the impact of adverse environments on children's outcomes. In this sense, self-regulation can be seen as a moderating factor. The optimal strategy for identifying a moderator factor is to test for both main effects of adverse environment and for self-regulation on later adolescent outcomes. More important, however, is to examine the interaction effect between self-regulation and adverse environments as it applies to adolescent outcomes. A significant statistical interaction suggests that self-regulation serves as a moderator of environmental experiences. These possibilities will be examined using a multiethnic sample of adolescents residing within a metropolitan community.

STUDY METHODS

Sample and Design

In 1996 and 1998, two cohorts of sixth-grade youth were invited to participate in a randomized prevention trial referred to as Project Alliance. The total sample consisted of 999 adolescents randomized at the individual level to a family-centered service within the public schools versus public schools as usual. The intervention strategy, referred to as the Adolescent Transitions Program (ATP), and specifics about the sample are described in detail in the book by Dishion and Kavanagh.[17]

The youth were assessed yearly at ages 11, 12, 13, 14 years, and again at ages 16–17 and 18–19 years. In the initial years, the assessments were exclusive to self-report and teacher report of family management, peer relations, and problem behavior. At ages 16–17 years, the participants were given the attention network task developed by Posner and colleagues, as well as the Child Behavior Questionnaire developed for adolescents.[14] In addition, at ages 18–19 years they were assessed on the Composite International Diagnostic Interview (CIDI) measure of psychopathology used by the World Health Organization.[18]

A PRIORI SUBGROUPS

Three groups were formed to capture developmental patterns as identified by longitudinal data from the youth's self-reports. The three groups are the following:

(i) Early-starter and persistent: High rates of problem behavior in each assessment were reported for these youth beginning at age 11 years and continuing through age 16 years. This group of 40 youth was equally distributed between male and female who fit this description, and all but one had been arrested.

(ii) Late-starter: Low rates of problem behavior were reported for these youth until age 16 years, and their rates were above the median at that point.

Again, 40 youth equally distributed between male and female were classified as late starters.

(iii) Successful adolescents: Low rates of problem behavior were reported for these youth from early through late adolescence.

Self-Regulation Construct

Three scales comprise the multiagent, multimethod self-regulation construct. The mother and youth reports were derived from the Rothbart scale. These consist of three subscales referred to as activation control (e.g., finishes homework before due dates), attention scale (e.g., good at keeping track of several different things that are happening at once), and inhibitory control (e.g., able to stop doing something when told). These same items and scales constitute both the youth and the mother report. Internal consistency was higher for the mother ($\alpha = 0.76$) than for the youth scale ($\alpha = 0.62$). The teacher rating of self-control was used as an indicator of self-regulation at school. These items consisted primarily of behaviors that are relevant to the school context such as thinking ahead of time about consequences, following through on tasks even if unpleasant, planning ahead of time before acting, finishing homework on time, working toward goals, paying attention to what he or she is doing, and doing homework accurately and completely. This scale showed high internal consistency ($\alpha = 0.95$). The youth report scale correlated significantly with both the parent scale ($r = 0.31, P < 0.05$) and the teacher scale ($r = 0.34, P < 0.05$), while the parent report correlated significantly with the teacher report ($r = 0.39, P < 0.05$).

Finally, the attention network task developed by Posner and colleagues assessed basic attentional functions such as alerting, orienting, and executive control. The task was administered via laptop computers primarily in the laboratory setting but occasionally in the home setting. The score used as an indicator of self-regulation was the executive control scale. This score consisted of the difference in reaction times in tasks that involve perceptual conflict (i.e., Stroop) versus those that involve simple reaction times. However, at this time the attention task did not covary with child, parent, and teacher report. Thus, the self-regulation construct consisted of the global reports of self-regulation. To create the composite score, z-scores for mother, youth, and teacher scales were calculated, and the self-regulation composite scale was calculated as the mean of these z-scores.

Peer Deviance

Deviant peer affiliation at ages 16–17 years was measured by adolescent, parent, and teacher reports on four items that assess the number of the youths' peers who engage in a variety of deviant behaviors, including misbehaving, breaking rules, and substance use. Items were rated on a 5-point scale, with higher scores reflecting more frequent affiliation with deviant peers. Internal consistency of this scale was acceptable for all reporters (youth: $\alpha = 0.69$; parent: $\alpha = 0.66$; teacher: $\alpha = 0.84$). The youth report scale correlated significantly with both the parent scale ($r = 0.31$, $P < 0.05$) and the teacher scale ($r = 0.34$, $P < 0.05$), and the parent report correlated significantly with the teacher report ($r = 0.39$, $P < 0.05$). To create the composite score, z-scores for mother, youth, and teacher scales were calculated, and the peer deviance composite scale was calculated as the mean of these z-scores.

Stress Exposure

Stress exposure at ages 16–17 years was measured via self-report on two questionnaires. The victimization questionnaire contained 12 items reflecting the number of times youth reported experiencing victimization events in the past year, including theft, physical assault, and sexual assault. A 37-item stressful life events measure based on Holmes & Rahe's measure[19] was also used. This item assessed the number of times youth reported experiencing a variety of stressful events in the past year. This measure assessed a wide array of stressors, including work-related difficulties, financial pressures, deaths/illnesses, relationship problems, and so forth.

Antisocial Behavior at Ages 16–17 Years

Adolescent antisocial behavior at ages 16–17 years was measured via self-report of nine items that assess frequency of antisocial behaviors during the past month. Internal consistency of this scale was also acceptable at T6, $\alpha = 0.67$. For a subset of analyses, individuals were grouped into one of three antisocial behavior patterns on the basis of self-report of these nine items at earlier assessment waves. Reliability analyses indicated that internal consistency of this scale was strong for each of the earlier waves of assessment: T1 (6th grade; $\alpha = 0.83$), T2 (7th grade; $\alpha = 0.84$), and T3 (8th grade; $\alpha = 0.77$).

Antisocial Behavior at Ages 18–19 Years

In late adolescence, antisocial behavior was measured via self-report on the Adult Self-Report (ASR) questionnaire.[20] Items that measure age 16–17 years antisocial behavior were not collected at T7. To maximize content similarity across these waves of data collection, we used the DSM-IV Antisocial Behavior scale score from the ASR. This scale consists of 20 items that assess youth engagement in antisocial behaviors (e.g., "I break rules at work or elsewhere," "I don't feel guilty after doing something I shouldn't," "I get in many fights"), with items measured on a 3-point scale (0 = not true, 1 = sometimes true, 2 = often true).

Internalizing Symptoms at Ages 16–17 Years

Internalizing symptoms at ages 16–17 years were measured via self-report on the Depression and Anxiety symptom scales from the Brief Symptom Inventory (BSI),[21] a widely used and well-validated measure that assesses the frequency of mental health symptoms during the prior week on a 4-point scale. The Depression and Anxiety scales consist of six items each.

Internalizing Symptoms at Ages 18–19 Years

In late adolescence, internalizing symptoms were measured via self-report on the ASR questionnaire. The DSM-IV Depressive problems and Anxiety problems scales were used. The Depressive problems scale consists of 14 items, and the Anxiety problems scale consists of 7 items, measured on a 3-point scale (0 = not true, 1 = sometimes true, 2 = often true).

RESULTS

Differentiating Subgroups

FIGURE 1 reveals the average level of self-regulation for early starters, late starters, and successful adolescents. The three groups were reliably distinguished on the measure of self-regulation $F(2, 115) = 19.0$, $P < 0.01$. Note from the box plots in FIGURE 1 that the distribution on self-regulation is quite normal; the early-starting youth have the lowest levels of self-regulation, and the successful youth have the highest levels.

Self-Regulation and Antisocial Behavior

Extensive literature links peer deviance and antisocial behavior.[22] The details of this study are reported in Gardner, Dishion, and Connell.[23] It is expected that the self-regulation construct would moderate the influence of deviant peers on antisocial behavior. To test this effect, we ran a multiple regression including intervention, gender of the child, ethnicity, wave antisocial behavior at age 16 years, peer deviance at age 16 years, self-regulation at age 16 years, and the interaction between peer deviance and self-regulation. The results are shown in TABLE 1. As can be seen, the major factors that predict antisocial behavior

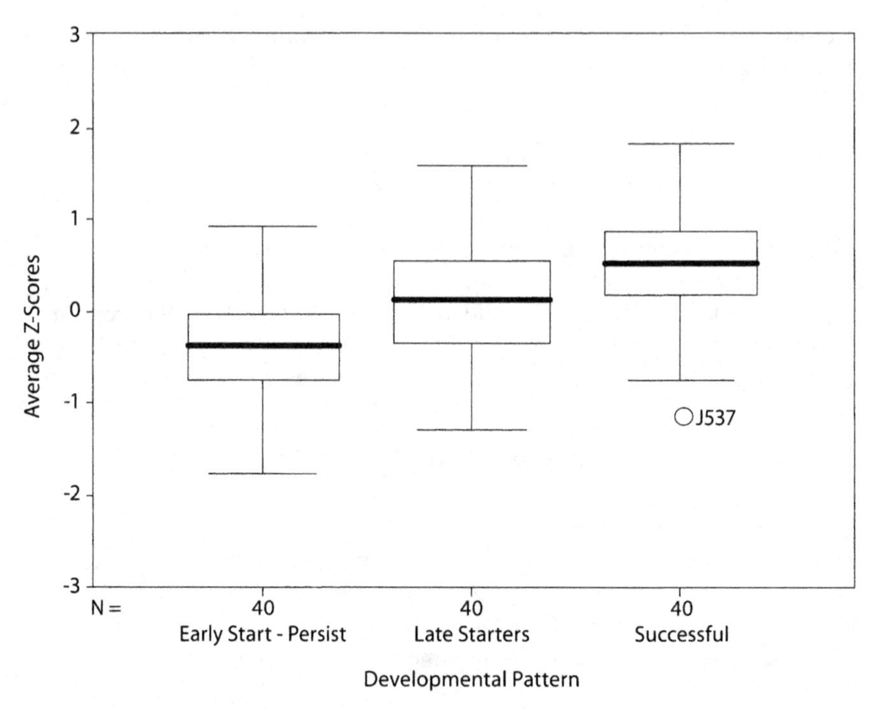

FIGURE 1. A composite measure of self-regulation differs by the developmental pattern of antisocial behavior.

at age 19 years are earlier antisocial behavior, peer deviance, self-regulation, and the interaction between peer deviance and self-regulation.

Following procedures described by Aiken and West,[24] simple slopes were plotted for the relation between deviant peer affiliation and self-reported antisocial behavior at high, mean, and low levels of effortful control (high = +1 SD; low = −1 SD). As shown in FIGURE 2, the youth defined as low in self-regulation were much more influenced by peer deviance with respect to

TABLE 1. Results for antisocial behavior

Predictor	Beta
Treatment	−0.03
Gender	−0.03
Ethnicity	0.01
Wave 6 antisocial	0.21*
Peer deviance	0.08*
Self-regulation	−0.26*
Peer deviance × self-regulation	−0.08*
Total $r^2 = 0.20$	

*$P < 0.05$.

later antisocial behavior. The lower boundary for the significance of the simple slopes was just below the mean level of self-regulation (self-regulation = −0.05), indicating that for youth at or above the mean on self-regulation, peer deviance was not significantly related to their own level of antisocial behavior at ages 18–19 years. Note that this multivariate relationship exists even when controlling for the youths' earlier antisocial behavior at ages 16–17 years.

Internalizing Symptoms and Self-Regulation

The results of work in this area are reported in more detail by Connell and Dishion.[16] To predict the youths' level of internalizing symptoms as assessed on the ASR, a strategy similar to that described above was used, although this analysis was carried out as a latent variable model in Mplus 4.01.[25] Two models were run, including a main effects–only model and a second interaction model. All models included three demographic control variables, including intervention, gender, ethnicity, and earlier internalizing symptoms. The main-effects model included self-regulation and stress exposure variables. The interaction model included an interaction between the stress exposure and self-regulation latent variables.

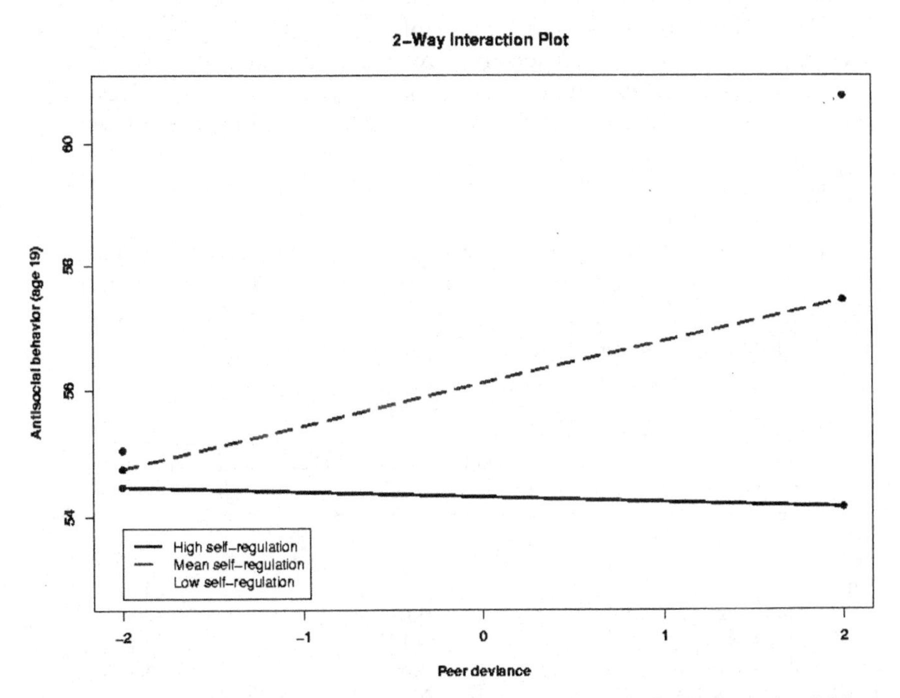

FIGURE 2. Interaction between self-regulation and peer deviance for antisocial behavior.

The main-effects model provided reasonable fit to the data, although the nonsignificant chi-square is likely due to the large sample size ($\chi^2 = 124.82$, $P < 0.05$, CFI = 0.94, RMSEA = 0.05, SRMR = 0.05). Because latent variable interaction models require numerical integration, typical model fit indices are not available. The results of this analysis are summarized in TABLE 2. As can be seen, the interaction term was again significant as were main effects for earlier depression, stress, and self-regulation.

FIGURE 3 reveals the interaction term between stress and self-regulation. Again, as can be seen from FIGURE 3, youth low in self-regulation were highly vulnerable to stressful experiences with respect to their later depressed mood. The r^2 for this group was 0.60 in comparison with youth with low self-regulation ($r^2 = 0.00$). Thus, it appears that self-regulation serves to moderate the influence of stress on youths' development of depressed mood.

CONCLUSIONS AND SUMMARY

These findings suggest that resilience in adolescence can indeed be studied as a process by using measurement and statistical techniques that emphasize continuous distributions.[5] The central role of motivated attention processes in both emotional and behavioral regulation is strongly supported by these data. The findings showing a moderating role of self-regulation with respect to deviant-peer exposure and antisocial behavior replicate and extend the work of Goodnight *et al.*[26] These findings are a salient signal that this line of research on self-regulation as a resiliency process is a promising venue for linking developmental and intervention science.

Challenges remain to realizing the potential for findings such as these. However, articulating them could help inform and improve programs and policies designed to promote positive adaptation in youth. The first challenge is to further refine neurocognitive tasks of attention regulation that map onto individual differences as revealed by global reports. The attention network task in early childhood has worked quite well with respect to established convergent

TABLE 2. Results for internalizing problems

Predictor	Beta from main-effects model	Beta from interaction model
Treatment	0.11	−0.16
Gender	1.43*	1.53*
Ethnicity	0.01	0.01
Wave 6 internalizing	3.03*	1.52*
Wave 6 stress exposure	0.12*	0.19
Self-regulation	−1.56*	−5.99*
Peer deviance × self-regulation	N/A	−3.71*

*$P < .05$

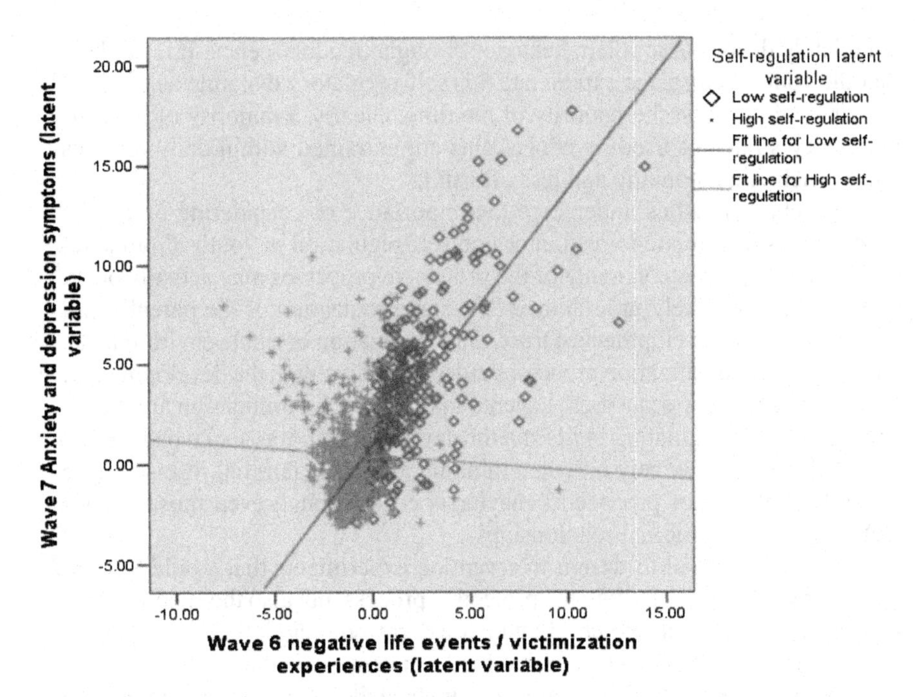

FIGURE 3. Interaction between self-regulation and stress exposure for internalizing problems.

validity with parent reports of the same construct.[12] Our research group is currently considering strategies for establishing individual differences in attention regulation as assessed using carefully designed neurocognitive tasks that are validated by means of imaging techniques. This validation process is a critical step in the current program of research because it reveals the mechanism that underlies self-regulation and therefore, provides clues regarding how this set of behaviors can be optimized during adolescent development.

The second challenge is that the youth report on self-regulation showed limited internal consistency. This trend may in part stem from using the shorter form of the Child Behavior Questionnaire for youth. More items will increase the liability. However, we also realize that much of self-regulation is probably unconscious and automatic.[27] Fitzsimons and colleagues suggested that even though self-regulation may be an effortful process, many basic components of self-regulation likely play out in a very automatic, unconscious fashion.[28] Self-regulation in adolescence undoubtedly depends on an infrastructure of diurnal behavioral routines that are conducive to overall self-control. For example, sleep, diet, and automatic daily routines provide a basis for the avoidance of pathogenic environments and resistance to peer pressures and stress when it does occur. It is compelling that 60% of youth who live in the same neighborhoods, walk through the same school halls, and attend the same classes are completely devoid of problem behavior throughout adolescence. It is unlikely that the youth themselves experience this self-regulatory dynamic as effortful and difficult, at least the majority of the time. Clearly, a majority of the self-regulatory strategies used by adolescents are entrained within daily routines and as such, are automatic and less effortful.

These characteristics underscore the importance of considering protective processes as they relate to resilience and self-regulation in youth. From a developmental perspective, many of the protective processes may actually occur quite early, most likely in infancy.[29] The synchronization of the parent–child relationship, the development of trust, the organization of stable environments, and successful socialization processes indeed must result in the development of basic self-regulatory strategies. Layered upon this solid foundation are the refinement of self-regulatory skills and the development of prosocial behavior.[30] Much of the work we rely on when thinking about the familial infrastructure for self-regulation of prosocial behavior is correlational, even those studies that establish longitudinal relationships.

It would be helpful to design intervention experiments that would test not only the hypotheses regarding the protective process, but also the specific family dynamics that promote child and adolescent self-regulation. Intervention experiments are advantageous in that they can demarcate the intervention targets, examine the mediating factors, and analyze the long-term outcomes. The analysis of this chain of events in an intervention strategy provides a compelling case for identifying a causal structure and designing comprehensive programs and policies that promote youth development. Finally, all interventions that target youth either explicitly or implicitly promote self-regulation. The advantage of a developmental analysis is that interventions such as these can improve the performance by targeting the specific brain behavior mechanisms at various points in development that are most germane to the child's emerging maturity and self-control. It is likely that many of the psychosocial interventions from diverse theoretical perspectives have valid intervention targets; however, their timing and application may at times be ill conceived.

Motivational interviewing is a technique that has resulted from a careful analysis of therapist–client processes related to change.[31] Motivational interviewing[32] emphasizes an interpersonal transaction that is Socratic in nature and that builds awareness in the client regarding his or her capacity and need to change under certain circumstances. A self-regulatory model is inherent in the motivational interviewing strategy. A comprehensive analysis of the role of self-regulation and change in the process of prevention research is discussed in detail by Higgins and Spiegel.[33] At this point, we hope that the next 10 years will provide a better understanding of the developmental patterns underlying self-regulation, the mechanisms accounting for self-regulation, and the individual difference factors that effect self-regulation to improve our ability to tailor and adapt interventions to the needs of children and adolescents in the context of varying family and community environments. We currently have a unique vantage point in that the developmental literature on resilience, the neuroscience of self-regulation, and intervention science are converging nicely to suggest future directions for improving the lives of children and adolescents.

REFERENCES

1. WERNER, E.E. 1995. Resilience in development. Curr. Dir. Psychol. Sci. **4:** 81–85.
2. KAUFMAN, A., A. COOK, L. ARNY, *et al.* 1994. Problems defining resiliency: illustrations from the study of maltreated children. Dev. Psychopathol. **6:** 215–229.
3. MASTEN, A.S., K.M. BEST & N. GARMEZY. Resilience and development: contributions from the study of children who overcome adversity. Dev. Psychopathol. **2:** 425–444.
4. MASTEN, A.S. 2006. Developmental psychopathology: pathways to the future. Int. J. Behav. Dev. **30:** 47–54.
5. LUTHAR, S.S. 2006. Resilience in development: a synthesis of research across five decades. *In* Developmental Psychopathology: Risk, Disorder, and Adaptation. D. Cicchetti & D.J. Cohen, Eds.: 740–795. Wiley. New York.
6. MASTEN, A.S. & J. COATSWORTH. 1998. The development of competence in favorable and unfavorable environments: lessons from research on successful children. Am. Psychol. **53:** 205–220.
7. LENGUA, L.J. & I.N. SANDLER. 1996. Self-regulation as a moderator of the relation between coping and symptomatology in children of divorce. J. Abnorm. Child Psychol. **24:** 681–701.
8. COMPAS, B., J. CONNER-SMITH, H. SALTZMAN, *et al.* 2001. Coping with stress during childhood and adolescence: problems, progress, and potential in theory and research. Psychol. Bull. **127:** 87–127.
9. ROTHBART, M.K. & J.E. BATES. 1998. Temperament. *In* Handbook of Child Psychology (5th edition): Social, Emotional, and Personality Development, Vol. 3. W. Damon & N. Eisenberg, Eds.: 105–176. Wiley. Hoboken, NJ.
10. FRITH, U. & C. FRITH. 2001. The biological basis of social interaction. Curr. Dir. Psychol. Sci. **10:** 151–155.
11. POSNER, M.I. & M.K. ROTHBART. 2000. Developing mechanisms of self-regulations. Dev. Psychopathol. **12:** 427–441.
12. RUEDA, M.R., M.I. POSNER & M.K. ROTHBART. 2004. Attentional control and self-regulation. *In* Handbook of Self-Regulation: Research, Theory, and Applications. R.F. Baumeister & K.D. Vohs, Eds.: 283–300. Guilford. New York.
13. EISENBERG, N., C.L. SMITH, A. SADOVSKY, *et al.* 2004. Effortful control: relations with emotion regulation, adjustment, and socialization in childhood. *In* Handbook of Self-Regulation: Research, Theory, and Applications. R.F. Baumeister & K.D. Vohs, Eds.: 259–282. Guilford. New York.
14. ELLIS, B.H. 2000. Relations between emotion language and emotion regulation in maltreated preschoolers. Unpublished doctoral dissertation. University of Oregon. Eugene.
15. DISHION, T.J., F. GARDNER & A. CONNELL. Self-regulation and the moderation of deviant peer influence in middle adolescence: a replication and extension. Manuscript submitted for publication.
16. CONNELL, A. & T.J. DISHION. Self-regulation and depression: buffering the effects of exposure to stressful events in adolescence. Manuscript in preparation.

17. DISHION, T.J. & K. KAVANAGH. 2003. Intervening in Adolescent Problem Behavior: A Family-Centered Approach. Guilford. New York.
18. WORLD HEALTH ORGANIZATION. 1997. Composite International Diagnostic Interview (CIDI, ver. 2.1). World Health Organization. Geneva, Switzerland.
19. HOLMES, T.H. & R.H. RAHE. 1967. The social readjustment rating scale. J. Psychosom. Res. **11:** 213–218.
20. ACHENBACH, T. 2003. Adult Self-Report for Ages 18–59. University of Vermont. Burlington.
21. DEROGATIS, L.R. 1993. Brief Symptom Inventory (BSI). Administration, Scoring, and Procedures Manual. National Computer Systems. Minneapolis, MN.
22. DISHION, T.J. & G.R. PATTERSON. 2006. The development and ecology of antisocial behavior in children and adolescents. *In* Developmental Psychopathology. Vol. 3: Risk, Disorder, and Adaptation. D. Cicchetti & D.J. Cohen, Eds.: 503–541. Wiley. New York.
23. GARDNER, F., T.J. DISHION & A. CONNELL. Adolescent self-regulation as resilience: resistance to antisocial behavior within the developing peer context. Manuscript submitted for publication.
24. AIKEN, L.S. & S.G. WEST. 1991. Multiple Regression: Testing and Interpreting Interactions. Sage. Newbury Park, CA.
25. MUTHÉN, L.K. & B.O. MUTHÉN. 2006. Mplus User's Guide, 4th ed. Muthén & Muthén. Los Angeles.
26. GOODNIGHT, J.A., J.E. BATES, J.P. NEWMAN, *et al.* 2006. The interactive influences of friend deviance and reward dominance on the development of externalizing behavior during early and middle adolescence. J. Abnorm. Psychol. **34:** 573–583.
27. BARGH, J.A. & M.J. FERGUSON. 2000. Beyond behaviorism: on the automaticity of higher mental processes. Psychol. Bull. **126:** 925–945.
28. FITZSIMONS, G.M. & J.A. BARGH. 2004. Automatic self-regulation. *In* Handbook of Self-Regulation: Research, Theory, and Applications. R.F. Baumeister & K.D. Vohs, Eds.: 151–170. Guilford. New York.
29. SHAW, D.S., M. GILLIOM, E.M. INGOLDSBY, *et al.* 2003. Trajectories leading to school-age conduct problems. Dev. Psychol. **39:** 189–200.
30. EISENBERG, N. & R.A. FABES. 1998. Prosocial development. *In* Handbook of Child Psychology: Social, Emotional, and Personality Development. W. Damon & N. Eisenberg, Eds.: 701–779. Wiley. New York.
31. PATTERSON, G.R. & M.S. FORGATCH. 1985. Therapist behavior as a determinant for client resistance: a paradox for the behavior modifier. J. Consult. Clin. Psychol. **53:** 846–851.
32. MILLER, W.R. & S. ROLLNICK. 2002. Motivational Interviewing: Preparing People for Change, (2nd edition) Guilford. New York.
33. HIGGINS, E.T. & S. SPIEGEL. 2004. Promotion and prevention strategies for self-regulation: a motivated cognition perspective. *In* Handbook of Self-Regulation: Research, Theory, and Applications. R.F. Baumeister & K.D. Vohs, Eds.: 171–187. Guilford. New York.

Promoting Resilience in Children and Youth

Preventive Interventions and Their Interface with Neuroscience

MARK T. GREENBERG

Prevention Research Center, Pennsylvania State University, University Park, Pennsylvania, USA

ABSTRACT: **Preventive interventions focus on reducing risk and promoting protective factors in the child as well as their cultural ecologies (family, classroom, school, peer groups, neighborhood, etc). By improving competencies in both the child and their contexts many of these interventions promote resilience. Although there are now a substantial number of preventive interventions that reduce problem behaviors and build competencies across childhood and adolescence, there has been little integration with recent findings in neuropsychology and neuroscience. This article focuses on the integration of prevention research and neuroscience in the context of interventions that promote resilience by improving the executive functions (EF); inhibitory control, planning, and problem solving skills, emotional regulation, and attentional capacities of children and youth. Illustrations are drawn from recent randomized controlled trials of the Promoting Alternative Thinking Strategies (PATHS) curriculum. The discussion focuses on the next steps in transdisciplinary research in prevention and social neuroscience.**

KEYWORDS: **prevention; intervention; neuroscience; children; youth; frontal lobe**

PROMOTING RESILIENCE IN CHILDREN AND YOUTH: PREVENTIVE INTERVENTIONS AND THEIR INTERFACE WITH NEUROSCIENCE

As a psychologist interested in creating change in communities and influencing public policy, I am often asked questions about developmental processes and trajectories in children. For example, "How can we help children resist

Address for correspondence: Dr. Mark T. Greenberg, Prevention Research Center, Henderson Building, South Room 109, Penn State University, University Park, PA 16802. Voice: 814-863-0112; fax: 814-865-2530.
e-mail: mxg47@psu.edu

**Ann. N.Y. Acad. Sci. 1094: 139–150 (2006). © 2006 New York Academy of Sciences.
doi: 10.1196/annals.1376.013**

negative influences when they live in high-risk neighborhoods?" "How can we improve children's academic outcomes when their families have experienced an intergenerational history of school failure?" "How can we help children control their emotions when their peers are bringing out the worst in them through teasing and taunting?" All of these questions imply the notion that many children are exposed to high-risk situations and the implication is that unless something is done, the probability of a poor outcome for some children is relatively high. Such situations are ripe for efforts to attempt to prevent difficulties that may spiral into longer-term poor outcomes across childhood, adolescence, and even adulthood. Beginning with the War on Poverty and the emergence of Head Start in the 1960s, preventive interventions have become central to our nation's public policy. As a result of the increased rate of both adolescent delinquency and drug use seen in the ensuing decades, the development of both preventive intervention programs and social/legislative policy initiatives has dramatically increased. The role of developmental science in public policy making has never been greater or more influential.

Improving the public's health, especially for those at greatest risk, is a complex problem that involves interventions at the level of economic and social policy as well as the ability to strengthen the skills of educators, parents, and youth themselves. Macrolevel interventions focused on changing community-level ecologies, attitudes, and behavior have ranged from large experiments in economic policy (e.g., earned income tax credits, TANF), changes in housing patterns,[1] social legislation ranging from raising the age at which youth can drive to building community partnerships to reduce youth problem behaviors and build positive youth development at the community level.[2] At a more microlevel, attempts to improve the culture, attitudes, and relations in families, peer groups, and schools have focused on building communication skills and values that promote positive developmental outcomes. Finally, there has been recognition that some attributes inside the individual, including skills, cognitions, and behaviors, may be malleable in response to preventive efforts. The enormous scope of activities undertaken is a testimony to our implicit understanding that child and youth outcomes are multidetermined and that various levels of influence impact developmental trajectories. Although at times these initiatives seem (or are) both random and chaotic, at another level they clearly reflect the combination of our growing basic knowledge of both the ecology of human development,[3] the advances made in developmental psychopathology,[4] and the emergent development of the field of prevention science.[5]

The study of resilience emerges out of the large research endeavor of public health epidemiology and the study of risk and protective factors and how they impact development. A number of guiding principles have emerged both from epidemiology and developmental psychopathology.[6,7] First, it is unlikely that there is a single "cause" of many of the preventable outcomes (e.g., mental disorders, substance abuse, school failure, delinquency); even in the case of disorders in which a biochemical or genetic mechanism has been discovered, the expression of the disorder is influenced by other biological or environmental events.[8,9] Second, there are multiple pathways both to and from risk and problem outcomes; for example, there are different combinations of risk factors that might lead to the same disorder. Third, no single cause may be either necessary or sufficient[10] and the effect of a risk factor will depend on its timing and relation to other risk factors. Fourth, many risk factors are not disorder-specific, but instead relate to a variety of outcomes. Finally, risk factors may vary in influence with host factors, such as gender, ethnicity, and culture.

Resiliency is commonly defined as positive or protective processes that reduce maladaptive outcomes under conditions of risk. That is, they are protective factors that may be especially important under conditions of risk. Although much less is known about protective factors and their operation,[7,11] at least three broad types of protective factors have been identified. These include characteristics of the individual (e.g., temperamental qualities and intelligence/cognitive ability), the quality of the child's relationships, and broader ecological factors, such as quality schools, safe neighborhoods, and regulatory activities.

An essential question related to adversity and resilience is the individual's development of an effective set of responses to stress. Central components of the stress response include the initial appraisal of the event and its emotional meaning, the ability to sufficiently regulate one's emotions and arousal to initiate problem solving and gather more information, the fuller cognitive-affective interpretation of the event, and one's behavioral response. Masten[12] has noted that among the most important resiliency factors are these very cognitive and emotion regulation skills.

Prospective longitudinal designs are critical to understanding the role of resiliency as they can identify (*a*) which risk factors are predictive of different developmental stages of a problem, (*b*) the dynamic relation between risk and protective factors in different developmental periods, and (*c*) what factors are most likely to "protect" or buffer persons under risk conditions from negative outcomes. In addition, randomized trials of preventive interventions can test these theories by examining how behavior changes are mediated.

THE INTERFACE OF PREVENTION, DEVELOPMENTAL PSYCHOPATHOLOGY, AND NEUROSCIENCE

Although developmental psychopathology, prevention, and neuroscience have developed in isolation, integrated research on protective factors and resilience has the potential to answer central questions regarding plasticity and the role of environmental and genetic process. While the primary goal of prevention science is to change behavior, behavior can be broadly defined as action, emotion, and cognition. Further, biological substrates underlie all of these processes and may serve as moderators, mediators, or outcomes of

TABLE 1. Levels and measures of the biological substrate

I. Neural processes	II. Autonomic nervous system
1. Structural aspects	1. Parasympathetic activity
A. Neuronal development and connections	A. Cardiac vagal tone
B. Localization of action	
2. Functional aspects	2. Sympathetic nervous system
A. Neurochemical systems (dopamine, noradrenaline, serotonin, brain-derived neurotrophic factor)	A. Resting heart rate
3. Neurocognitive function	3. Neuroendocrine function
A. Neuropsychological testing	A. HPA axis–Glucocorticoids
	4. Immunological function
	A. T cells/antibody titers to vaccines

preventive interventions.[13] A broad vision of the integration of prevention and neuroscience would examine how a variety of biological processes play a role in a deeper understanding of the processes and effects of preventive interventions. TABLE 1 provides a list of some of the biological substrates that would be of interest at the levels of both the brain and autonomic nervous system.

A central task for the next decade is to understand in much greater detail the relations between the multiple levels of the biological substrate and these resilience processes involved in cognitive processes and emotional regulation. With transdisciplinary collaboration involving neuroscientists and the use of multilevel models of measurement driven by the theory/logic model, prevention research has the potential to make a major contribution to understanding the developing interplay of biology and behavior.

Many preventive interventions focus on supporting improved emotion regulation and problem-solving skills in which executive functions (EF) and the actions of the prefrontal lobes play a central role. EF generally refers to the psychological processes that are involved in the conscious control of thought. Examples of processes include inhibition, future time orientation, consequential thinking, and the planning, initiation, and regulation of goal-directed behavior.[14] Substantial data indicate that EF skills as assessed by neuropsychological tasks are related to childhood maladaptation.[13,15] However, there has been little evidence in childhood between the performance of EF tasks (inhibitory control, working memory, planning) and neuroanatomical localization of activity in areas of the frontal lobe.[16,17] Due to the methodological requirements for valid Functional Magnetic Resonance Imaging (fMRI) assessments with young children, few data are available before the age of 10 years, although recent work using high-density Event Related Potential (ERP) assessments are particularly promising.[18] A series of methodological and conceptual challenges still have to be solved in order to fully assess the specific brain localization of neurocognitive and affective skills in children.[19] Further, there is a need to broaden methods to understand how childhood cognitive and affective processing (especially under conditions of stress) are related to other biological processes, including action in the autonomic nervous systems that include correlates of the hypo-pituitary-adrenal (HPA) axis,[20,21] immunological function, the parasympathetic system (vagal tone), as well as functional analysis of brain action (neurotransmitter release).

Pioneering work with children has already begun to show the potential yield of this vision in which interventions use measurement models and theories based on our rapidly developing knowledge of neuroscience. Research has indicated that there is correspondence between improved reading skills and changes in brain activity in reading-deficient children.[22] An intervention to improve the outcomes of children in the foster care system has indicated changes in both behavior and children's salivary cortisol.[23] Computer-based training for children with Attention-Deficit Hyperactivity Disorder (ADHD) has indicated changes in EF and behavior.[16] Meditation training in adults has been shown to alter both frontal brain activity (hemispheric laterality) and immunological response.[24] Further, a number of studies has shown the moderating role of biological variables, including how EF moderates the effect of a brief intervention on high-risk teens[25] and how the hypoactivity of anterior cingulate cortex predicts poor response to treatment for depression.[26]

Although neuroanatomical findings on cognitive and emotion regulation skills in childhood are sparse, there is a burgeoning literature on adults regarding brain localization of EF that can judiciously guide theory and action with children. The field of social–cognitive neuroscience (studies with lesion patients, patients with psychopathologies, and normally developing adults) has clearly implicated the orbital/dorsolateral/limbic circuit in the processing of emotional stimuli and the cognitive control and regulation of behavior.[27,28] Findings indicate a clear role for the anterior cingulate in the processing of emotions, executive attention processes, and working memory.[29–31] The role of the dorsolaternal prefrontal area has been shown in cognitive control and inhibition of emotional arousal.[32,33] Further, the orbital frontal area has been related to emotion processing and regulation.[34] Although research has attempted to completely localize processes in single neuroanatomical areas, it is clear that there is strong and rapid connectivity between these areas during decision making and there are sometimes contradictory findings between studies of specific loci.[35] As most of this work is less than a decade old, conclusions regarding specific loci may be premature. Further, noradrenaline, serotonin, and dopamine are projected to all these areas and thus energize action across systems. Double dissociation[36] and lesion studies as well as intervention trials[24] will play substantial roles in further differentiation.

THE DEVELOPMENT OF EF

Although infancy and toddlerhood provide a basis for critical aspects of later coping,[21,37] much of the child's more complex cognitive processes, coping, and regulation skills arise with neurocognitive maturation in the frontal lobes. This maturation proceeds from the preschool years through late adolescence. Although numerous linguistic and cognitive processes are developing, the development of EF appears crucial to healthy development and deficiencies in EF have been related to numerous poor outcomes. These outcomes involve cognitive processes related to effective emotional regulation and behavioral performance, including aggression, delinquency, depression, and disorders of attention.[13,38]

INTERVENTION AND EF: ILLUSTRATIONS FROM THE PROMOTING ALTERNATIVE THINKING STRATEGIES (PATHS) CURRICULUM

During the past few decades our research group has been involved in the development, implementation, evaluation, and refinement of a social and emotional learning curriculum based on neuroscientific principles that focus on promoting emotional awareness and effective cognitive control. The PATHS curriculum is a universal school-based prevention curriculum aimed at reducing aggression and behavior problems by promoting the development of social–emotional competence in children during the preschool and elementary school years.[39] PATHS is based on the affective-behavioral-cognitive-dynamic (ABCD) model of development.[40] The ABCD model focuses on how cognition, affect, language, and behavior become integrated in the developing child. A fundamental concept is that as youth mature, emotional development precedes most forms of cognitive development. That is, young children experience emotions and react to them long before they can verbalize their experiences. Early in life, emotional development is an important precursor to other ways of thinking and must be integrated with cognitive and linguistic abilities, which are much slower to develop. Then, during the elementary years, further developmental integration occurs among affect, behavior, and cognition/language through maturation of the prefrontal circuit. These processes of brain maturation are important in achieving socially competent action and healthy peer relations.

The PATHS curriculum places special attention on neurocognitive models of development.[41] Of significant importance are the concepts of *vertical control* and *verbal processing of action* (e.g., horizontal control). Vertical control refers to the process of higher-order cognitive processes exerting control over lower-level limbic impulses vìs-a-vìs the development of frontal cognitive control.[14] PATHS attempts to consciously teach children the processes of vertical control by providing opportunities to practice conscious strategies for self-control. This is achieved via instruction with curriculum lessons and a variety of cognitive/behavioral techniques that are developmentally appropriate from the ages of 4 to 11 years. One central example is the use of a control signals poster that teaches children the steps for problem solving in social contexts.

The curriculum also has an intentional and intensive focus on helping children to verbally identify and label feelings in order to manage them. This is achieved through curriculum lessons and the integration of "feeling faces" that children use throughout the day to identify their feelings and those of others.

A series of outcome trials have indicated that effective implementation of the PATHS curriculum leads to decreases in externalizing and internalizing problems by both teacher and self-report and to increases in social and emotional competence.[42–45] However, as with many preventive interventions, there has been little investigation of how such change is mediated. Although some aspect of this mediation may be due to changes external to the child (improved classroom environment, warmer teacher–student relations), we believe that the curriculum promotes more effective inhibitory control, emotion regulation, and planning skills. The curriculum logic model is based on the idea that the intervention will lead children (1) to become less impulsive and more planful in their social interactions, and (2) to recruit language to regulate behavior and communicate effectively with others.

We recently tested this mediation model in a randomized controlled study of 318 second-and third-grade children.[46] Schools were randomized to receive the PATHS intervention or to control status. Intervention teachers received both a 3-day initial training workshop as well as ongoing weekly coaching in curriculum implementation. The PATHS lessons were taught approximately three times per week, with each lesson lasting 20–30 min. In addition, teachers used techniques to generalize PATHS skills with the goal of supporting students to apply the PATHS skills in the "hot" naturally occurring contexts of their school day. These situations of high emotional arousal usually occurred during conflictual interactions with peers, with their teachers, or when feeling academic frustration. Students were assessed at pretest, posttest (7 months later), and follow-up (1 year after the curriculum ended).

Outcome findings examined teachers' ratings of both internalizing and externalizing behavioral problems using the Child Behavioral Checklist (CBCL[47]). EF were assessed by two well-known measures validated to activate anterior cingulate and dorsolateral prefrontal cortex.[48] Inhibitory control was assessed with the Stroop Test and verbal fluency was assessed using the Verbal Fluency Subtest of the McCarthy Scales of Children Abilities. To test a mediational model, it was first necessary to demonstrate that the intervention affected both behavior and EF. Results indicated that there were significant differences at posttest showing greater improvements in both inhibitory control and verbal fluency in the intervention children. At the 1-year follow-up, intervention children also were rated by teachers as lower in externalizing and internalizing problems. Further, posttest changes in both inhibitory control and verbal fluency were significantly related to teacher ratings of behavior problems at follow-up.

The specific mediational hypothesis we tested was that EF would mediate the relationship between prevention/control group assignment and teacher-reported externalizing and internalizing behavior problems. The findings indicated that improvements in inhibitory control at posttest significantly mediated the relation between experimental condition and both teacher-reported externalizing and internalizing behavior at 1-year follow-up. In addition, improvements in verbal fluency significantly mediated the relation between experimental condition and teacher-reported internalizing behavior. However, improvements in verbal fluency showed only a trend toward explaining change in teacher-reported externalizing behavior.

These findings provide empirical support for the conceptual theory of action that underlies the PATHS curriculum model. That is, child neurocognitive functioning plays a key role in children's social and emotional adaptation and changes in EF directly relate to reductions in behavioral problems. However, a broader view and greater incorporation of the biological substrate into our understanding of the processes would begin to assess less peripheral systems of mediation than only the use of neuropsychological tests.

Although our own work with the PATHS intervention is very preliminary, I use it as a case example of how we might develop transdisciplinary connections between prevention scientists and neuroscientists. A clear logic model of the intervention might hypothesize that such behavioral changes would lead to greater activation in the anterior cingulate and dosolateral prefrontal areas. Although such assessments could not be readily accomplished using fMRI at these younger ages, EEG–ERP assessments might be used. One might also hypothesize that such an intervention might impact the child's stress reactivity (HPA axis) or their parasympathetic activity under moderately stressful testing conditions. Finally, if such an intervention impacted both frontal activity and stress-reactivity, one might hypothesize that over time it might impact overall bodily health as assessed by immunological function.

The point here is that effective preventive models that have more fully articulated logic models of action should begin to ask "deeper" questions about the neuroscientific underpinnings of either change processes or obstacles to intervention impact. That is, how might measures of the biological substrate serve as mediators, moderators, and outcomes?

Of course, there are some important caveats at this stage in the scientific enterprise. First, children may recruit different brain regions than do adults to accomplish the same task and extrapolated theories from research on adults should be used with caution.[49] Further, even when fMRI can be used with older children, there are substantial conceptual and methodological challenges in interpreting such findings.[19] Finally, although some aspects of the effects of preventive interventions may be better understood by taking a neuroscientific perspective, much of the action of some prevention models occurs primarily through changes in the environment (quality of the classroom or community) or in the context of social interactions that may not be well-captured by current models of neuroscience.

These findings and others in neuroscience point to the importance of considering social–emotional development as best understood within broader theories that take into account how children's experiences and relationships affect their brain organization, structuralization, and development.[38] As such, there is a need for an extensive research agenda in which there is a transdisciplinary collaboration among prevention scientists, developmental psychopathologists, and neuroscientists. However, this will require not only clearer logic models of change and possibly more potent preventive interventions, but substantial advances in basic research in childhood neuroscience including improvements in both measurement and conceptualization. Through such work, carefully developed studies should take us past the "black box" outcome to more fully understand the cognitive and neural mediators and moderators of change.

ACKNOWLEDGMENTS

This work was supported by the National Institute of Mental Health (NIMH) grant R01MH42131. Dr. Greenberg is one of the developers of the PATHS curriculum program and has a publishing agreement with Channing–Bete Publishers.

REFERENCES

1. LEVENTHAL, T., R.C. FAUTH & J. BROOKS-GUNN. 2005. Neighborhood poverty and public policy: a 5-year follow-up of children's educational outcomes in the New York City moving to opportunity demonstration. Dev. Psychopath. **43:** 933–952.
2. HAWKINS, J.D. & R.F. CATALANO, JR. 1992. Communities that Care: Action for Drug Abuse Prevention. Jossey-Bass. San Francisco.
3. BRONFENBRENNER, U. 1977. Toward an experimental ecology of human development. Am. Psych. **32:** 513–531.
4. CICCHETTI, D. & D. TUCKER. 1994. Development and self-regulatory structures of the mind. Dev. Psychopath. **6:** 533–549.
5. COIE, J.D., N.F. WATT, S.G. WEST, *et al.* 1993. The science of prevention: a conceptual framework and some directions for a national research program. Am. Psych. **48:** 1013–1022.
6. CICCHETTI, D. & D.J. COHEN. 1995. Developmental Psychopathology: Vol 2. Risk, Disorder, and Adaptation. Wiley. New York.
7. MASTEN, A.S. 2001. Ordinary magic: resilience processes in development. Am. Psych. **56:** 227–238.
8. CASPI, A., T.E. MOFFITT, M. CANNON, *et al.* 2005. Moderation of the effect of adolescent onset cannibus use on adult psychosis by a functional polymorphism in the Catechol-O-Methyltransferase gene. Bio. Psych. **57:** 1117–1127.
9. RUTTER, M. Implications of resilience concepts for scientific understanding. Ann. N. Y. Acad. Sci. This volume.
10. GREENBERG, M.T., M.L. SPELTZ & M. DEKLYEN. 1993. The role of attachment in the early development of disruptive behavior problems. Dev. Psychopath. **5:** 191–213.

11. LUTHAR, S.S. 1993. Annotation: methodological and conceptual issues on research on childhood resilience. Pediatric Annals **20:** 501–506.
12. MASTEN, A.S. Competence and resilience in development. Ann. N. Y. Acad. Sci. This volume.
13. RIGGS, N.R. & M.T. GREENBERG. 2004. The role of neuro-cognitive models in prevention research. *In* The Science, Treatment, and Prevention of Antisocial Behaviors (Vol. 2). D. Fishbein, Ed.: Civic Research Institute. Kingston, NJ.
14. LURIA, A.R. 1966. Higher Cortical Functions in Man. Basic Books. New York.
15. RAINE, A. 2002. Annotation: the role of prefrontal deficits, low autonomic arousal, and early health factors in the development of antisocial and aggressive behavior in children. J. Child Psych. Psy. **43:** 417–434.
16. KLINGBERG, T., E. FERNELL, P.J. OLESEN, *et al.* 2005. Computerized training of working memory in children with ADHD: a randomized, controlled trial. J. Am. Acad. Child Adol. Psy. **44:** 177–186.
17. CASEY, B.J., N. TOTTENHAM, C. LISTEN, *et al.* 2005. Imaging the developing brain: What have we learned about cognitive development? Trends in Cog. Sci. **9:** 104–110.
18. LEWIS, M. Behavioral differences in aggressive children linked with neural mechanisms of emotional regulation. Ann. N. Y. Acad. Sci. This volume.
19. PETERSEN, B.S. 2003. Conceptual, methodological, and statistical challenges in brain imaging studies of developmentally based psychopathologies. Dev. Psychopath. **15:** 811–832.
20. BLAIR, C. 2002. School readiness: integrating cognition and emotion in a neurobiological conceptualization of children's functioning at school entry. Am. Psych. **57:** 111–127.
21. GUNNAR, M.R. & D.M. VAZQUEZ. 2001. Low cortisol and a flattening of expected daytime rhythm: potential indices of risk in human development. Dev. Psychopath. **13:** 515–538.
22. SHAYWITZ, B.A., S.E. SHAYWITZ, B.A. BLACHMAN, *et al.* 2004. Development of left ocipitotemporal systems for skilled reading in children after a phonologically-based intervention. Bio. Psy. **55:** 926–933.
23. FISHER, P., M.R. GUNNAR, P. CHAMBERLAIN, *et al.* 2000. Preventive intervention for maltreated preschool children: impact on children's behavior, neuroendocrine activity, and foster parent functioning. J. Am. Acad. Child Adol. Psy. **39:** 1356–1364.
24. DAVIDSON, R.J., J. KABAT-ZINN, J. SCHUMACHER, *et al.* 2003. Alterations in brain and immune function produced by mindfulness meditation. Psycho. Med. **65:** 564–570.
25. FISHBEIN, D., C. HYDE, D. ELDRETH, *et al.* 2006. Neurocognitive skills moderate urban male adolescent responses to preventive intervention materials. Drug Alcohol Depend. **82:** 47–60.
26. PIZZGALLI, D.A., J.B. NITSCHKE, T.R. OAKES, *et al.* 2001. Anterior cingulate activity as a predictor of degree of treatment response in major depression: evidence from brain electrical tomography analysis. Am. J. Psy. **158:** 405–415.
27. BECHARA, A. 2005. Decision making, impulse control, and loss of willpower to resist drugs: a neurocognitive perspective. Nat. Neurosci. **8:** 1458–1463.
28. OCHSNER, K.N. 2004. Current directions in social cognitive neuroscience. Cur. Op. Neurobiol. **14:** 254–258.

29. BUSH, G., P. LUU & M.I. POSNER. 2000. Cognitive and emotional influences in the anterior cingulate cortex. Trends Cog. Sci. **4:** 215–222.
30. DREVETS, W.C. & M.E. RAICHLE. 1998. Reciprocal suppression of regional cerebral blood flow during emotional versus higher cognitive processes: implications for interactions between emotion and cognition. Cog. Emo. **12:** 353–385.
31. STERZER, P., C. STADLER, A. KREBBS, *et al.* 2005. Abnormal neural responses to emotional visual stimuli in adolescents with conduct disorder. Biol. Psy. **57:** 7–15.
32. OCHSNER, K.N., S.A. BUNGE, J.J. GROSS, *et al.* 2002. Rethinking feelings: an fMRI study of the cognitive regulation of emotion. J. Cog. Neurosci. **14:** 1215–1229.
33. PHAN, K.L., D.A. FITZGERALD, P.J. NATHAN, *et al.* 2005. Neural substrates for voluntary suppression of negative affect: a functional magnetic resonance imaging study. Bio. Psy. **57:** 210–219.
34. BEER, L.S., E.A. HEERY, D. KLETNER, *et al.* 2003. The regulatory function of self-conscious emotion: insights from patients with oribitofrontal damage. J. Pers. Soc. Psych. **85:** 594–604.
35. FARRAH, M.J. & L.K. FELLOWS. 2005. Is anterior cingulate cortex necessary for cognitive control. Brain **205:** 788–799.
36. CHAMBERLAIN, S.R., U. MULLER, A.D. BLACKWELL, *et al.* 2006. Neurochemical modulation of responses inhibition and probabilistic learning in humans. Science **311:** 861–863.
37. GREENBERG, M.T. 1999. Attachment and psychopathology in childhood. *In* Handbook of Attachment: Theory, Research, and Clinical Applications. J. Cassidy & P.R. Shaver, Eds.: 469–496. Guilford. New York.
38. FISHBEIN, D. 2001. The importance of neurobiological research to the prevention of psychopathology. Prev. Sci. **1:** 89–106.
39. KUSCHÉ, C.A. & M.T. GREENBERG. 1994. The PATHS (Promoting Alternative Thinking Strategies) Curriculum. Channing-Bete. South Deerfield, MA.
40. GREENBERG, M.T. & C.A. KUSCHÉ. 1993. Promoting Social and Emotional Development in Deaf Children: The PATHS Project. University of Washington Press. Seattle.
41. KUSCHÉ, C.A. & M.T. GREENBERG. 2006. Brain development and social emotional learning: an introduction for educators. *In* The Educator's Guide to Emotional Intelligence and Academic Achievement. M. Elias & H. Arnold, Eds.: Corwin Press. Thousand Oaks, CA.
42. CONDUCT PROBLEMS PREVENTION RESEARCH GROUP. 1999. Initial impact of the Fast Track prevention trial for conduct problems: II. Classroom effects. J Cons. Clin. Psych. **67:** 648–657.
43. GREENBERG, M.T. & C.A. KUSCHÉ. 2002. Promoting Alternative Thinking Strategies. Blueprint for Violence Prevention (Book 10), Institute of Behavioral Sciences, University of Colorado. CO
44. KAM, C., M.T. GREENBERG & C.A. KUSCHÉ. 2004. Sustained effects of the PATHS curriculum on the social and psychological adjustment of children in special education. J. Emot. Behav. Disorders **12:** 66–78.
45. RIGGS, N.R., M.T. GREENBERG, C.A. KUSCHÉ, *et al.* 2006. The mediational role of neurocognition in the behavioral outcomes of a social-emotional prevention program in elementary school students: effects of the PATHS Curriculum. Prev. Sci. **7:** 91–102.

46. RIGGS, N.R., C. BLAIR & M.T. GREENBERG. 2003. Concurrent and 2-year longitudinal relations between executive function and the behavior of 1st and 2nd grade children. Child Neuropsych. **9:** 267–276.
47. ACHENBACH, T.M. 1991. Manual for the Child Behavior Checklist and 1991 Profile. Department of Psychiatry, University of Vermont. Burlington, VT.
48. RAVNKILDE, B., P. VIDEBECH, R. ROSENBERG, *et al.* 2002. Putative tests of frontal lobe function: a PET-study of brain activation during Stroop's Test and verbal fluency. J. Clin. Exp. Neuropsychol. **24:** 534–547.
49. BUNGE, S.A., N.M. DUDUKOVIC, M.E. THOMANSON, *et al.* 2002. Immature frontal lobe contributions to cognitive control in children: evidence from fMRI. Neuron **33:** 1–20.

Prevention Approaches to Enhance Resilience among High-Risk Youth

Comments on the Papers of Dishion & Connell and Greenberg

KAROL L. KUMPFER AND JULIA FRANKLIN SUMMERHAYS

Department of Health Promotion and Education, University of Utah, Salt Lake City, Utah, USA

ABSTRACT: This article synthesizes research on resilience theory and its implications for prevention interventions to increase resilience in high-risk children and adolescents. In addition, this response to both the articles by Drs. Greenberg and Dishion summarizes their key points. Their papers discuss the neuroscience substrate behind two major mediators of antisocial behaviors, namely lack of self-regulation and executive function problems. In addition, we present an overall Resilience Framework that will help the reader organize the aspects of resilience discussed by these two researchers into a transactional process model. This article extends prior researchers' suggestion that resilience is the product of the interaction of genetic, biological, and environmental precursors to a further consideration of higher-level cognitive precursors, such as purpose in life and existential meaning. The relevance of resilience to the prevention of negative outcomes in high-risk children of alcoholics (COAs) and substance abusers is covered. Within this third wave of resilience research on prevention interventions, we present data suggesting that family strengthening approaches have the greatest impact on increasing resilience.

KEYWORDS: resilience; theory; prevention; substance abuse; high-risk adolescents

INTRODUCTION

Resilience has been defined as the achievement of competence or positive developmental outcomes under conditions that are adverse or that challenge adaptation.[1] In a fast-paced, stressful world providing children with fewer

Address for correspondence: Dr. Karol Kumpfer, Department of Health Promotion and Education, University of Utah, Salt Lake City, Utah 84112. Voice: 801-581-7718; fax: 801-581-5872.
e-mail: kkumpfer@xmission.com

Ann. N.Y. Acad. Sci. 1094: 151–163 (2006).
doi: 10.1196/annals.1376.014

interpersonal and family supports, the prevention field promotes increased resilience and positive developmental outcomes for children. No child today is beyond risk; no child is, or could be, completely protected. Exposure to moderate stressors, challenges, and risks can help children develop effective coping responses and resilience. Wise parents naturally titrate a child's temperament, capabilities, and resilience with levels and types of stressors before allowing or encouraging new challenges. Poor cognitive executive functioning and lack of self-regulation leading to a thrill-seeking temperament are also major hazards, as so well described in the papers by both Drs. Dishion and Greenberg. Parents or caring adults who fail to recognize these developmental deficits in a child may be the greater hazard to positive youth development. Emmy Werner's 40 years of research on resilience in a cohort of children born on the island of Kauai, Hawaii, discovered that "one caring adult in a child's life" is possibly the most critical protective factor in resilience.[2] Growing levels of adolescent problems suggest that far too few parents are caring and wise.

OVERVIEW OF RESPONSE TO GREENBERG AND DISHION PAPERS

Prevention research seeks knowledge about prevention interventions to help parents, teachers, and other caring adults in their efforts to promote resilience and positive outcomes in children. Many evidence-based interventions have supported positive child development by increasing resilience to negative life stressors.[3,4] This response to Drs. Greenberg and Dishion summarizes their key points concerning the application of research on etiology and prevention interventions toward supporting resilience in youth. Their papers discuss the

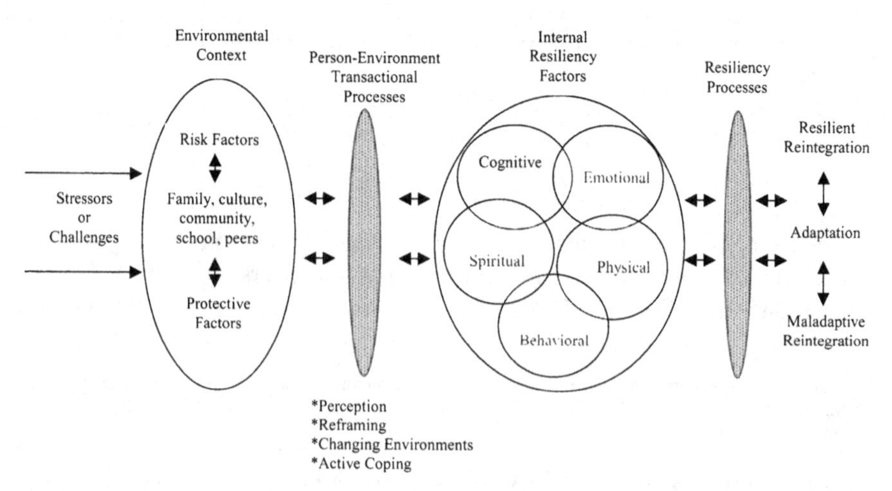

FIGURE 1. The Resilience Framework (Kumpfer, K.L.[7]).

neuroscience substrate behind two major mediators of antisocial behaviors, namely lack of self-regulation[5] and executive function problems.[6] In addition, we will present an overall Resilience Framework (see FIG. 1) that will help the reader organize the aspects of resilience discussed by these two researchers into a transactional process model.[7]

We will also extend observations made by Greenberg and Dishion and others about resilience as the product of the interaction of genetic, biological, and environmental precursors to a further consideration of higher-level cognitive precursors, such as purpose in life and existential meaning. We will argue that resilience is not a new concept but has been recognized since recorded time in the indigenous wisdom of our ancestors. This article will also discuss the relevance of resilience to the prevention of negative outcomes in the very high-risk children of alcoholics (COAs) and substance abusers. Within the third wave of resilience research on prevention interventions,[8] we present data suggesting that family strengthening approaches have the greatest impact on increasing resilience. Wise and mindful parenting results in not only stronger cognitive executive functioning and self-regulation in children, discussed as essential features of resilience by Greenberg and Dishion, but also in meaning in life and indigenous wisdom.[9]

RESILIENCE AND INDIGENOUS WISDOM

According to the ancient Greek view of medicine in the Hippocratic tradition, sickness resulted from being out of harmony with your world. Both mind and body and beauty in your world contributed to health. Perfection and good character were to be sought after as constant goals. Both Eastern and Western traditions of medicine and mental health agreed on this point. Our studies of resilience among Native Americans also support this indigenous wisdom. Being in harmony with nature and interpersonal relationships are considered critical to resilience to disease and social ills.[10] The natural circle of life includes a balance between physical, mental, social and spiritual needs and realms, which are the paths to a long, happy, and healthy life. Avoiding excess or addictions was part of this indigenous wisdom or secret of resilience.

HIGH-RISK CHILDREN OF ALCOHOL AND DRUG ABUSERS

Too many children today are born to parents with various addictions (e.g., psychoactive substances, food, sex, gambling, or work) whose lives are out of balance and have little time or inclination to be wise and caring parents. For example, about a quarter of all children under 17 years of age in the United States (19 million) have a parent who is an alcoholic. Because of the intergenerational transmission of genetic and environmental risk factors for alcoholism, these COAs are at very high risk for many neuropsychological and limbic system deficits that lead to reduced resilience, such as (*a*) behavioral and emotional self-regulation problems and (*b*) reduced executive functioning.[11] Sons of early onset (before the age of 15 years) male alcoholics who have many alcoholic relatives across generations, a characteristic of a highly heritable type of alcoholism called Type II Male Limited Alcoholism, have been reported to be genetically vulnerable to two major syndromes: (1) the Overstressed Youth Syndrome (e.g., poor emotional regulation, difficult temperament, autonomic hyperreactivity, rapid brain waves) and (2) prefrontal cognitive deficits in verbal and abstract reasoning and verbal learning. Heritable dysfunctions of the prefrontal cortex and limbic systems have been posited as causing these self-regulation and executive functioning dysfunctions;[12] however, cognitive impairments may also stem from environmental neglect or fetal alcohol exposure. Alcohol and drugs serve as self-medication because they smooth out the overactive autonomic nervous system (ANS) stress response[12] and increase essential neurotransmitters (dopamine, serotonin, noradrenalin) to reduce depression and anxiety.

Luthar found similar adverse circumstances are present for children whose parents abuse illegal drugs.[13] She concludes from her research, however, that maternal drug abuse *per se* is not as damaging to children's resilience as maternal stress, depression, and anxiety disorders.[14] Addicted parents have been found to spend about half as much time with their children, use lax or excessive punishment, but more often just neglect their children. With parents working more and fewer extended family supports, parental neglect is occurring in homes of both the rich and the poor. Neglect is possibly even more devastating than physical punishment to children's brain development as well as social and emotional development. Like Suomi's peer-raised monkeys,[15] children who do not feel protected by caring adults tend to cluster into strong peer groups, such as gangs. They exhibit increased levels of stress, anxiety, and insecure attachment leading to reduced exploratory behaviors needed to develop self-control and executive functioning.

FRAMING GREENBERG AND DISHION'S RISK FACTORS WITHIN A TRANSACTIONAL RESILIENCE FRAMEWORK

Greenberg[6] has summarized guiding principles of the development of resilience, concluding that multiple hereditary and environmental factors interact to produce multiple pathways to resilience that are not disorder specific but rather their salience varies depending on timing, age, gender, and ethnicity. Tested etiological theories help to order risk and protective factors into developmental pathways that help prevention scientists design more effective prevention interventions. For instance, the author's Pathways Model[16] found that there are three primary developmental mediating pathways to positive life adaptation: (1) a family environment pathway (parent–child attachment, supervision, and communication of positive behaviors and values impacting choice of peers) that was the most influential pathway, (2) a secondary pathway that appeared to reflect more the child's temperament or biological factors, such as self regulation that linked primarily to school performance and peer–teacher acceptance, and (3) a very weak pathway from the community environment to the problem behavior. Girls were slightly more impacted by family protective factors and boys and American Indians by community environment, but in general the strength of these pathways was significant and similar by gender, ethnicity, and age.

THE TRANSACTIONAL FRAMEWORK OF RESILIENCE

Luthar and associates[17] argue, "future empirical studies on resilience must be presented within cogent theoretical frameworks (p. 553)." The authors' Transactional Framework of Resilience[7] proposes that parent–child transactional processes are extremely important in mediating or moderating biological and environmental risk and promoting resilience. Greenberg defines resilience as "positive or protective processes that reduce maladaptive outcomes under conditions of risk." Greenberg[6] discusses three broad types of protective factors—the child's characteristics, quality of relationships, and broader environmental or ecological factors. Similarly, the Resilience Framework[7] identifies three major types of resilience processes (e.g., the child's personal strengths, the family or interpersonal dynamics, and the environmental or community context of stressors) within a single transactional model. This model builds on prior social ecology, transactional, and integrated models to create a metatheory or inclusive framework of characteristics and processes impacting resilience.

Internal Strength or Resilience Characteristics

In the first wave of resilience research different personality characteristics were found to be associated with resilience.[8] These were conceptually clustered by Kumpfer into seven primary resilience characteristics, namely: happiness, wisdom and insight, humor, empathy, intellectual competencies, purpose in life, and perseverance.[7] Collette Evans' qualitative research on resilience with two American Indian tribes suggests that these same qualities are often prized by American Indians as indicators of resilience, but named differently.[10] For instance, "purpose in life" is somewhat analogous to the indigenous concept of "Right Path." An indicator of high self-esteem is "walking tall." Four dissertations using structural equations modeling (SEM) involving different populations (adult COAs, college students, working women in several states) suggest that the most important characteristic promoting resilience is purpose in life or existential meaning.[9] Creating meaning for one's life through goals, dreams, and a desire to use one's talents to make the world a better place helps people be resilient survivors in times of severe adversity. More recently, the field of positive psychology has further studied some of the cognitive–spiritual resilience factors including happiness, optimism, faith, creativity, hope and dreams, wisdom, and excellence.[18] The Resilience Framework also recognizes that developmental trajectories can be changed by active individual choices in which the child or advocates can help a child to change environments. In this way a limited type of "free will" can occur within our stimulus/response, deterministic worldview.

Transactional Intra- and Interpersonal Resilience Enhancing Processes

While the first wave of research on resilience focused on discovering resilience qualities, the second wave of research focused on resilience as an interactional or transactional process.[7,8] Few resilience researchers have focused until the last 10 years on these transactional relationships in research. Many of these dynamic concepts are employed in psychotherapy or have been studied in child development under the notions of coping with stress. Germane to this concept is Greenberg's thesis that: "An essential question related to adversity and resilience is the individual's development of an effective set of responses to stress." He identifies five central transactional processes between the stress stimulus in the environment at the left side and the final resulting behavioral response, namely: (*a*) perceptions or the initial appraisal of the stressor and its emotional meaning, (*b*) the ability to regulate one's emotional arousal, (*c*) effective problem solving, and (*d*) the cognitive–affective interpretation of the event. Unfortunately, he does not elaborate on these critical transactional processes, although they are very important for a better understanding of what processes can be brought to bear in designing prevention interventions to enhance resilience in children. The Transactional Resilience Framework[7] discusses these processes that should be enhanced when designing prevention interventions. *Cognitive reframing* of a stressor into a challenge or a growth experience may be one of the perception processes that facilitate the initial emotional appraisal of the stressor. Parents who encourage children to seek out new challenges may do so by using phrases similar to "No pain, no gain." They encourage children to stretch themselves from their comfort zone and also reward their positive stress-coping approaches. When children do fail, they do not see it as a failure to "make lemonade out of lemons," but they encourage the child to consider what they could do better the next time to achieve their goals and dreams. They encourage them to dream and scheme. Perseverance is encouraged within healthy or realistic bounds. As summarized by Masten, parents and mentors use processes of modeling, coaching, teaching, advising, supporting, reinforcing, advocating, providing opportunities, nurturance, and encouraging the attempt of reasonable challenges to facilitate child development.[19]

According to the Resilience Framework[7] parents or caretakers should use these socialization processes to improve their children's resiliency characteristics in all five resilience areas:[20]

1. Spiritual/motivation—support development of talents, uniqueness, goal-orientation, perseverance, internal locus of control, and purpose in life
2. Cognitive—support development of self-esteem, provide knowledge and academic skills
3. Behavioral—model, coach, and reinforce behavioral competence
4. Emotional—reflect feelings, model and reinforce mood management
5. Physical—teach and reinforce good health and healthy choices

Other transactional processes noted include: active environmental modification by the child or caring adults to get rid of or reduce the stressor, and parent facilitation of emotional regulation. These are discussed below in more detail and in Kumpfer and Bluth.[20]

ACTIVE MODIFICATIONS OF NEGATIVE ENVIRONMENTS

Determinism proposes that children merely respond to their environments. New transactional–ecological models of child development are challenging this notion. The child and any "caring other" can team together to perceive or interpret stressors and problem-solve better environments. Some resilient children have been discussed in resilience studies as finding "surrogate parents" to provide the love and learning opportunities that they need to become resilient and grow to be happy and healthy adults. To help a child find a better fit with their environment, some parents move so the child can attend a school better for them.

PARENTAL FACILITATION OF EMOTIONAL REGULATION

Parents and caring adults use many parenting strategies to help children control their emotions and develop behavioral self-control or regulation. They can model these self-restraint behaviors themselves by never "losing control," not using physical or emotional outbursts, reinforcing good self-regulation and control, and discussing stories or examples in children's literature, movies, or videos where the characters showed great emotional control over fear, anxiety, or anger to attain their goals.

Of course, as discussed in both the Greenberg and Dishion papers, some children have a more difficult time with self-control possibly because of genetic or environmental risk factors. Some children have developmental delays or dysfunctions in their orbital/dorsolateral/limbic systems in the processing of emotional stimuli and self-regulation of their behavioral response. Greenberg discusses the new neuroscience research that helps to locate the areas of the developing brain that are responsible for self-regulation and executive functioning in problem solving. Recent brain imaging techniques as summarized by Volkow[21] suggest that children's brains are still developing until 25 to 30 years of age primarily in their higher cortical areas of the dorsal/lateral prefrontal cortex that anticipates consequences of different responses to stimuli. These brain areas also help a child to anticipate possible negative consequences of responses and to override the most likely or most rewarded stimulus/response (S-R) connection. Hopefully, the child has seen through vicarious learning possible negative reactions to that strongest S-R situation. This is a hallmark of good self-regulation—stifling bad habits or not doing a behavior that is most probable, but thinking ahead about consequences.

Richardson[9] believes the third wave of resilience research should focus on a metatheoretical integration that includes self-righting forces within individuals that promote or energize the resilience process, such as biological, moral, and spiritual survival. New developments in higher-level physics and string theory provide glimpses into complex energy and social forces that could impact resilience processes. These concepts support indigenous wisdom of our ancestors (whether American Indian or Western culture) that internal strivings for harmony or balance is what leads to resilience, health, and well-being.

EFFECTIVE PREVENTION APPROACHES INCREASE RESILIENCE

Greenberg categorized effective prevention approaches according to Bronfenbrenner's social ecology theory as targeting: (1) *macrosystem level* environment changes through community coalitions, media campaigns, and policy changes impacting national, community, or school-level ecologies, norms, and behaviors and (2) *microsystem level* environmental changes in families and children through skills training in communication and other interpersonal skills. Parent training can also impact at an *exosystem* level parental social support and at a *mesosystem level* parental monitoring of peers. The greater the number of risk factors compared to the number of protective or resilience factors, the greater the child's risk of developmental psychopathology. A number of different prevention approaches have been developed and found effective because the causes of children's outcomes are multidetermined.[3,4] Combining prevention interventions to address more risk and protective factors has been found to result in even better developmental outcomes. Thus combining a parenting and family intervention, such as the authors' *Strengthening Families Program (SFP)* with a child-only skills training program, Spivack and

Shure's *I Can Problem Solve,* resulted in larger effect sizes roughly equivalent to adding together the individual program effect sizes.[22]

Given the etiological theories presented here suggesting the primary importance of parent/child attachment in reducing developmental psychopathology, one disappointing omission within the papers of Dishion and Greenberg is their lack of mention of the critical importance of family strengthening interventions, although both of these researchers have developed evidence-based family interventions. Dishion has excellent results from his *Adolescent Transitions Program*[23] and Greenberg is conducting a massive, multisite, two-state study (PROSPER) of the implementation of the seven-session *SFP for 10 to 14 Year Olds* (formerly called the Iowa SFP). The Foxcroft and associates' Cochrane Collaboration Review of school-based alcohol prevention[24] concluded this family intervention was twice as effective as the next best prevention program (a parenting program) based on longitudinal randomized control trials.[25] Spoth and Trudeau reported at the 2005 Society for Prevention Research conference on 10-year follow-up results.[26,27] They reported two to three times reduced mental health diagnoses (depression, anxiety, social phobia, and personality disorder) by the age of 22 years in the youth who participated. Such a large impact on mental health disorders with such a short seven-session family intervention is truly amazing and very cost-effective to society as a whole. A cost-benefit analysis has found a $9.60 cost return for every dollar spent to schools alone that implement *SFP* 10–14 years.[25] Culturally adapted *SFP* versions for ethnic families have resulted in similar positive outcomes, with recruitment and retention improved by 40%.[28]

MEDIATING MECHANISMS UNDERLYING EVIDENCE-BASED PREVENTION PROGRAMS

The mechanisms of effectiveness of evidence-based prevention programs are only beginning to be explored, but the Greenberg and Dishion research studies suggest these prevention interventions are effective because they improve behavioral and emotional self-regulation and executive cognitive functioning. Almost all evidence-based prevention programs teach children what Greenberg calls *vertical control* and *horizontal control.* Vertical control is the use of higher-order frontal cognitive processes to control lower-level limbic emotional impulses. Horizontal control refers to verbal processing of emotional and behavioral action. For instance, youth are taught conscious strategies for self-control including verbal mediation (self-talk) and inhibitory control. One example of inhibitory would be a control signals poster with "Red = Stop, Yellow = Think, Green = Go" strategy. Feeling charades or pictures are used to teach cognitive labeling of emotions. Because of increased neglect, children of substance abusers are frequently not taught by parents to reflect on feelings. Hence, they are more frequently diagnosed with "alexithemia" or an inability to identify feelings. The authors' *SFP* includes a technique called "Child's Game" that teaches parents to watch in a play situation for their children's expression of feelings and to describe the body cues and label the feeling for the child. In this manner, parents are taught to help the children learn a full feelings vocabulary beyond just "sad, mad, and glad."

Greenberg tested a specific mediational hypothesis that the executive functions would mediate behavioral control. His hierarchical linear modeling analysis of 1-year follow-up data on 318 third graders found that increased inhibitory control at posttest because of the Promoting Alternative Thinking Strategies (PATHS) curriculum resulted in decreased teacher reported child externalizing and internalizing behavior problems. Hence, his prevention intervention impact on increasing inhibitory control helped to also test and confirm the mediating mechanisms in his theory.[6]

CONCLUSION

Both the Greenberg and Dishion prevention papers focus on the biological substrate that underlie resilience, which they seek to enhance in their prevention interventions. Greenberg's school-based, teacher-led PATHS program seeks to increase emotional control by increasing self-talk through teaching verbal mediation in problem solving and the identification of feelings.[6] Dishion also seeks to increase self-control or self-regulation by teaching youth steps to improving resistance to pressures in the environment to act in damaging ways.[5] Both papers discuss the brain sites or neurological functions that underlie these problem behaviors. This article identifies one group of children who are at higher risk for these self-regulation and executive functioning problems that can lead to reduced resilience, namely children of substance abusers. Their genetic risk can lead to increased use of alcohol and drugs that further damage their prefrontal cognitive development. Recovery can take up to 2 years according to brain scan studies by Volkow, now the Director of National Institute on Drug Abuse (NIDA).[21]

In the final analysis, while breakthroughs in neurosciences and physiological functioning will help us to better understand why we behave the way we do, improving these behaviors to support resilience in high-risk children will come from the testing of prevention interventions. Effective prevention interventions are designed based on theories of resilience and mediators of child development, but randomized control trials of prevention interventions can be used as pointed out by Greenberg[6] "to test these theories by examining how behavior changes are mediated." Transactional models, such as Wills and Dishion's proposed model of the interaction of temperament and self-control as resilience constructs with parenting and parent risk factors,[30] could be tested using SEM with prevention interventions data. For instance, the Center for Substance Abuse Prevention (CSAP) High-Risk Youth Prevention data were used to test the earlier Kumpfer and Turner's Social Ecology Model in the Pathways Model. The results showed that parent–child attachment and effective parenting significantly moderates lack of self-control to improve academic competency.[16] In the future, increased use of more sophisticated transactional data analysis of longitudinal studies as advocated by Werner[29]should be used to further explore the transactional processes of resilience and to design even more effective prevention interventions.

Already considerable research has demonstrated effective prevention approaches increase resilience by improving impulse control and executive functioning. Programs like *Project PATHS* or *I Can Problem Solve* that instruct teachers to work with high-risk children or the *SFP* that teaches parents to work with their own children, have been demonstrated to be effective in increasing high-risk youths' resilience and positive development.

At the level of public policy, evidence-based prevention approaches, such as family-strengthening approaches (www.strengtheningfamilies.org) should be supported because they have enduring impact on increased resilience and improving child outcomes.[4] Other child and family friendly policy approaches, such as WIC, childcare, early preschool, and family support programs, should be supported nationally. Parents and other caring adults need all the help they can get from prevention scientists, wise politicians, and a supportive citizenry in raising resilient youth.

Because families are primarily responsible for child rearing functions including providing for physical necessities, emotional support, learning opportunities, moral guidance, and building self-esteem and resilience, the failure of families to parent children can mean a failure to pass on knowledge and values to the next generation. A massive failure of a culture, society, or nation to parent and socialize children is clearly a recipe for disaster. Development of scientific knowledge about effective ways to support resilience and improve developmental outcomes in high-risk children is critically important. The application of this knowledge to major public health, social, and education initiatives is no less important.

REFERENCES

1. MASTEN, A. & D. COATSWORTH. 1998. The development of competence in favorable and unfavorable environments. Am. Psychol. **53:** 205–220.
2. WERNER, E. & R. SMITH. 1992. Overcoming the odds: high risk children from birth to adulthood. Cornell University Press. Ithaca, NY.
3. BIGLAN, A. & T.K. TAYLOR. 2000. Increasing the use of science to improve child-rearing. J. Primary Prevention **21:** 207–226.
4. KUMPFER, K.L. & R. ALVARADO. 2003. Family strengthening approaches for the prevention of youth problem behaviors. Am. Psychol. **58:** 457–465.
5. DISHION T. Adolescents' resilience as a self-regulatory process. Ann. N. Y. Acad. Sci. This volume.

6. GREENBERG, M.T. Promotion reslience in children and youth: preventive interventions and their interface with neuroscience. Ann. N. Y. Acad. Sci. This volume.
7. KUMPFER, K.L. 1999. Factors and processes contributing to resilience: the resilience framework. *In* Resilience and Development: Positive Life Adaptations. M.D. Glantz & J.L. Johnson, Eds.: 179–224. Kluwer Academic/Plenum Publishers. New York.
8. O'DOUGHTERY WRIGHT, M. & A.S. MASTEN. 2005. Resilience processes in development. *In* Handbook of Resilience in Children. S. Goldstein & R.B. Brooks, Eds.: 17–38. Kluwer Academic/Plenum Publishers. New York.
9. RICHARDSON, G.E. 2002. The metatheory of resilience and resiliency. J. Clin. Psychol. **58:** 307–321.
10. EVANS, C.M. 1997. There needs to be somebody: An exploration of the ways Great Basin Indian youth get through difficult times (substance abuse resiliency). University of Utah, Dissertation Abstracts International, 57(10-A) 5068.
11. CHASSIN, L., A. CARLE, D. NISSIM-SABAT & K.L. KUMPFER. 2004. Fostering resilience in children of alcoholic parents. *In* Investing in Children, Youth, Families, and Communities: Strengths-Based Research and Policy. K.I. Maton, Ed.: APA Books. Washington, DC.
12. SCHUCKIT, M. 1991. A longitudinal study of children of alcoholics. *In* Recent Developments in Alcoholism. Vol. 9: Children of alcoholics. M. Galanter, H. Begleiter *et al.* Eds.: 5–19. Plenum Press. New York.
13. LUTHAR, S., G. CUSHING, K. MERIKANGAS & B. ROUNSAVILLE. 1998. Multiple jeopardy: risk and protective factors among addicted mothers' offspring. Dev. Psychopathol. **10:** 117–136.
14. LUTHAR, S. S., K. D'Avanzo & S. HITES. 2005. Maternal drug abuse versus other psychological disturbances. *In* Resilience and Vulnerability: Adaptation in the Context of Childhood Adversities. S.S. Luthar, Eds.: Cambridge University Press. Cambridge, UK.
15. SUOMI, S. 2006. Risk, resiliency, and gene-environment interactions in rhesus monkeys. Ann. N. Y. Acad. Sci. This volume.
16. KUMPFER, K.L., R. ALVARADO & H.O. WHITESIDE. 2003. Family-based interventions for substance use and misuse prevention. Substance Use Misuse **38:** 1759–1789.
17. LUTHAR, S.S., D. CICCHETTI & B. BECKER. 2000. The construct of resilience: A critical evaluation and guidelines for future research. Child Dev. **71:** 543–562.
18. SELIGMAN, M.E.P. & M. CSIKSZENTMIHALYI. 2000. Positive psychology. Am. Psychol. **55:** 5–14.
19. MASTEN, A.S. 1994. Resilience in individual development: successful adaptation despite risk and adversity. *In* Educational Resilience in Inner-City America. M.C. Wang & E.W. Gorden, Eds.: 3–25. Erlbaum. Hillsdale, NJ.
20. KUMPFER, K.L. & B. BLUTH. 2004. Parent/child transactional processes predictive of resilience or vulnerability to substance abuse disorders. Substance Use Misuse. **39:** 721–748.
21. VOLKOW, N. 2006. Paper presented at meeting "Resilience in Children" Sponsored by New York Academy of Science, held Feb. 28, 2006.
22. KUMPFER, K.L., R. ALVARADO, C. TAIT & C. TURNER. 2002. Effectiveness of school-based family and children's skills training for substance abuse prevention among 6-8 year old rural children. Psychol. Addictive Behav. **16** (4S): S65–S71.
23. DISHION, T.J. & D.W. ANDREWS. 1995. Preventing escalation in problem behaviors with high risk young adolescents: Immediate and 1-year outcomes. J. Consult. Clin. Psychol. **63:** 538–548.

24. FOXCROFT, D.R., D. IRELAND, D.J. LISTER-SHARP, *et al.* 2003. Longer-term primary prevention for alcohol misuse in young people: A systematic review. Addiction **98:** 397–411.
25. SPOTH, R., M. GUYLL & S. DAY. 2002. Universal family-focused interventions in alcohol-use disorder prevention: cost-effectiveness and cost-benefit analyses of two interventions. J. Studies Alcohol **63:** 219–228.
26. SPOTH, R., C. REDMOND, A. MASON, R. KOSTERMAN, K. HAGGERTY, & J.D. HAWKINS. 2005. Ten-year follow-up assessment of brief, family-focused intervention effects on lifetime conduct and antisocial personality disorders: Preliminary results. Poster presented at the Society for Prevention Research 13th Annual Meeting, Washington, D.C. (PRS 186).
27. TRUDEAU, L. & R. SPOTH. 2005. Universal family-focused preventive intervention effects on non-targeted adolescent outcomes: generalization of effects. Presented in organized paper symposia at the Society for Prevention Research 13th Annual Meeting, Washington, D.C. (PRS 184).
28. KUMPFER, K.L., R. ALVARADO, P. SMITH & N. BELLAMY. 2002. Cultural sensitivity in universal family-based prevention interventions. Prevention Science (Special Issue). **3:** 241–244.
29. WERNER, E. 2005. What can we learn about resilience from large-scale longitudinal studies? *In* Handbook of Resilience in Children. S. Goldstein & R.B. Brooks, Eds.: 91–106. Kluwer Academic/Plenum Publishers. New York.
30. WILLS, T.A. & T.J. DISHION. 2004. Temperament and adolescent substance use: a transactional analysis of emerging self-control. J. Clin. Child Adol. Psychol. **33:** 69–81.

Behavioral Differences in Aggressive Children Linked with Neural Mechanisms of Emotion Regulation

MARC D. LEWIS,[a] ISABELA GRANIC,[b] AND CONNIE LAMM[a]

[a] *Department of Human Development and Applied Psychology, University of Toronto, Toronto, ON, Canada*

[b] *Community Health Systems Resource Group, Hospital for Sick Children, Toronto, Canada*

ABSTRACT: Children with aggressive behavior problems may have difficulties regulating negative emotions, resulting in harmful patterns of interpersonal behavior at home and in the schoolyard. Ventral and dorsal regions of the prefrontal cortex (PFC) have been associated with response inhibition and self-control—key components of emotion regulation. Our research program aims to explore differences among aggressive and normal children in the activation of these cortical regions during emotional episodes, to the extent possible using electrophysiological techniques, to identify diagnostic subtypes, gain insights into their interpersonal difficulties, and help develop effective treatment strategies. This report reviews several recent studies investigating individual and developmental differences in cortical mechanisms of emotion regulation, corresponding with different patterns of interpersonal behavior. Our methods include event-related potentials (ERPs) and cortical source modeling, using dense-array electroencephalography (EEG) technology, as well as videotaped observations of parent–child interactions, with both normal and aggressive children. By relating patterns of brain activation to observed behavioral differences, we find (i) a steady decrease in cortical activation subserving self-regulation across childhood and adolescence, (ii) different cortical activation patterns as well as behavioral constellations distinguishing subtypes of aggressive children, and (iii) robust correlations between the activation of cortical mediators of emotion regulation and flexibility in parent–child emotional communication in children referred for aggressive behavior problems. These findings point toward models of developmental psychopathology based on the interplay among biological, psychological, and social factors.

KEYWORDS: aggression; cortical source modeling; emotion; psychopathology; event-related potentials (ERPs)

Address for correspondence: Marc D. Lewis, Department of Human Development and Applied Psychology, University of Toronto, 252 Bloor St. West, Toronto, ON M5S 1V6, Canada. Voice: 416-923-6641 x2443.
e-mail: mlewis@oise.utoronto.ca.

**Ann. N.Y. Acad. Sci. 1094: 164–177 (2006). © 2006 New York Academy of Sciences.
doi: 10.1196/annals.1376.017**

INTRODUCTION

The capacity to regulate emotional impulses effectively is critical for normal development, and children lacking these skills often develop serious behavior problems. Specifically, aggressive children may not adequately regulate the thoughts, feelings, and actions arising from negative emotional states such as anger and anxiety, and this may greatly diminish the quality of their relationships, first with their parents and later with their peers. Yet research on emotion regulation in child clinical populations has not made much progress. This may be due, in part, to the problems inherent in assessing emotion regulation using behavioral measures, which inevitably conflate emotional expression, regulation, and behavior itself. Thanks to the new tools of cognitive neuroscience, however, the biological substrates of emotion regulation can now be explored in the laboratory and related to individual differences in interpersonal behavior. Linking neural indices of emotion regulation with observed behavioral differences has been the goal of our research over the last few years, and we have pursued these objectives through the use of dense-array electroencephalography (EEG) and videotaped observations of parent–child interactions. By examining these measures for clinically referred children, and by comparing them with data from age-matched controls, we are advancing a model of developing emotion regulation capacities—a model that can help explain typical and atypical developmental trajectories and guide prevention and intervention policies.

In this report we outline the theoretical and empirical considerations that guide the search for brain mechanisms of emotion regulation in children, relate them to research on aggressive behavior problems, review the methods we have developed for analyzing brain and behavior patterns, and highlight results from several recent studies. Our most interesting finding to date is that reduced neural activity related to emotion regulation corresponds with an overall decrease in behavioral flexibility in children with aggressive behavior problems.

Scope of the Problem

Approximately half of all referrals to children's mental health agencies are for oppositional or aggressive behaviors.[1] Childhood aggression is associated with a host of serious difficulties. Most notably, early onset of aggression predicts later delinquency and adult criminality[1] and is linked to severe psychosocial maladjustment across several domains including peer relations[2] and academic functioning.[3] Adolescent antisocial behavior is predictive of later occupational instability, unemployment, marital problems, depression, and substance abuse.[1,3] Moreover, it is widely accepted that childhood anxiety and aggression problems co-occur.[4] Several studies suggest that children with both aggression and anxiety problems are at higher risk for a number of negative outcomes, compared with "pure" aggressive children.[5]

Emotion Regulation and Child Psychopathology

Clinically significant aggression and anxiety problems can be understood as disorders of emotion regulation.[6,7] Children with these problems may have failed to develop the capacity to appropriately modulate their feelings of anger and anxiety and the behaviors that flow from them. Research with young children indicates an association between poor emotion regulation and aggressive outcomes. Young children who are less able to voluntarily shift their attention and inhibit their emotional impulses have higher levels of aggression.[8] In contrast, children with good emotional control are able to shift attention away from anger-inducing cues and use nonhostile verbal methods.[9] In these and related studies, behavior regulation and emotion regulation are sometimes considered extensions of a more fundamental capacity for executive or "effortful" control.[10]

Neurocognitive Mechanisms of Emotion Regulation

Individual differences in emotion regulation become deeply entrenched, they reliably predict psychopathological outcomes, and they become increasingly resistant to intervention as children mature. For these reasons, most investigators assume that different styles of emotion regulation express distinct biological mechanisms.[11] Developmental psychologists are becoming increasingly interested in the neurobiological substrates of these mechanisms. Neural approaches use imaging techniques, lesion studies, and electrophysiological methods to specify cortical regions and activation profiles that mediate them. Research with adults has made progress linking these control mechanisms with normal and abnormal emotional processes. However, *developmental* neuroscience is only beginning to tackle emotion and its regulation, despite wide agreement on the importance of this agenda.

Neuroimaging and lesion studies have focused on prefrontal systems that mediate appraisal, inhibitory control, and self-monitoring, which may all be critical components of emotion regulation. The dorsal anterior cingulate cortex (ACC), on the medial wall of each frontal lobe, is a key structure for selecting among competing choices, making judgments, monitoring one's performance, and learning.[12,13] The ACC can also be involved in processing emotion, and it is specifically implicated when individuals are in control of their emotional responses or judgments.[14] The orbitofrontal cortex (OFC), on the ventral surface of the prefrontal cortex (PFC), is responsible for assigning emotional significance, especially in social situations, and for maintaining a response set such as avoidance or inhibition in anticipation of emotional consequences.[15] Thus, dorsal and ventral prefrontal systems have unique cognitive styles: dorsal systems (e.g., dorsal ACC) appear to mediate the smooth, deliberate control of behavior in a supervisory or top-down fashion, whereas ventral systems (e.g., ventral ACC and OFC) control impulses rigidly, in anticipation of negative consequences. Importantly, both children and adults show increased activation in both the ACC and OFC during response inhibition.[16] Hence, both structures may play a role in emotion regulation in children as well as adults.[17]

In adults, externalizing and internalizing psychopathologies are linked with emotion dysregulation corresponding to anomalies in both these frontal systems. Aggressive individuals typically show deficits in both ACC and OFC activation,[18] implying under-regulation of behavior. Blair[15] suggests that the OFC is especially important for the regulation of reactive aggression, and Hoptman[19] found aggression to be associated with decreased metabolism in anterior, inferior, and medial–frontal systems. Conversely, anxious and depressed individuals show greater-than-normal activation in ventral systems including the OFC and ventral ACC.[20]

EEG methods are particularly appealing for clinical research because they are noninvasive, versatile, and relatively inexpensive. EEG or electrical brain wave activity is recorded at the scalp from an array of electrodes. Event-related potentials (ERPs) are computed by averaging EEG data over many trials on a given task. Several ERP components recorded over the PFC are thought to tap aspects of cognitive control. The frontal N2 is seen 200–400 msec post-stimulus on trials requiring participants to withhold a prepotent response, and it is often assumed to tap inhibitory control mechanisms. Negative emotional evaluations predict higher amplitude N2s[21] and the N2 is enhanced by negative feedback concerning one's performance.[22] Thus, greater N2 amplitudes may reflect the ramping up of inhibitory controls when negative emotions arise. Another ERP component, the error-related negativity (ERN), is recorded approximately 50–100 msec postresponse and is thought to tap action monitoring or response control.[23] The ERN has been linked to anxiety and negative affect. Less impulsive, more controlled individuals show enhanced ERNs[24] as do individuals with obsessive-compulsive styles.[23] Similarly, individuals with negative mood or trait negative affect show higher amplitude ERNs,[25,26] whereas undersocialized individuals show lower amplitude ERNs.[27] Thus, the cognitive controls tapped by the N2 and ERN may be recruited, to different degrees by different individuals, for the regulation of emotion and emotional behavior. Researchers have now begun to examine these ERP components in children,[17] but few studies to date have investigated their role in children's emotional processes.

Dense-array EEG techniques (e.g., recording from 128 channels rather than just a few) allow researchers to model the generators of ERPs using source analysis methods. Source modeling programs place hypothetical generators in a model of the cortex and test for goodness-of-fit against the fine-grained scalp data provided by multiple electrodes. We are particularly interested in this methodology, because it allows us to test hypotheses about the approximate location of cortical activities that may underpin unique mechanisms of emotion regulation. Source analyses of medial–frontal ERPs (including the N2 and ERN) indicate a key generator in the region of the ACC for adults.[28,13] Similarly, the region of the OFC, particularly in the right hemisphere, has been identified as a generator of the N2 in studies of adults and children.[28,29] Source analysis of scalp EEG cannot provide definitive anatomical information, but we have utilized source modeling to examine the *relative* contributions of global prefrontal systems to ERP variables that may differentiate styles of emotion regulation.

Parent–Child Interactions and the Development of Psychopathology

Poor parent–child interactions are one of the central causal factors implicated in the development of childhood psychopathology.[30] Most notably, decades of direct observational studies conducted in the home and the laboratory have established a clear link between particular patterns of parent–child relations and childhood aggression.[31,32] Our recent work[33] points to the flexibility versus rigidity of parent–child relations as an especially relevant dimension for predicting clinical disorders. Both aggressive and anxious children tend to have inflexible parent–child interactions (they become "stuck" in habitual emotional exchanges) in contrast to nonclinical family interactions that flexibly shift to accommodate contextual demands.

Linking Parent–Child Interactions with Neurocognitive Mechanisms of Emotion Regulation

How might parent–child interaction patterns that contribute to aggressive behavior problems be associated with distinct neurobiological constellations of impaired emotion regulation? According to our model, aggressive children who are "pure" externalizers (EXT) cannot control their angry impulses when confronted with blocked goals because they do not anticipate negative consequences from their overly permissive parents. We hypothesize that these children fail to recruit both dorsal and ventral frontocortical controls, and thus their angry emotions remain unregulated. However, children who are comorbid for internalizing and externalizing problems (MIXED) may have parents who are intermittently permissive and punitive, and they may attempt to regulate their resultant anxiety through excessive reliance on ventral control systems. Thus, compared with age-matched controls, both subpopulations may be unable to control their emotional impulses in a smooth, deliberate manner using the dorsal ACC, and such differences should show up in ERPs associated with specific cortical regions and specific regulatory functions.

In conclusion, our working hypothesis is that unique regulatory dysfunctions depend on particular cortical modes of control that develop in parallel with distinct parent–child interaction styles and predict distinct constellations of behavior problems. These modes may preclude flexible, top-down self-regulation and thus contribute to the behavioral rigidity that characterizes the parent–child interactions of aggressive children.

REVIEW OF METHODS AND SELECTED EMPIRICAL FINDINGS

Development of State Space Grid Methodology

We have recently developed state space grid (SSG) analysis, a graphical and quantitative tool based on dynamic systems (DS) principles. This method allows researchers to examine several coexisting interaction patterns and explore movement from one to the other in real time. DS theorists use the concept of a state space to represent the range of behavioral habits, or attractors, for a given system. Behavior is conceptualized as moving along a real-time trajectory on this hypothetical landscape, being pulled toward certain attractors and freed from others.[34] Based on these abstract formalisms, Lewis *et al.*[35] developed a graphical approach that utilizes observational data and quantifies these data according to two ordinal variables that define the state space for any individual psychobehavioral system. Granic and Lamey extended this methodology to represent dyadic behavior (e.g., parent–child interactions).[36] The dyad's trajectory (i.e., the sequence of emotional states) is plotted on a grid representing all possible combinations (FIG. 1). Much like a scatterplot, one dyad member's (e.g., parent's) coded behavior is plotted on the x-axis and the other member's (e.g., child's) behavior is plotted on the y-axis. Thus, each point on the grid represents a simultaneously coded parent–child event (i.e., a dyadic state).

Differences in Parent–Child Interactions

We began our investigation of the etiology and treatment of clinical subtypes by trying to discover the distinct parent–child interaction patterns that differentiate pure EXT and MIXED children.[36] Parents and clinically referred children were asked to discuss a problem for 4 min and then try to "wrap up" in response to a signal (or perturbation). The perturbation was intended to increase the emotional pressure on the dyad, triggering a reorganization of their behavioral system. It was hypothesized that, as a function of differences in the underlying structure of their relationships, EXT and MIXED dyads would be differentially sensitive to the perturbation and would reorganize to different regions of the state space. Subtyping was determined by scores on parent- and

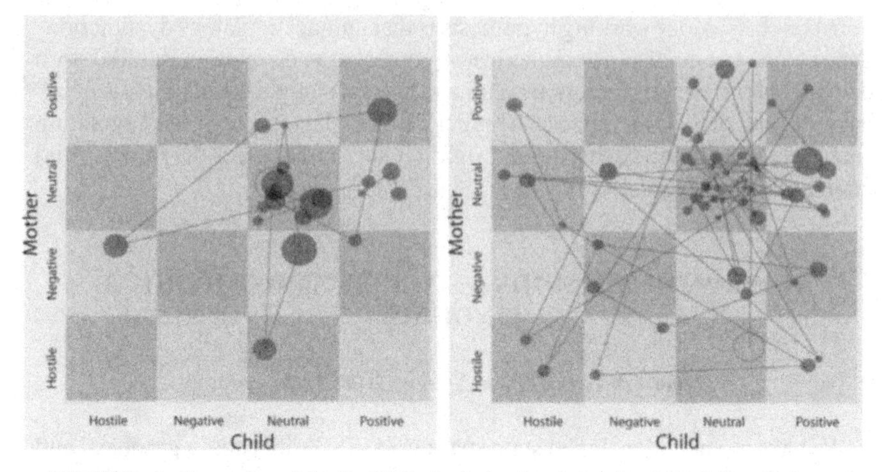

FIGURE 1. Examples of dyadic SSGs depicting low behavioral flexibility (left panel) and high behavioral flexibility (right panel).

teacher-rated behavior scales: EXT children were those with externalizing scores in the clinical range, whereas MIXED children scored in the clinical range on the internalizing *and* externalizing scales. Separate grids were constructed for the pre- and postperturbation interaction sessions. Both EXT and MIXED dyads tended toward the permissive region of the SSG (child hostile–parent neutral/positive), as well as other regions (i.e., mutual neutrality and negativity), *before* the perturbation. After the perturbation, EXT dyads tended to stabilize in the permissive region. MIXED dyads, however, tended toward the mutual hostility or mutual negativity region of the grid. These graphical observations were subsequently confirmed by case-sensitive, multivariate analyses including log-linear modeling.

Emotion-Induction ERP Methodology

We then developed a novel ERP paradigm that integrates an emotion induction process with a go/no-go procedure. On standard go/no-go tasks, participants respond as quickly as possible with a button-click on most trials but withhold clicking given particular cues. ERPs recorded during successful no-go trials (e.g., the N2) are seen as tapping cognitive processes involved in response inhibition, whereas ERPs following errors (e.g., the ERN) are thought to tap cognitive processes recruited for performance monitoring. In our task, the children are shown desirable toys or gift certificates prior to the procedure, and they are reminded several times that they need to earn a high number of points to receive one of these rewards. They are then instructed to click each time a letter appears but to avoid clicking when the same letter appears twice.

The stimulus presentation speed is adjusted dynamically to maintain an error rate (on no-go trials) of approximately 50%.[37] This innovation ensures that task difficulty is consistent across children, regardless of age and concentration skills. The task is divided into three blocks, and points (displayed on-screen every 20 trials) rise steadily for all children during block A. However, due to an adjustment in the algorithm, points begin to drop sharply in block B and end up back at zero. This block induces negative emotions such as anxiety, anger, and distress, as confirmed by emotion rating scales administered following the task. Finally, points rise again during block C so that a prize can be awarded, but negative emotions are presumed to remain active.

Developmental Differences in Cortical Mechanisms of Emotion Regulation

In the first complete study using the new task, we examined developmental differences in two inhibitory ERPs, the N2 and frontal P3, before and after the negative emotion induction (block A vs. blocks B and C).[17] Fifty-eight normal children, 5–16 years of age, were tested. We hypothesized that ERP amplitudes would diminish with age, consistent with fMRI and ERP studies suggesting that cortical efficiency improves with development, but that amplitudes would increase with the emotion induction in blocks B and C, indicating greater efforts at inhibitory control. Indeed, both the frontal N2 and frontal P3 components decreased in amplitude as well as latency across five age points in a fairly linear profile, $F(4,48) = 2.66, P = 0.04$ and $F(4,49) = 4.75, P = 0.003$ for the main effect of age on amplitudes. Amplitudes were also greater following the emotion induction phase of the task, suggesting increased inhibitory control in the service of emotion regulation. Source modeling indicated more central-posterior activation in younger children, giving way to medial–dorsal activation, suggestive of the dorsal ACC, as children matured. The finding of developmental "frontalization" is consistent with other recent work,[38] and it provides a useful backdrop for studying clinical groups.

Neurocognitive Differences among Subtypes of Aggressive Children

In our first study comparing clinically referred and normal children, we examined differences in the emotion regulatory mechanisms of subtypes of aggressive children.[39] Children (aged 8–12 years) were recruited from outpatient group treatment programs for aggressive children along with gender- and age-matched controls. Subtyping was determined by scores on parent- and teacher-rated behavior scales, as before. Only the MIXED children's N2s increased in response to the emotion induction, $F(2, 31) = 3.56$, $P < 0.05$, resulting in greater amplitudes than EXT children in block C, mean difference $= 4.08\ \mu V$, $P < 0.05$. As shown in FIGURE 2, ERN amplitudes were greatest for control children and smallest for EXT children, with MIXED children in between, but these differences were significant only prior to the emotion induction, $F(2, 33) = 3.68$, $P < 0.05$. These results suggest that anticipatory self-regulation recruited unusually high cortical activation for MIXED children in the presence of negative emotion, but that EXT children actually required negative emotion to recruit near-normal levels of activation following their errors. Also shown in FIGURE 2 are striking differences in the source models of peak ERN activity across the three groups. The black squares superimposed on the Brain Electrical Source Analysis (BESA) head models depict the two regions of interest: that of the dorsal ACC (above) and the ventral PFC (OFC and ventral ACC) (below). Across all blocks, normal children showed

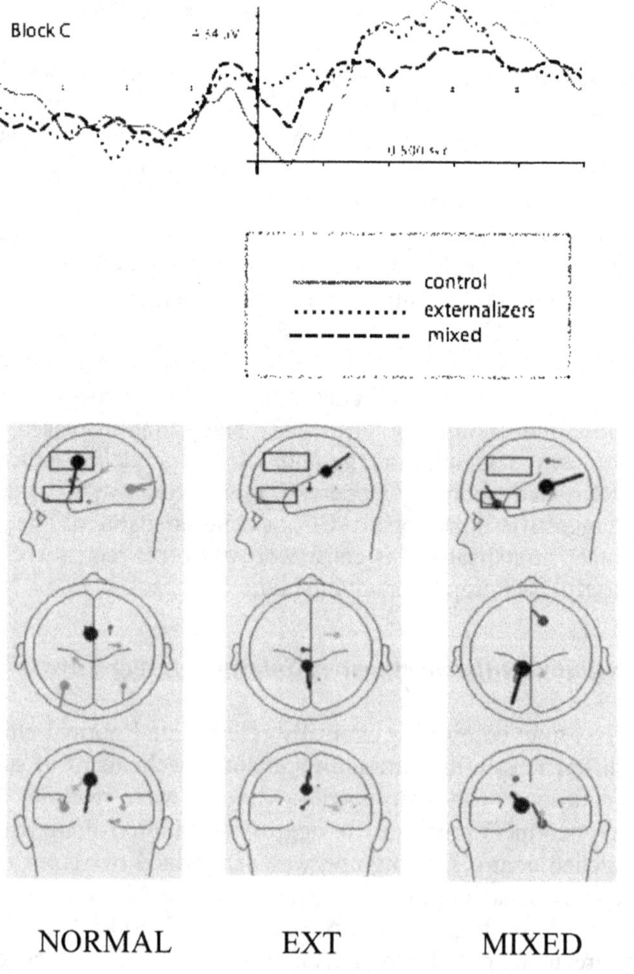

FIGURE 2. Grand-averaged waveforms and source models shown at peak ERN amplitudes, for normal, pure externalizing, and comorbid (externalizing/internalizing) children.

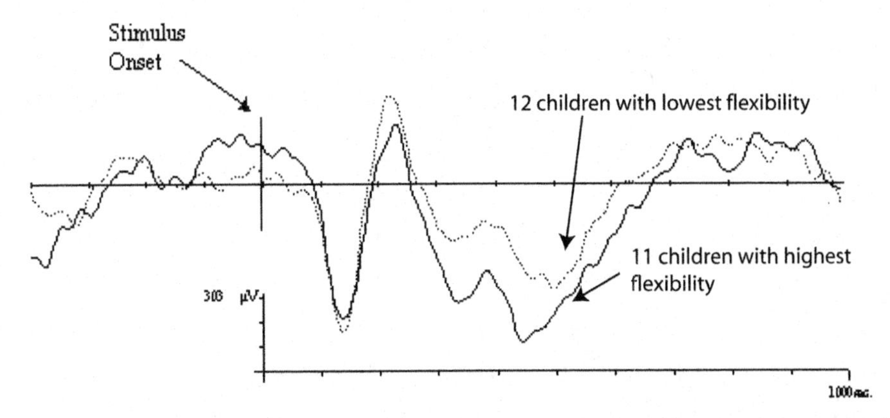

FIGURE 3. Grand-averaged waveforms for the most flexible and least flexible subgroups of children (n = 11 or 12). The N2, indicated by the arrow, shows greater mean amplitude for the flexible subgroup.

a strong source in the region of the dorsal ACC, consistent with models of adult brain activity during performance monitoring. EXT children showed no frontal activity whatever, but displayed a posterior source in the region of the posterior cingulate cortex. MIXED children demonstrated a similar posterior source and, importantly, a source in the region of the right OFC or right ventral ACC. These findings provide initial support for our model of subtype-specific differences in neurocognitive mechanisms of emotion regulation.

Neurophysiological Substrates of Behavioral Flexibility: Combining SSG and ERP Measures

Using the same sample of referred children, parent–child interactions were videotaped in the home before treatment. At each home visit, parents and children discussed consecutively: a positive topic, a mutually unresolved, anger-provoking problem, and another positive topic. Dyadic SSGs were constructed based on second-by-second codes derived from a modified version of the Specific Affect Coding System (SPAFF).[40] The flexibility of parent–child interactions was then assessed for the problem-solving discussion (the second topic) using three SSG measures: transitions—the number of movements from cell to cell, dispersion—the overall spread of behavior durations across the cells of the grid, and mean cell duration—the tendency for behavior to remain "stuck" within cells (a measure of rigidity, the converse of flexibility). We then examined associations between behavioral flexibility, tapped by these measures, and N2 amplitudes thought to tap neural mechanisms of emotion regulation derived from our task.

Values for children with complete observational and ERP data (n = 33) were entered into a three-step regression model, with N2 amplitudes as

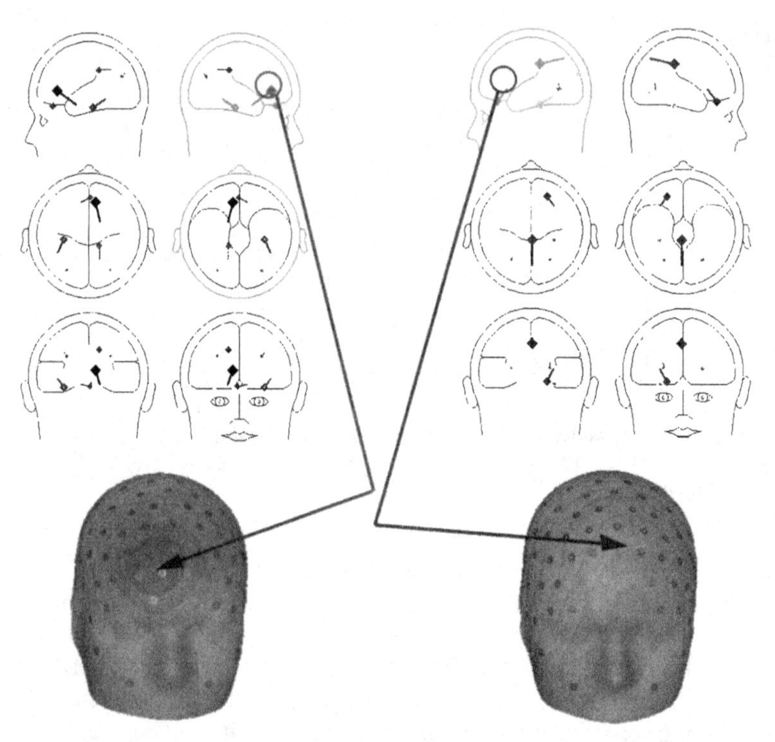

FIGURE 4. BESA head models for extreme groups (n = 7) of flexible (left panel) versus nonflexible (right panel) subgroups of aggressive children. A source in the region of the rostral ACC, at the peak of the N2, is evident for the flexible dyads only.

the dependent variable. The first step controlled for age, gender, ERP segment count, mean stimulus time, and medication (stimulant vs. nonstimulant). The second step controlled for the proportion of time spent in negative states, as negative emotion itself might be assumed to increase N2 amplitudes. In the third step, each of the three flexibility measures was entered in turn.

Flexibility measures did not predict N2 amplitudes in block A. However, these same measures predicted N2 amplitudes in block C (following the negative emotion induction; see FIG. 3): for transitions, $\Delta R^2 = 0.24$, $F(1, 25) = 10.26$, $P = 0.004$; for dispersion, $\Delta R^2 = 0.17$, $F(1, 25) = 6.52$, $P = 0.02$; for mean cell duration, $\Delta R^2 = 0.19$, $F(1, 25) = 7.57$, $P = 0.01$. In all analyses greater flexibility predicted greater amplitude N2s, suggesting greater recruitment of frontocortical control systems. A source analysis was performed on the most flexible and least flexible children (n = 7 in each group). As shown in FIGURE 4, a generator in the midline region of the PFC, corresponding to the rostral ACC, was observed for the flexible group but not for the nonflexible group. These results indicate higher amplitude cortical activations, probably mediated by anterior cingulate areas, following the induction of negative emotions, for children showing more flexible interpersonal behavior during emotionally challenging interactions with their parents. Although all children in this sample were referred for aggressive behavior problems, these differences in behavioral flexibility corresponding with biological mediators of emotion regulation may help determine which families are most likely to benefit from treatment. Current research activities are aimed at testing this prediction.

CONCLUSION

Developmentalists are increasingly interested in refining and testing models of brain-behavior relations that can help explain individual differences in socioemotional development in general and childhood psychopathology in particular. Our research represents one approach for linking neural mechanisms of emotion regulation with behavioral habits that differ both in emotional content and overall flexibility. The work reviewed in this article represents an early phase of a relatively untested research paradigm, based on the integration of DS thinking and methods of cognitive neuroscience. However, the results so far have been encouraging, and they suggest future research directions that may ultimately benefit troubled children, their families, and their communities.

REFERENCES

1. LOEBER, R. 1990. Development and risk factors of juvenile antisocial behavior and delinquency. Clin. Psychol. Rev. **10:** 1–41.
2. BEHAR, D. & M.A. STEWART. 1982. Aggressive conduct disorder of children. Acta. Psychiat. Scand. **65:** 210–220.
3. TREMBLAY, R.E. *et al.* 1994. Predicting early onset of male antisocial behavior from preschool behavior. Arch. Gen. Psychiat. **51:** 732–739.
4. ZOCCOLILLO, M. 1992. Co-occurrence of conduct disorder and its adult outcomes with depressive and anxiety disorders. J. Am. Acad. Child Adol. Psychiat. **31:** 547–556.
5. HARRINGTON, R. *et al.* 1991. Adult outcomes of childhood and adolescent depression: II. Links with antisocial disorders. J. Am. Acad. Child Adol. Psychiat. **30:** 434–439.
6. BRADLEY, S. 2000. Affect Regulation and the Development of Psychopathology. Guildford. New York.
7. CALKINS, S.D. 1994. Origins and outcomes of individual differences in emotion regulation. Monogr. Soc. Res. Child **59:** 53–72.
8. ROTHBART, M.K., S.A. AHADI & K.L. HERSHEY. 1994. Temperament and social behavior in childhood. Merrill-Palmer Quart. **40:** 21–39.
9. EISENBERG, N. *et al.* 1994. The relations of emotionality and regulation to children's anger-related reactions. Child Dev. **65:** 109–128.
10. POSNER, M.I. & M.K. ROTHBART. 2000. Developing mechanisms of self-regulation. Dev. Psychopathol. **12:** 427–441.

11. COLE, P.M., S.E. MARTIN & T.A. DENNIS. 2004. Emotion regulation as a scientific construct. Child Dev. **75:** 317–333.
12. FRITH, C.D. *et al.* 1991. A PET study of word finding. Neuropsychologia **29:** 1137–1148.
13. VAN VEEN, V. & C.S. CARTER. 2002. The timing of action-monitoring processes in the anterior cingulate cortex. J. Cognitive Neurosci. **14:** 593–602.
14. LANE, R.D. *et al.* 1998. Neural correlates of levels of emotional awareness. J. Cognitive Neurosci. **10:** 525–535.
15. BLAIR, R.J.R. 2001. Neurocognitive models of aggression, the antisocial personality disorders, and psychopathy. J. Neurol. Neurosur. Ps. **71:** 727–731.
16. CASEY, B.J. *et al.* 1997. A developmental functional MRI study of prefrontal activation during performance of a Go-No-Go task. J. Cognitive Neurosci. **9:** 835–847.
17. LEWIS, M.D. *et al.* 2006. Neurophysiological correlates of emotion regulation in children and adolescents. J. Cognitive Neurosci. **18:** 430–443.
18. DAVIDSON, R.J., K.M. PUTNAM & C.L. LARSON. 2000. Dysfunction in the neural circuitry of emotion regulation—a possible prelude to violence. Science **289:** 591–594.
19. HOPTMAN, M.J. 2003. Neuroimaging studies of violence and antisocial behavior. J. Psychiat. Pr. **9:** 265–278.
20. DREVETS, W.C. 2000. Neuroimaging studies of mood disorders. Biol. Psychiat. **48:** 813–829.
21. TUCKER, D.M. *et al.* 2003. Corticolimbic mechanisms in emotional decisions. Emotion **3:** 127–149.
22. LUU, P. *et al.* 2003. Activity in human medial frontal cortex in emotional evaluation and error monitoring. Psychol. Sci. **14:** 47–53.
23. GEHRING, W.J., J. HIMLE & L.G. NISENSON. 2000. Action monitoring dysfunction in obsessive-compulsive disorder. Psychol. Sci. **11:** 1–6.
24. PAILING, P.E. *et al.* 2002. Error negativity and response control. Psychophysiology **39:** 198–206.
25. HAJCAK, G., N. MCDONALD & R.F. SIMONS. 2004. Error-related psychophysiology and negative affect. Brain Cognition **56:** 189–197.
26. LUU, P., P. COLLINS & D.M. TUCKER. 2000. Mood, personality, and self-monitoring. J. Exp. Psychol. Gen. **129:** 43–60.
27. DIKMAN, Z.V. & J.J.B. ALLEN. 2000. Error monitoring during reward and avoidance learning in high- and low-socialized individuals. Psychophysiology **37:** 43–54.
28. BOKURA, H., S. YAMAGUCHI & S. KOBAYASHI. 2001. Electrophysiological correlates for response inhibition in a Go/NoGo task. Clin. Neurophysiol. **112:** 2224–2232.
29. PLISZKA, S.R., M. LIOTTI & M.G. WOLDORFF. 2000. Inhibitory control in children with attention-deficit/hyperactivity disorder. Biol. Psychiat. **48:** 238–246.
30. CUMMINGS, E.M., P. DAVIES, P. & S.B. CAMPBELL. 2000. Developmental Psychopathology and Family Process: Theory, Research, and Clinical Implications. Guildford. New York.
31. DUMAS, J.E. & P.J. LAFRENIERE. 1993. Mother-child relationships as sources of support or stress. Child Dev. **64:** 1732–1754.
32. PATTERSON, G.R. 1982. Coercive Family Processes. Castalia. Eugene, OR.
33. GRANIC, I. & G.R. PATTERSON. 2006. Toward a comprehensive model of antisocial development: a dynamic systems approach. Psych. Review. **113:** 101–131.
34. LEWIS, M.D. 2000. The promise of dynamic systems approaches for an integrated account of human development. Child Dev. **71:** 36–43.

35. LEWIS, M.D., A.V. LAMEY & L. DOUGLAS. 1999. A new dynamic systems method for the analysis of early socioemotional development. Dev. Sci. **2:** 458–476.
36. GRANIC, I. & A.V. LAMEY. 2002. Combining dynamic systems and multivariate analyses to compare the mother-child interactions of externalizing subtypes. J. Abnorm. Child Psych. **30:** 265–283.
37. GARAVAN, H., T.J. ROSS & E.A. STEIN. 1999. Right hemispheric dominance of inhibitory control. Proc. Natl. Acad. Sci. USA. **96:** 8301–8306.
38. BUNGE, S.A. *et al.* 2002. Immature frontal lobe contributions to cognitive control in children. Neuron **33:** 301–311.
39. STIEBEN, J. *et al.* Neurophysiological correlates of emotion regulation distinguish subtypes of antisocial children. Dev. Psychopath submitted.
40. GOTTMAN, J.M. *et al.* 1996. The Specific Affect Coding System (SPAFF) for Observing Emotional Communication in Marital and Family Interaction. Erlbaum. Mahwah, NJ.

Arousal Regulation, Emotional Flexibility, Medial Amygdala Function, and the Impact of Early Experience

Comments on the Paper of Lewis *et al.*

LINDA C. MAYES

Child Study Center, Yale University, 230 South Frontage Rd., New Haven, Connecticut, USA

ABSTRACT: The balance between optimal levels of emotional arousal and cognitive performance reflects the integration of several dopaminergically and adrenergically regulated neural systems. The amygdalar system is a key region for gating stimulation to cortical regions and the medial amygdala appears to play an especially key role in mediating the fear response. More generally, these arousal regulatory neural systems are key to frustration or stress impact prefrontal cortical function. Further, the threshold for when the level of stress is overwhelming and hence impairs cognitive function reflects minimally genetic and experiential influence. An important interface between Drs. Lewis and Davis's work is how early experience, especially through early parenting, may set the threshold of responsiveness for these arousal regulatory neural systems.

KEYWORDS: arousal regulation; emotional flexibility; medial amygdala

INTRODUCTION

The findings presented by Drs. Lewis and Davis contain several provocative possibilities for linking to the theme of resilience in children. I shall focus on two points from these papers: First is the relation of negative arousal or emotion and neurocognitive performance and second is the role of the medial nucleus of the amygdala (MeA) and the relation of opiate receptors in conditioned fear. I shall comment on possible neurobiological implications of the findings presented by Dr. Lewis and link these together with Dr. Davis's findings by suggesting that more research is needed on the sources of individual differences in these emotional regulatory strategies both in flexibility and impact

Address for correspondence: Linda C. Mayes, M.D., Yale University, Child Study Center, 230 South Frontage Rd., New Haven, CT 06520. Voice: 203-785-7205.
e-mail: linda.mayes@yale.edu

**Ann. N.Y. Acad. Sci. 1094: 178–192 (2006). © 2006 New York Academy of Sciences.
doi: 10.1196/annals.1376.018**

on neurocognitive performance. The threshold for negative impact of stress or anxiety on children's adaptive behavior and cognitive performance may be set at key developmental periods including in early infancy. Work on the impact of early parental care on stress response systems may be relevant to both of these lines of work.

THE RELATION OF NEGATIVE AROUSAL AND NEUROCOGNITIVE PERFORMANCE

Emotional flexibility is a central developmental construct and Dr. Lewis's conceptualization of this construct using nonlinear models is an important contribution to the study of emotional regulation in children. His findings regarding the relationship between stress (or specifically, frustration) and neurocognitive performance assessed both behaviorally and electrophysiologically are consonant with a growing body of preclinical work on the relation between emotional arousal and prefrontal cortical function. In both adults and children, monoaminergic-rich regions of the brain (e.g., locus coeruleus, raphe nuclei, substantia nigra, striatum, amygdala) are integral to arousal and attention regulation and have extensive ascending and descending connections with the prefrontal and posterior cortices and hippocampus.[1–5] Arousal or emotional regulation is a central concept for understanding how stimulation is gated to different cortical regions and particularly to the prefrontal cortex (PFC[6]). Current conceptualizations of arousal regulation describe several distinct yet interactive systems receiving neurochemical inputs from discrete neural groups especially within the amygdala and projecting to different regions and layers of the prefrontal and posterior cortex.[3,4,7] These interactive systems serve as multilevel gates that protect the prefrontal and posterior cortex from excessive stimulation and also facilitate coordination between attentional, executive, and sensory cortical systems. In relation to Dr. Lewis' findings, at least two components of these multilevel arousal systems are crucial. One involves primarily the noradrenergic (NE) system projecting from the locus coeruleus to the prefrontal and posterior cortex and hippocampus. Another involves the mesolimbic and mesostriatal dopaminergic (DA) systems that also have extensive cortical projections from the striatum and limbic region including the amygdala.[4,8]

Norepinephrine enhances the activation and function of many pre- and posterior cortical and subcortical brain regions[9,10] but different NE receptor systems have opposite effects in the PFC (as well as in other regions). In the prefrontal cortex, α_1 postsynaptic receptor stimulation in the PFC impairs function[11] while α_2 postsynaptic receptor stimulation markedly enhances PFC-based working memory function.[12] In contrast, α_1 (and β) stimulation enhances long-term memory consolidation in hippocampus,[13] in the entorhinal and parietal cortices,[14] and in the amygdala[13–17] while α_2 stimulation impairs memory consolidation mechanisms in the amygdala and hippocampus[18,19] as well as performance on attentional and orienting tasks.[20] Thus, at low levels of stimulation, α-2 systems are engaged and prefrontal cortical function is enhanced, while at higher levels of arousal or stimulation, α1 systems are more engaged, posterior cortical functions are enhanced, and the PFC is effectively "off-line". Dopaminergic systems also show a different effect on the PFC at different levels of activation or stimulation intensity. Generally, the D1 dopamine receptor family (D1 and D5) enhances PFC function.[21] However, under excessive stimulation/excessive catecholamine release, D1 stimulation impairs PFC function.

Thus, relations between arousal and prefrontal cortical function are mediated in part through the interdependent DA (D1 receptor) and NE α2 effects and balanced by an opposing, inhibitory NE α1 effect.[22,23] Within a range of activation, as the level of cortical activation increases with NE/DA stimulation, performance improves on a variety of prefrontal cortical functions, including anticipation (shifting of attention), planning, working memory, and sustained attention to relevant or salient stimuli.[24,25] But with increasing stress, catecholamine release—mediated in part through the amygdala[26]—is increased. With sufficient hyperarousal, the D1/α2 system in the PFC is taken off-line by increased α1 activity[21] while other more automatic functions are enhanced including α1 NE-related functions for vigilance in the posterior cortex and DA-related functions in the amygdala and hippocampus where basic circuitry for memory consolidation is based.

Termed a "neurochemical switch" by some investigators,[12] this mechanism may be quite useful in situations of danger and extreme stress when automatic responding is necessary. The threshold for activation of this neurochemical switch increases over the course of development as infants and children are able to tolerate more intense and more varied stimulation and experiences. But this threshold always remains individually variable and subject to enduring change based on overwhelmingly traumatic/stressful experiences and/or illness or environmental conditions at different phases of development. Indeed, several models are now proposed for how acute and chronic stress may lead to enduring alterations in the threshold for activation of the DA and NE arousal system[26,27] and thus altered thresholds for hyperarousal.[28] In this model, the notion of arousal regulation is better considered as a dynamic continuum of reactivity in increasingly novel or stressful situations with a switching at some point from more executive to more automatic functions. Impairments in arousal regulation would be those instances in which the child or adult switches from more executive to automatic functions either much earlier or much later than is adaptive or functionally necessary, a phenomenon that may be captured at the behavioral level by Dr. Lewis's concept of varying levels of emotional flexibility. We might suggest that Dr. Lewis's findings in his sample of conduct disordered children's changing performance in the face of increasing frustration may also suggest a different threshold for arousal-modulated decrease in prefrontal cortical function as measured in his sample. Or conversely, his finding of greater frontocortical activity (as measured by larger N2 amplitude on event-related potential) in the presence of negative emotion associated with greater behavioral flexibility suggests a more adaptive regulation of stress that maintains prefrontal cortical activity. (Parenthetically, others have suggested the N2/P3 components may reflect a combination of failed inhibition and continued processing of the error after the response is made.[29]) At least one question key to these findings is what might be the sources of individual variability in emotional flexibility in the face of stress and frustration, a question that provides the link to Dr. Davis's work.

ROLE OF MEDIAL NUCLEUS OF THE AMYGDALA AND OPIATE RECEPTORS IN CONDITIONED FEAR

The medial amygdala nucleus and opiates not only have a central role in fear conditioning and stress response/arousal regulation but also in the regulation of social and affiliative behaviors, and specifically parenting behaviors, among mammalian species. Drawing these lines of work together makes a case for a model of how social/affiliative systems involved in parenting share similar/overlapping circuitry with fear systems and to ask questions about how early rearing conditions and genetic substrate may shape later response to stress and fear and specifically emotional flexiblility or emotional regulation.

Postpartum maternal behavior in the rodent model involves heightened pup-directed behaviors including licking and grooming, nursing, retrieval along with heightened aggression toward intruders at the nest site, and a generalized decrease in fearfulness on a range of behavioral tests. It is this interplay between fearfulness or fearlessness and parental care at a critical developmental period that may form the link between Davis's findings and childhood resilience.

As Davis suggests, the medial nucleus of the amygdala has long been recognized as involved in sexual behavior in males and females. Indeed, the extended amygdala generally has been previously implicated in various aspects of affiliative behavior, including maintenance of physical proximity with adult conspecifics,[30] maternal behavior,[31] and facial recognition.[32,33] The medial nucleus specifically has been implicated in the control of social behavior[34,35] and there is accumulating evidence for the effect of the MeA on parental behavior. It may be that the MeA (along with other associated regions) plays a different role at different points in development, as in, for example, at the initiation of parenting compared to learned parental behaviors. In rodents, a key role of the MeA in the control of parenting (and possibly other social) behaviors is in the processing of olfactory cues.[35] The MeA receives direct input from the accessory olfactory bulb that in turn receives input from the vomeronasal organ, a region of the olfactory system key to pheromone detection and also input from the main olfactory bulb through the cortical amygdaloid nucleus. Hence, the MeA may be especially central in mediating olfactory cue-regulated affective changes to pups in the newly parturient animal. Nonpregnant, nulliparous female rats do not show maternal behavior unless sensitized by repeated pup exposure.[36] If the female is rendered anosmic, this period is considerably shortened suggesting that pup odors may actually inhibit the onset of maternal behavior.[37] Fleming and colleagues showed that in virgin females, lesions to the MeA or to olfactory projections to the MeA show significantly shorter latencies to the onset of maternal behavior.[34,38] Electrical stimulation of the MeA lengthens sensitization in estrous-cycling female rats.[39] Hence, the MeA may be responsible for an olfactory-based neophobia to pups at least prior to exposure and thus, the MeA inhibits maternal activity on early exposure. Even in experienced animals, MeA stimulation early inhibits maternal behavior as measured by the latency to retrieve or crouch over the pups.[39]

However, the initiation of maternal behavior, especially in the rodent model, involves a decrease in fearfulness and especially aversive response to pup-related stimuli as well as an increase in maternal behaviors. The reduction in fearfulness may be in part mediated by a number of hormones related to pregnancy and parturition including estrogen, progesterone, prolactin, and oxytocin.[40] For example, estrogen and progesterone seem to promote maternal responsiveness by promoting changes in the female's attraction to pup odors and reducing her withdrawal tendencies in the presence of the pup. Virgin rats given a hormonal regimen designed to mimic parturition exhibit preference for pup-related stimuli.[41,42] More broadly, though, recently parturient rats show a general decrease in fearfulness as evidenced by shorter latency to open-field exploration among recently parturient, primiparous compared to nulliparous females.[43] Similarly, ovarectomized rats treated with a hormone regimen known to facilitate maternal behavior are also generally less fearful.[44,45] Further, lactating female rats show increases in exploration of the open arms of an elevated plus maze when compared to diestrus, proestrus, ovariectomized, and pregnant females.[46]

Once parental behavior is established, however, MeA lesions do not disrupt maternal behavior[47,48] and indeed in some instances, MeA activity seems to facilitate parental behavior. Axon-sparing lesions of the corticomedial amygdala using the excitotoxin N-methyl-D,L-aspartic acid (NMA) with a highly affiliative species, the prairie vole, result in males who show significantly less contact with a familiar adult female and a pup when compared with males with lesions of the basolateral nucleus or with controls. A more selective, specific MeA lesion decreased paternal behavior but not contact with a familiar adult conspecific. In neither case were other behaviors impacted including exploratory behaviors or fearfulness in novel situations.[49] Further, other investigators have reported that selective lesions of the basolateral nucleus of the amygdala do not impact parental behavior.[50,51]

However, the role of the MeA in social behavior cannot be considered in isolation. As Davis presents, a major projection of the medial nucleus of the amygdala is to the hypothalamus and especially the medial preoptic area (MPOA). Indeed, the major efferents of the MeA are to both the anterior and ventromedial hypothalamus and the bed nucleus of the stria terminalis (BNST) and MPOA with minor projections to other limbic areas including the lateral septum and the hippocampus, areas implicated in social and memory processes and maternal behavior.[52–55] Pup exposure has been shown to increase the expression of fos peptide in both the medial nucleus and amygdala of the MPOA in male prairie voles[56] and in both virgin and experienced female rats.[39] The MeA also innervates other targets that have been implicated in female parental care. In the rat, both the peripeduncular nucleus and the ventral tegmental area (VTA) receive projections from cells in the MeA.[57] The peripeduncular nucleus is implicated in maternal aggression[58] and the VTA is involved in several aspects of maternal behavior, especially pup retrieval.[59]

The analysis of *fos* gene activation within neurons, as measured by the increased production of various Fos proteins, is an important advance in outlining the larger neural circuits that may be involved in either inhibiting or facilitating maternal behavior. Using the neural cFos response to pups in two groups of naïve females with no prior maternal experience with one group hormonally primed for maternal behaviors and pup care and the other not, Sheehan and colleagues identified putative inhibitory and excitatory regions within the forebrain.[54,60] Inhibitory regions included the anterior hypothalamic nuclei (AHN), ventral part of the lateral septum (LSv), dorsal premammillary nucleus (PMd), and the parvocellular part of the paraventricular hypothalamic nucleus (PVNp). The excitatory regions included the dorsal part of the MPOA, vBST, and intermediate part of the lateral septum (LSi). Importantly, the MeA was activated irrespective by pup exposure equally irrespective of maternal behavior in the animals. Thus, it may be that one circuit from the MeA to the AHN, PMd, LSv, and PVNp is a “central aversion system” that is not only activated by novel olfactory stimuli from pups leading to maternal withdrawal but more generally by a variety of stressful or threatening situations.[61,62]

There are also projections from the AHN and VMN to the MPOA, which may also serve to actively inhibit approach to pups.[63] However, when female rats are fully primed with maternal hormones, they are attracted to pup odors, the shift in behavior referred to earlier. It may be that the hormonal events of late pregnancy and parturition shut down the inhibitory MeA output system with projections to the AHN while promoting activity in an MeA output system to the MPOA and vBST that stimulates interest in and approach to pup olfactory cues. That is, one inhibitory MeA system is shut down leaving active a facilitatory MeA to MPOA/vBST system.[63] It may also be that in nonmaternal or inexperienced mothers, input from the MeA to the AHN inhibits maternal behavior while in experienced animals, olfactory cues activate an MeA to MPOA/BST circuit that facilitates approach and care, an area requiring considerable study.

How this potential change in the balance of inhibitory and facilitative MeA to hypothalamic circuits occurs is not clear but may involve mechanisms of conditioned or associative learning[64] in addition to hormone regulation. Indeed, considerably less is known about the control of maternal/parental behavior or the circuitry of learned or established parental behavior after the initial period of hormone priming and exposure. We know that long-lasting parental experience involves activation of both the somatosensory and olfactory systems and is mediated by some of the same neurochemical systems that underlie learning in other functional contexts,[65] in particular the noradrenalin system so key to learning in, for example, traumatic situations. With repeated pup exposure, could there be a change in neural structure in the amygdala consistent with learning an enhanced attraction to pups and diminished aversion to pup cues. Further, as discussed above, established maternal behavior is associated with a general reduction in fearfulness and a concomitant increase in aggression especially toward intruders posing danger to pups. Sensitization to pup cues and habituation to their withdrawal-eliciting properties on repeated exposure may be reflected in changes in medial amygdaloid nuclei as well as associated regions, especially hypothalamic connections. It may also be that true associative learning involving the pairing of conditioned and nonconditioned cues (along with the reinforcing effects of pup responsive behavior) plays a role in the maintenance of maternal behavior, and thus is especially relevant to the extended amygdaloid complex and the MeA. For example, there is difference in fos-Lir immunoreactivity between experienced and nonexperienced rat mothers in the medial preoptic area of the hypothalamus (MPOA), the basolateral nucleus of the amygdala, and the prefrontal cortex.[66] How continued exposure to pups changes the balance of inhibitory or facilitative activity in the MeA and how reducing or blocking MeA activity in the context of established parenting influences maternal behavior is an open question.

Important to the relation between the MeA and parenting is also the role of oxytocin in the amygdala generally and the MeA specifically. Oxytocin, and a related neuropeptide vasopressin, are intimately involved in the initiation of parenting behavior.[67] Oxytocin is primarily synthesized in the magnocellular secretory neurons of two hypothalamic nuclei, the paraventricular and supraoptic nuclei that project to the pituitary. Oxytocin fibers from the PVN project to areas of the limbic system including the amygdala, lateral septum, and bed nucleus of the stria terminalis, each region involved in regulating parental behavior.[68] Oxytocin receptors are located in the central and medial amygdala and oxytocin's action on the central nucleus of the amygdala produces an anxiolytic effect.[69] Further, oxytocin influences olfactory-related processes in the medial amygdala that are a part of social recognition and also may be a part of maternal aggression toward intruders.[70,71] It may be that the anxiolytic effect of oxytocin moderates the initial pup aversion as mediated through the MeA and is a part of the shift between initial fearfulness to pup cues to attraction and caring behavior—a hypothesis needing detailed study especially as related to the MeA and parenting.

Turning to opiates and social behavior, the brain opiod theory of social attachment has accumulating empirical support. Lines of evidence indicate that (1) opioids diminish the reaction to social separation; (2) opioids are released during bouts of social contact; (3) opioids are rewarding and can induce odor and place preferences; and (4) low basal levels of opioids induce motivation to seek social contact. Like the neuropeptides, oxytocin and vasopressin,[67,72,73] the endogenous opioid system may be shared by different forms of attachment. It has been hypothesized that a release of endogenous opioids mediates the rewarding properties of attachment and a reduction results in emotional distress and a need to seek and maintain proximity with the attachment object.[74] Thus, exogenous opiates, such as morphine, should reduce the motivation to seek social contact and opiate blockers, such as naltrexone, should increase social contact—hypotheses demonstrated now by many studies across nonprimate, mammalian species[73,75] in adult and offspring–parent attachment. For example, opiate agonists decrease separation-induced distress among infant offspring[76] and these effects of endogenous opioids on infant attachment-related behavior have been primarily linked to the mu receptors.[77] Further, mice lacking the mu-opioid receptor gene show marked reduction in attachment-related behaviors including reduction in vocalization and preference for maternal cues.[78] Additionally, several studies have indicated that endogenous opioids are released in response to somatosenory contact and milk transfer, both of special relevance to infant care and parent–infant attachment.[73] In situations of rough and tumble play, common to nearly all mammalian species, there is an increase in the release of endogenous opioids.[79] Blocking this release reduces levels of play and physical contact among rats.[80]

Fewer studies have examined the effect of endogenous or exogenous opiates or opiate antagonists on maternal attachment behaviors toward the infant though much more work has been done on infant to mother attachment.[73] The MPOA is rich in both fibers and receptors for opioid peptides[81] and the major receptor for β-endorphin, the mu receptor, is found specifically in the MPOA.[82] In lactating females, morphine injected directly into the MPOA reduced maternal behavior, including pup grouping and pup retrieval; this effect was blocked by naloxone[83] and the morphine effects appeared to be mediated by the mu receptor.[84] In one study examining mother–infant separation and reunion in rhesus macaques, morphine decreased clinging with the infant upon reunion whereas naltrexone increased clinging.[85] Conversely, in the VTA, another region involved in parenting behavior, opiods appear to facilitate maternal responsiveness.[86] It may be that maternal experience impacts the balance between the inhibitory and facilitative aspects of the opioid system on maternal behavior such that with experience, the inhibitory effect on the MPOA is decreased and the facilitative effect on the VTA increased.[63] Finally, there is considerable evidence that drug abuse, cocaine or opiates, disrupt the neural mechanisms, especially those regulated by the MPOA, which contribute to maternal motivation and care.[86–88]

While there is much more work to be done, we might hypothesize that in situations of established parenting, on separation from her offspring, a mother experiences a reduction in endogenous opiates with an increase in her conditioned fear response to the distress calls of her infant mediated in part through the MeA and a parallel drive to increase contact and increase endogenous opiates. Upon contact, there is an increase in endogenous opiates and a reduction in MeA activity as well as a reduction in anxiety. There may well be a parallel with oxytocin and the related anxiolytic properties though there is much to be explored in this hypothesis for the circuitry may be specific to different types of stress. For example, a recent study using restraint as a stressor showed that the MeA was unaffected by oxytocin infusion and was the only area of the amygdala to show activation under restraint stress[89] though these studies were not done with parturient animals.

How then to tie these bodies of work that potentially link the MeA, opiates, and parental attachment with emotional flexibility/regulation and theme of resilience? First, there is considerable evidence now linking early maternal behavior and separation/loss to HPA axis dysfunction in offspring, and conversely, animals exposed to increased handling as pups show reduced glucocorticoid response to stress well into adulthood. Prenatally stressed rats also show longer adult sensitization latencies to their new pups, suggesting a longer period of pup aversion and general fearfulness before the onset of maternal behavior.[90] Some of the more compelling work comes from Meaney and colleagues who have studied naturally occurring variations in maternal care in terms of the amounts of licking and grooming a mother provides her pup.[91–93] The value of these models is the demonstration that long-term changes in both behavior and stress reactivity—or more generally, in threat-response mechanisms—can be produced by natural variations in maternal care.

Pups of so-called low licking and grooming mothers show, as adults, similar patterns of parenting behavior as well as an increase in the adult offspring's emotional reactivity to novelty and stress as mediated through a change in HPA axis function.[92] Offspring of high licking and grooming mothers show reduced plasma ACTH and cortocosterone responses to restraint stress.[94] These effects on stress regulation appear mediated through gene expression in those brain regions that regulate behavior and endocrine response to stress. As adults, pups who have been either handled or cross-fostered to high licking and grooming mothers show increased hippocampal glucocorticoid receptor mRNA expression, increased central benzodiazepine receptor levels in the central and basolateral nuclei of the amygdala, and decreased corticotrophin-releasing factor mRNA in the paraventricular nucleus of the hypothalamus.[91] These same pups as new mothers also show shorter latency to pup sensitization (and conversely, pups of low licking and grooming mothers show, as adults, longer latency to sensitization),[95] presumably because of reduced or increased MeA regulation of aversion to pup-related olfactory stimuli—a hypothesis yet to be studied in the models using naturally occurring variations in maternal care—and perhaps also because of an alteration in the balance of inhibitory and excitatory efferent activity of the MeA. The role of endogenous opiates in mediating this shift in inhibitory and excitatory efferent activity of the MeA in maternal behavior has also not been studied.

Among the questions that may be modeled in the laboratory are (1) What is the impact of opiates on the conditioned fear response in pregnant and recently parturient animals? and (2) How does early neglect/separation impact the conditioned fear response in the MeA and the impact of opiates? While there is much to be worked out, it is possible that naturally occurring variations in maternal care convey to offspring not only the now well-documented variations in stress reactivity but also a different developmental trajectory in the initiation of parenting behaviors conveyed in part through different sensitivity of the MeA–AHN and MeA–MPOA systems. Such a different sensitivity may make it more difficult for new parents to care for their infants, especially in circumstances of heightened stress, poor environmental support, or drug addiction. In these instances, parents may not be able to buffer their infants sufficiently against the stress and chaos of their environments. In this way, the excitatory/inhibitory balance among arousal systems necessary for optimal cortical function may be distorted and in turn, convey to the offspring heightened sensitivity to stress or frustration, poor emotional regulation, and limited emotional flexibility.

REFERENCES

1. LeDoux, J.E. 1987. Emotion, *In* Handbook of Physiology: 1. The Nervous System: Vol. 5: Higher Functions of the Brain. E. Plum, Ed.: American Psychological Society. Bethesda, MD.
2. Gonzalez-Lima, F. 1989. Functional brain circuitry related to arousal and learning in rats. *In* Visuomotor Coordination. J. Ewert & M. Arbib, Eds.: Plenum. New York.
3. Robbins, T.W. & B.J. Everitt. 1995. Arousal systems and attention. *In* The Cognitive Neurosciences. M. Gazzaniga Ed.: 703–720. MIT Press. Cambridge, MA.
4. Robbins, T.W., S. Granon, J.L. Muir, *et al.* 1998. Neural systems underlying arousal and attention. Ann. N. Y. Acad. Sci. **846:** 222–237.
5. Coull, J.T. 1998. Neural correlates of attention and arousal: insights from electrophysiology, functional neuroimaging, and psychopharmacology. Prog. Neurobiol. **55:** 343–361.
6. Damasio, A.R. 1995. On some functions of the human prefrontal cortex. *In* Structure and Functions of the Human Prefrontal Cortex. J. Grafman & K.J. Holyoak, Eds.: 241–251. New York Academy of Sciences. New York.
7. Marrocco, R.T., E.A. Witte & M.C. Davidson. 1994. Arousal systems. Curr. Opin. Neurobiol. **4:** 166–170.

8. Robbins, T.W. 1984. Cortical noradrenaline, attention, and arousal. Psychol. Med. **14:** 13–21.
9. Foote, S.L., F.E. Freedman & A.P. Oliver. 1975. Effects of putative neurotransmitters on neuronal activity in monkey auditory cortex. Brain Res. **86:** 229–242.
10. Waterhouse, B.D., H.C. Moises & D.J. Woodward. 1998. Phasic activation of the locus coeruleus enhances responses of primary sensory cortical neurons to peripheral receptive field stimulation. Brain Res. **790:** 33–44.
11. Arnsten, A.F.T., R. Matthew, R. Ubriani, *et al.* 1999. Alpha-1 noradrenergic receptor stimulation impairs prefrontal cortical cognitive function. Biol. Psychiatry **45:** 26–31.
12. Arnsten, A.F.T. 2000. Through the looking glass: differential noradrenergic modulation of prefrontal cortical function. Neural Plasticity **7:** 133–146.
13. Hopkins, W.F. & D. Johnston. 1988. Noradrenergic enhancement of long-term potentiation at mossy fiber synapses in the hippocampus. J. Neurophysiol. **59:** 667–687.
14. Ardenghi, P., D. Barros, L.A. Izquierdo, *et al.* 1997. Late and prolonged post-training memory modulation in entorhinal and parietal cortex by drugs acting on the cAMP/protein kinase A signaling pathway. Behav. Pharmacol. **8:** 745–751.
15. Cahill, L. & J.L. McGaugh. 1996. Modulation of memory storage. Curr. Opin. Neurobiol. **6:** 237–242.
16. Cahill, L., B. Prins, M. Weber, *et al.* 1994. Beta-adrenergic activation and memory for emotional events. Nature **371:** 702–704.
17. Packard, M.G. & L.A. Teather. 1998. Amygdala modulation of multiple memory systems: hippocampus and caudate-putamen. Neurobiol. Learn. Memory **69:** 163–203.
18. Genkova-Papazova, M., B.P. Petkova, M. Lazarova-Bakarova, *et al.* 1997. Effects of flunarizine and nitrendipine on electroconvulsive shock- and clonidine-induced amnesia. Pharmacol. Biochem. Behav. **56:** 583–587.
19. Sirvio, J., P. Riekkinnen, I. Vajanto, *et al.* 1991. The effects of guanfacine, alpha 2-agonist, on the performance of young and aged rats in spatial navigation task. Behav. Neur. Biol. **56:** 101–107.
20. Witte, E.A. & R.T. Marrocco. 1997. Alterations of brain noradrenergic activity in rhesus monkeys affects the altering component of covert orienting. Psychopharmacology **132:** 315–323.
21. Arnsten, A.F.T. 1998. Catecholamine modulation of prefrontal cognitive function. Trends Cog. Sci. **2:** 436–447.
22. Grace A.A., C.R. Gerfen & G. Aston-Jones. 1998. Catecholamines in the central nervous system. Adv. Pharmacol. **42:** 655–670.
23. Arnsten A.F.T. 1997. Catecholamine regulation of the prefrontal cortex. J. Psychopharmacol. **11:** 151–162.
24. Wilkins A.J., T. Shallice & R. McCarthy. 1987. Frontal lesions and sustained attention. Neuropsychologia **25:** 359–365.
25. Robbins T.W. 1996. Dissociating executive functions of the prefrontal cortex. Phil. Transac. Royal Soc. Lond.–Series B: Biol. Sci. **351:** 1463–1470.
26. Field, T., B. Healy, S. Goldstein, *et al.* 1988. Infants of depressed mothers show "depressed" behavior even with nondepressed adults. Child Dev. **59:** 1569–1579.
27. Davis, M. & Y. Lee. 1998. Fear and anxiety: possible roles of the amygdala and bed nucleus of the stria terminalis. Cog. Emot. **12:** 277–305.

28. Valentino, R.J., A.L. Curtis, M.E. Page, *et al.* 1998. Activation of the locus coeruleus brain noradrenergic system during stress: circuitry, consequences, and regulation. Adv. Pharmacol. **42:** 781–784.
29. Ramautar, J.R., A. Kok & K.R. Ridderinkhof. 2004. Effects of stop-signal probability in the stop-signal paradigm: the N2/P3 complex further validated. Brain Cog. **56:** 234–252.
30. Kling, A. 1972. Effects of amygdalectomy on social-affective behavior in nonhuman primates. *In* The Neurobiology of the Amygdala. B.E. Eleftheriou, Ed.: Plenum. Oxford, UK.
31. Fleming, A.S., M. Miceli & D. Moretto. 1983. Lesions of the medial preoptic area prevent the facilitation of maternal behavior produced by amygdala lesions. Physiol. Behav. **31:** 503–510.
32. Brothers, L., B. Ring & A. Kling. 1990. Response of neurons in the macaque amygdala to complex social stimuli. Behav. Brain Res. **41:** 199–213.
33. Everitt, B.J. 1990. Sexual motivation: a neural and behavioral analysis of the mechanisms underlying appetitive and copulatory responses of male rats. Neurosci. Biobehav. Rev. **14:** 217–232.
34. Fleming, A.S., F. Vaccarino & C. Luebke. 1980. Amygdaloid inhibition of maternal behavior in the nulliparous female rat. Physiol. Behav. **25:** 731–743.
35. Lehman, M.N. & S.S. Winans. 1982. Vomeronasal and olfactory pathways to the amygdala controlling male hamster sexual behavior: autoradiographic and behavioral analysis. Brain Res. **240:** 27–41.
36. Rosenblatt, J.S. 1967. Nonhormonal basis of maternal behavior in the rat. Science **156:** 1512–1514.
37. Fleming, A.S. & J.S. Rosenblatt. 1974c. Olfactory regulation of maternal behavior in rats: II. Effects of peripherally induced anosmia and lesions of the lateral olfactory tract in pup-induced virgins. J. Comp. Physiol. Psychol. **86:** 233–246.
38. Fleming, A.S., F. Vaccarino, L. Tambosso, *et al.* 1979. Vomeronasal and olfactory system modulation of maternal behavior in the rat. Science **203:** 372–374.
39. Morgan, H.D., J.A. Wachtus, N.W. Milgram, *et al.* 1999. The long lasting effects of electrical stimulation of the medial preoptic area and medial amygdala on maternal behavior in female rats. Behav. Brain Res. **99:** 61–73.
40. Numan, M. & M.J. Numan. 1994. Expression of Fos-like immunoreactivity in the preoptic area of maternally behaving virgin and postpartum rats. Behav. Neurosci. **108:** 379–394.
41. Fleming, A.S., U. Cheung, N. Myhal, *et al.* 1989. Effects of maternal hormones on "timidity" and attraction to pup-related odors in female rats. Physiol. Behav. **46:** 449–453.
42. Fleming, A.S., C. Kuchera, A. Lee, *et al.* 1994. Olfactory-based social learning varies as a function of parity in female rats. Psychobiology **22:** 37–43.
43. Fleming, A.S., F. vaccarino & C. luebke. 1981. Timidity prevents the nulliparous female from being a good mother. Physiol. Behav. **27:** 863–868.
44. Bridges, R.S. 1984. A quantitative analysis of the roles of dosage, sequence, and duration of estradiol and progesterone exposure in the regulation of maternal behavior in the rat. Endocrinology **114:** 930–940.
45. Picazo, O. & A. Fernandez-Guasti. 1993. Changes in experimental anxiety during pregnancy and lactation. Physiol. Behav. **54:** 295–299.
46. Bitran, D., R.J. Hilvers & C.K. Kellogg. 1991. Ovarian endocrine status modulates the anxiolytic potency of diazepam and the efficacy of y-aminobutyric

acid-benzodiazepine receptor-mediated chloride ion transport. Behav. Neurosci. **105:** 653–662.
47. Fleming, A.S., K. Gavarth & J. Sarker. 1992. Effects of transections to the vomeronasal nerves or to the main olfactory bulbs on the initiation and long-term retention of maternal behavior in primiparous rats. Behav. Neural. Biol. **57:** 177–188.
48. Kolunie, J.M. & J.M. Stern. 1995. Maternal aggression in rats: effects of olfactory bulbectomy, ZnS04-induced anosmia, and vomeronasal organ removal. Horm. Behav. **29:** 492–518.
49. Kirkpatrick, B., C. Carter, S. Newman, *et al.* 1994a. Axon sparing lesions of the medial nucleus of the amygdala decrease affiliative behaviors in the prairie vole (Microtus ochrogaster): behavioral and anatomic specificity. Behav. Neurosci. **108:** 501–513.
50. Numan, M., M.J. Numan & J.B. English. 1993. Excitotoxic amino acid injections into the medial amygdala facilitate maternal behavior in virgin female rates. Horm. Behav. **27:** 56–81.
51. Slotnick, B.M. & B.J. Nigrosh. 1975. Maternal behavior of mice with cingulate, cortical, amygdala, or septal lesions. J. Comp. Physiol. Psychol. **88:** 118–127.
52. Kalinichev, M., J.S. Rosenblatt, Y. Nakabeppu, *et al.* 2000b. Induction of c-Fos-like and FosB-like immunoreactivity reveals forebrain neuronal populations involved differentially in pup-mediated maternal behavior in juvenile and adult rats. J. Comp. Neurol. **416:** 45–78.
53. Numan, M. & M.J. Numan. 1997. Projection sites of medial preoptic area and ventral bed nucleus of the stria terminalis neurons that express Fos during maternal behavior in female rats. J. Neuroendocrinol. **9:** 369–384.
54. Sheehan, T.P. 2000. An investigation into the neural and hormonal inhibition of maternal behavior in rats. unpublished doctoral dissertation, Boston College.
55. Numan, M. 2004. Maternal behaviors: central integration or independent parallel circuits? Theoretical comment on Popeski and Woodside. Behav. Neurosci. **118:** 1469–1472.
56. Kirkpatrick, B. & T.R. Insel. 1993. Fos immunoreactivity increases in the medial nucleus of the amygdala after pup exposure in prairie vole males. Soc. Neurosci. Abstracts **661:** 1.
57. deOlmos, J., G.F. Alheid & C.A. Beltramino. 1985. Amygdala. *In* The Rat Nervous System, Vol. 1. Forebrain and Midbrain. Academic Press: Orlando, FL. 223–334.
58. Factor, E.M., A.D. Mayer & J.S. Rosenblatt. 1993. Peripeduncular nucleus lesions in the rat: I. Effects on maternal aggression, lactation, and maternal behavior during pre- and postpartum periods. Behav. Neurosci. **107:** 166–185.
59. Hansen, S., C. Harthon, E. Wallin, *et al.* 1991b. The effects of 6-OHDA-induced dopamine depletions in the ventral or dorsal striatum on maternal and sexual behavior in the female rat. Pharmacol. Biochem. Behav. **39:** 71–77.
60. Sheehan, T.P., J. Cirrito, M.J. Numan, *et al.* 2000. Using c-Fos immunocytochemistry to identify forebrain regions that may inhibit maternal behavior in rats. Behav. Neurosci. **114:** 337–352.
61. Canteras, N.S., S. Chiavegatto, L.E. Ribeiro Do Valle, *et al.* 1997. Severe reduction in rat defensive behavior to a predator by discrete hypothalamic chemical lesions. Brain Res. Bull. **44:** 297–305.

62. DIELENBERG, R.A., G.E. HUNT & I.S. MCGREGOR 2001. When a rat smells a cat: The distribution of Fos immunoreactivity in rat brain following exposure to a predatory odor. Neuroscience **104:** 1085–1097.
63. NUMAN, M. & T.R. INSEL. 2003. The Neurobiology of Parental Behavior: Springer.
64. NUMAN, M. & T.P. SHEEHAN. 1997. Neuroanatomical circuitry of mammalian maternal behavior. Ann. N. Y. Acad. Sci. **807:** 101–125.
65. MORGAN, H.D., A.S. FLEMING & J.M. STERN. 1992. Somatosensory control of the onset and retention of maternal responsiveness in primiparous Sprague-Dawley rats. Physiol. Behav. **51**: 541–555.
66. FLEMING, A.S. & M. KORSMIT. 1996. Plasticity in the maternal circuit: effects of maternal experience on Fos-Lir in hypothalamic, limbic, and cortical structures in the postpartum rat. Behav. Neurosci. **110:** 567–582.
67. INSEL, T.R. 1997. A neurobiological basis of social attachment. Am. J. Psychiatry **154:** 726–735.
68. SOFRONIEW, M.V. & A. WEINDL. 1981. Central nervous system distribution of vasopressin, oxytocin, and neurophysin. *In* Endogenous Peptides and Learning and Memory Processes. J.L. Martinex, *et al.* Eds.: Academic Press. New York.
69. BALE, T.L., A.M. DAVIS, A.P. AUGER, *et al.* 2001. CNS region-specific oxytocin receptor expression: importance in regulation of anxiety and sex behavior. J. Neurosci. **21:** 2546–2552.
70. FERGUSON, J.N., J.M. ALDAG, T.R. INSEL, *et al.* 2001. Oxytocin in the medial amygdala is essential for social recognition in the mouse. J. Neurosci. **21:** 8278–8285.
71. FERREIRA, A., L. DAHLOF & S. HANSEN. 1987. Olfactory mechanisms in the control of maternal aggression, appetite, and fearfulness: effects of lesions to olfactory receptors, mediodorsal thalamic nucleus, and insular prefrontal cortex. Behav. Neurosci. **101:** 709–717.
72. CARTER, C.S. 1998. Neuroendocrine perspectives on social attachment and love. Psychoneuroendocrinology **23:** 779–818.
73. NELSON E.E. & J. PANKSEPP. 1998. Brain substrates of infant mother attachment: contributions of opioids, oxytocin, and norepinephrine. Neurosci. Biobehav. Rev. **22:** 437–452.
74. PANKSEPP, J. 1981. Hypothalamic integration of behavior. Handbook of the hypothalamus, behavioral studies of the hypothalamus, 3, part b: 289–431.
75. PANKSEPP, J., E. NELSON & S. SIVIY. 1994. Brain opiods and mother-infant social motivation. Acta Paediatrica **83**(Suppl. 397): 40–46.
76. CARDEN, S.E., G.A. BARR & M.A. HOFER. 1991. Different effects of specific opioid receptor agonists on rat up isolation cells. Behav. Brain Res. **62:** 17–22.
77. CARDEN, S.E., G.A. BARR, L. DAVACHI, *et al.* 1994. U50, 488 increases ultrasonic vocalizations in 3-, 10-, and 18-day old rat pups in isolation and the home cage. Dev. Psychobiol. **27:** 65–83.
78. MOLES, A., B.L. KIEFFER & F.R. D'AMATO. 2004. Deficit in attachment behavior in mice lacking the mu-opiod receptor gene. Science **304:** 1983–1986.
79. PANKSEPP, J. 1981. Brain opioids: a neurochemical substrate for narcotic and social dependence. *In* Theory in Psychopharmacology. J.S. Cooper, Ed.: 149-175. Academic Press. London.
80. PANKSEPP, J., S. SIVIY & L.A. NORMANSELL. 1984. The psychobiology of play: theoretical and methodological perspectives. Neurosci. Biobehav. Rev. **8:** 465–492.

81. SIMERLY, R.B., R.A. GORSKI & L.H. SWANSON. 1986. Neurotransmitter specificity of cells and fibers in the medial preoptic nucleus: an immunohistochemical study in the rat. J. Comp. Neurol. **246:** 343–363.
82. HAMMER, R.J. & R.S. BRIDGES. 1987. Preoptic area opioids opiate receptors increase during pregnancy and decrease during lactation. Brain Res. **420:** 48–56.
83. RUBIN, B.S. & R.S. BRIDGES. 1984. Disruption of ongoing maternal responsiveness by central administration of morphine sulfate. Brain Res. **307:** 91–97.
84. MANN, P.E., C.H. KINSLEY & R.S. BRIDGES. 1991. Opioid receptor subtype involvement in maternal behavior in lactating rats. Neuroendocrinology **53:** 487–492.
85. KALIN, N.H., S.E. SHELTON & D.E. LYNN. 1995. Opiate systems in mother and infant primates coordinate intimate contact during reunion. Psychoneuroendocrinology **20:** 735–742.
86. THOMPSON, A.C. & M.B. KRISTAL. 1996. Opioid stimulation in the ventral tegmental area facilitates the onset of maternal behavior in rats. Brain Res. **743:** 184–201.
87. BRIDGES, R.S. 1996. Biochemical basis of parental behavior in the rat. Adv. Study Behav. **25:** 215–242.
88. ELLIOTT, J.C., D.A. LUBIN, C.H. WALKER, *et al.* 2001. Acute cocaine alters oxytocin levels in the medial preoptic area and amygdala in lactating rat dams: implications for cocaine-induced changes in maternal behavior and maternal aggression. Neuropeptides **35:** 127–134.
89. WINDLE, R.J., Y.M. KERSHAW, N. SHANKS, *et al.* 2004. Oxytocin attenuates stress-induced c-fos mRNA expression in specific forebrain regions associated with modulation of hypothalamo-pituitary-adrenal activity. J. Neurosci. **24:** 2974–2982.
90. KINSLEY, C.H. & R.S. BRIDGES. 1988. Prenatal stress and maternal behavior in intact virgin rats: response latencies are decreased in males and increased in females. Horm. Behav. **22:** 76–89.
91. FRANCIS, D., J. DIORIO, D. LIU, *et al.* 1999. Non-genomic transmission across generations of maternal behavior and stress responses in the rat. Science **286:** 1155–1158.
92. LIU, D., J. DIORIO, B. TANNENBAUM, *et al.* 1997. Maternal care, hippocampal glucocorticoid receptors, and hypothalamic-pituitary-adrenal responses to stress. Science **277:** 1659–1662.
93. CALDJI, C., B. TANNENBAUM, S. SHARMA, *et al.* 1998. Maternal care during infancy regulates the development of neural systems mediating the expression of fearfulness in the rat. Proc. Natl. Acad. Sci. **95:** 5335–5340.
94. FRANCIS, D.D. & M.J. MEANEY. 1999. Maternal care and the development of stress responses. Curr. Opin. Neurobiol. **9:** 128–134.
95. BREDY, T., I. WEAVER, F. CHAMPAGNE, *et al.* 2001. Stress, maternal care, and neural development in the rat. *In* Toward a Theory of Neuroplasticity. C.A. Shaw & J.C. McEachern, Eds.: New York.

Genetic and Environmental Influences on the Development of Alcoholism

Resilience vs. Risk

MARY-ANNE ENOCH

Laboratory of Neurogenetics, National Institute on Alcohol Abuse and Alcoholism, NIH, Bethesda, Maryland, USA

ABSTRACT: The physiological changes of adolescence may promote risk-taking behaviors, including binge drinking. Approximately 40% of alcoholics were already drinking heavily in late adolescence. Most cases of alcoholism are established by the age of 30 years with the peak prevalence at 18–23 years of age. Therefore the key time frame for the development, and prevention, of alcoholism lies in adolescence and young adulthood. Severe childhood stressors have been associated with increased vulnerability to addiction, however, not all stress-exposed children go on to develop alcoholism. Origins of resilience can be both genetic (variation in alcohol-metabolizing genes, increased susceptibility to alcohol's sedative effects) and environmental (lack of alcohol availability, positive peer and parental support). Genetic vulnerability is likely to be conferred by multiple genes of small to modest effects, possibly only apparent in gene–environment interactions. For example, it has been shown that childhood maltreatment interacts with a monoamine oxidase A (MAOA) gene variant to predict antisocial behavior that is often associated with alcoholism, and an interaction between early life stress and a serotonin transporter promoter variant predicts alcohol abuse in nonhuman primates and depression in humans. In addition, a common Met158 variant in the catechol-O-methyltransferase (COMT) gene can confer both risk and resilience to alcoholism in different drinking environments. It is likely that a complex mix of gene(s)—environment(s) interactions underlie addiction vulnerability and development. Risk–resilience factors can best be determined in longitudinal studies, preferably starting during pregnancy. This kind of research is important for planning future measures to prevent harmful drinking in adolescence.

KEYWORDS: **MAOA; HTTLPR; COMT; polymorphism; adolescents**

Address for correspondence: Dr. Mary-Anne Enoch, NIH/NIAAA/DICBR/LNG, 5625 Fishers Lane, Room 3S32, MSC 9412, Bethesda, MD 20892. Voice: 301-496-2727; fax: 301-480-2839.
e-mail: maenoch@niaaa.nih.gov

Ann. N.Y. Acad. Sci. 1094: 193–201 (2006).
doi: 10.1196/annals.1376.019

INTRODUCTION

Adolescent alcohol misuse is a major factor in teen car crashes, homicides, and suicides, the three leading causes of death for 15–24-year olds. Drinking tends to start in the teenage years; the average age of the first drink is 11 years for boys and 13 years for girls. In 2004, 19%, 35%, and 48% of 8th, 10th, and 12th graders, respectively, admitted drinking in the previous month.[1] Binge drinking (≥5 drinks/occasion in any 2-week period) is common at this age. Approximately 60% of all adolescents who drink alcohol indulge in this harmful drinking pattern: in 2004 the percentages of binge drinkers were 11%, 22%, and 29%, respectively, for 8th, 10th, and 12th graders.[1] The main reasons teenagers give for drinking to excess are sheer enjoyment and the relief of social anxiety: that is, the perceived improvement of social skills. Thankfully, not all adolescent heavy drinkers become addicted to alcohol: the prevalence of 12-month alcohol use disorders (abuse + dependence) (AUD) is 5% in both boys and girls aged 12–17 years with a peak prevalence at age 18–23 years: 20% in men and 10% in women.[2] By the ages of 23–30 years, 50–75%, respectively, of all AUDs have been diagnosed.[3] Thus the key time frame for the development of alcoholism lies in adolescence and young adulthood.

HERITABILITY OF ALCOHOLISM

Alcoholism has been described as the interminable cycling of preoccupation and anticipation, binge–intoxication, and withdrawal–negative affect.[4] A recent meta-analysis of twin studies has shown that the heritability (the genetic component of interindividual variability) of all addictive substances ranges from 40% to 60%.[5] The heritability of alcoholism, derived from nearly 10,000 twin pairs, is 50%.[5] Thus genetic and environmental factors are almost equally important in alcoholism risk, although the proportions will vary in different populations. Genetic vulnerability to alcoholism is likely to be due to numerous genes of small to modest effects in many neurotransmitter systems (e.g., opioid, serotonin, dopamine, GABA, glutamate, and cannabinoid) and signal transduction pathways within the mesolimbic dopamine reward pathway[6] and interacting stress response systems.[7] Some individuals may be more vulnerable to the development of long-term or permanent neurobiological changes in response to heavy alcohol use resulting in addiction.

RISK FACTORS FOR THE DEVELOPMENT OF ALCOHOLISM

Alcoholism runs in families. A child with an alcoholic parent has a 4- to 10-fold increased risk of developing alcoholism themselves. This can be due to both genetic and environmental factors. Environmental influences, such as alcohol availability, parental attitudes, and peer pressure, strongly influence if and when a child starts to drink. Not surprisingly, frequent drinking in adolescence has been shown to independently increase the risk for alcoholism (OR = 3 [95% CI: 1–8]).[8] Starting to drink before the age of 15 years is associated with a fourfold increased risk for lifetime alcoholism compared with starting at the age of 21 years.[9] One reason for this may be that heavy drinking during adolescence can impair brain development (particularly the hippocampus) and function (particularly learning and memory).[10,11] Animal studies have demonstrated permanent changes in adult brain resulting from adolescent binge drinking.[12] Two important neurotransmitter systems that are affected by alcohol consumption and undergo substantial changes during adolescence are dopamine, implicated in the rewarding effects of alcohol, and GABA, implicated in alcohol's sedating effects and the development of tolerance.[11] For developmental reasons, adolescents are less influenced by the sedating effects of alcohol than adults. Longitudinal studies starting with young adults have shown that a heritable trait, a low level of response to the sedating effects of alcohol, predicts a fourfold increased risk of future alcoholism.[13] Thus vulnerable, low-response individuals who start drinking when very young may be at even greater risk for addiction.

Severe childhood stressors, especially emotional (harsh, inconsistent discipline, hostility, rejection), physical, and sexual abuse, have been associated with increased vulnerability to addiction. Childhood sexual abuse is associated with a fourfold increase in the lifetime prevalence of alcoholism and other drugs of abuse in women.[14] Among female drug users, 70% report childhood sexual abuse.[15] In populations, such as some American Indian tribes that have a high prevalence of both adverse childhood events and alcoholism, childhood abuse and neglect is associated with a twofold increase in risk for alcoholism for one exposure, increasing to a three- to sevenfold increased risk for $\geq$4 exposures.[16]

Children of depressed mothers experience increased antisocial behavior and conduct problems, thought to be predominantly due to impoverished nurturing.[17] Teacher-rated hyperactive and conduct problems in boys aged 8 years have been shown to predict frequent drunkenness 10 years later.[18] Childhood antisocial behavior predicts regular alcohol use in early adolescence and the development of alcoholism later on.[8]

In rodents it has been shown that poor maternal contact in early life results in several neurobiological changes that persist into adulthood. These include effects on the hippocampus that are due to alterations in gene transcription.[19] It is not known whether these same permanent changes occur in humans but if so, the combination of these epigenetic effects and drinking at a young age may account for some aspect of increased addiction vulnerability.

Not all children who experience adverse events subsequently develop psychopathology predictive of alcoholism or take up drinking. What makes some children resilient, despite experiencing severe stressors?

RESILIENCE FACTORS

Genetic: Alcohol-Metabolizing Enzymes

Genetic variation in alcohol-metabolizing genes, seen in Asian and Jewish populations, provides protection against the development of heavy drinking and subsequent alcoholism (FIG. 1). Alcohol dehydrogenases (ADH) metabolize ethanol to acetaldehyde, a toxic intermediate, which is then converted to acetate by aldehyde dehydrogenases (ALDH). Approximately half of Japanese, Chinese, and Koreans, together with other East Asian individuals, have functional polymorphisms at four different genes: ADH2, ADH3, ALDH1, and ALDH2. The most important genetic variants are ALDH2*2 (Glu487Lys), which dominantly inactivates ALDH2, the mitochondrial enzyme responsible for most acetaldehyde metabolism in cells, and ADH2*2 (Arg47His), a superactive variant. ADH2*2 and ALDH2*2 act independently and additively to increase acetaldehyde levels: ADH2*2 increases the rate of synthesis and ALDH2*2 decreases the rate of metabolism.[20,21] Therefore when individuals with the ALDH2*2 and ADH2*2 genotypes drink even small amounts of alcohol they experience a very unpleasant reaction characterized by facial flushing, headache, hypotension, palpitations, tachycardia, nausea, and vomiting. The ALDH2*2 variant causes a stronger flushing reaction than ADH2*2; the ALDH2*2/2 homozygous genotype is nearly completely protective against heavy drinking and the heterozygous genotype is partially protective. The ADH2*2 allele has been shown to account for 20–30% of the alcohol intake variance between light drinking and heavy drinking Jews, and it has been suggested that the relatively high frequency of the ADH2*2 allele might be implicated in the lower levels of alcohol consumption and increased sensitivity to alcohol observed among Jews.[22,23]

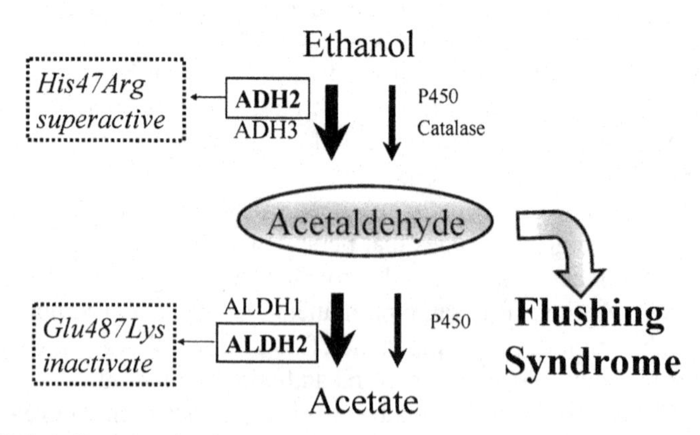

FIGURE 1. Functional polymorphisms in ethanol metabolism confer resilience to the development of alcoholism.

Environmental Factors

Parental mental health and family interaction strongly influence the child's own mental health. Good family functioning, good parent–child relationships and close parental monitoring, higher socioeconomic status, and educational aspiration have been shown to protect against heavy drinking in adolescence.[24]

Gene × Environment Interactions

There are likely to be multiple genes, as well as gene–gene and gene–environment interactions, underlying a complex, heterogeneous disorder, such as alcoholism (FIG. 2). So far, relatively few common, functional genetic polymorphisms have been discovered. However, recent studies have demonstrated that three common polymorphisms that have significant effects on central nervous system (CNS) availability of the neurotransmitters serotonin, dopamine, and norepinephrine, interact with childhood environmental factors to predict alcoholism and associated psychopathology.

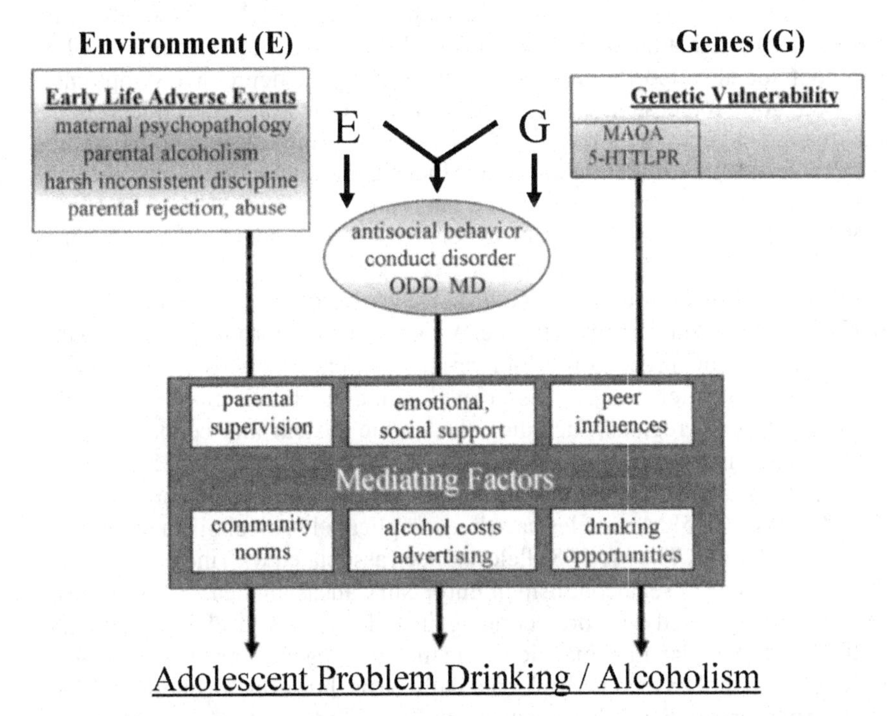

FIGURE 2. Individual and interactive effects of genetic vulnerability and early childhood adverse events on the development of problem drinking and alcoholism in adolescence. MD = major depression, ODD = oppositional defiant disorder.

The neurotransmitter serotonin (5-HT) plays an important role in mood control and is implicated in impulsivity, anxiety–dysphoria, and alcoholism. Monoamine oxidase A (MAOA) is primarily responsible for 5-HT degradation. Recent studies have shown that maltreatment (parental rejection, harsh discipline, physical and sexual abuse) and family adversity (interparental violence, neglect) experienced by young boys interact with a genotype conferring low levels of MAOA expression to predict childhood conduct disorder and adult antisocial behavior, often antecedents for addiction.[25,26] Thus the gene variant that produces high MAOA levels confers resilience against the development of alcoholism-related psychopathology in maltreated boys.

5-HT actions are terminated by the serotonin transporter (5-HTT) through reuptake at the synaptic cleft. 5-HTTLPR is a common 44-base-pair insertion/deletion in the 5-HTT promoter region; the short "S" allele is associated with an approximately 50% reduction in transporter availability and consequent increase in synaptic 5-HT compared with the longer "L" allele. Individuals with the S allele show greater amygdala activation in response to fearful stimuli[27] as well as greater coupling between the amygdala and the ventromedial prefrontal cortex,[28] a limbic brain area implicated in major depression.[29] Depression is predicted by the interaction between the S allele and cumulative stressful life events in young adults and adolescents.[30,31] In addition, it has been shown that maltreatment combined with the S allele in children who had poor social support was associated with increased depressive symptoms, however, good social support protected children from the adverse effects of the maltreatment–genotype interaction.[32] Depressive symptoms in childhood are often antecedents for adult alcoholism. Indeed, the interaction between early life stress (emotional deprivation) and the S allele has been shown to predict increased alcohol consumption in female rhesus macaque monkeys.[33] Thus the 5-HTTLPR L allele can be regarded as a resilience factor.

Catechol-O-methyltransferase (COMT) plays a major role in the metabolism of CNS dopamine and norepinephrine. A common polymorphism, Val158Met, is responsible for three- to fourfold variation in enzyme activity. The lower activity Met158 allele has been associated with greater activation in emotion-modulating brain regions, including the limbic system and connected prefrontal areas, in response to unpleasant visual stimuli.[34] COMT Met158 has also been associated with a more anxious, sensitive, cautious personality.[35–37] Both COMT Val158Met alleles have been implicated in alcoholism but in different populations. The Met158 allele has been associated with increased social drinking and late onset alcoholism in European Caucasian men.[38–40] However, Met158 is associated with protection against alcoholism in Plains American Indians.[41] The explanation may lie within the differing drinking environments. European alcoholics tend to drink on a daily basis, however, alcoholics within many American Indian tribes, such as the Plains Indians, tend to drink heavily but episodically.[41] Thus the Met158 allele may be a vulnerability factor for anxiety-relieving maintenance drinking in some societies, such as Europeans, but in other societies, such as American Indians, the anxious, cautious personality associated with the Met158 allele may protect against excessive bouts of heavy drinking. Adolescents tend to have the same binge-drinking pattern; it remains to be seen whether COMT Met158 is a resilience factor against heavy drinking in adolescents.

FUTURE DIRECTIONS

Longitudinal research is the best way of tracking the influences of parental psychopathology and other early childhood adverse events on the emergence of behavioral problems and psychopathology in the child as well as the child's own eventual alcohol use. We are undertaking gene–environment interaction studies in a cohort of 7,500 children from Avon, UK, intensively followed from conception in 1991–1992 onward (Avon Longitudinal Study of Parents and Children (ALSPAC)) (www.alspac.bris.ac.uk). Results will be forthcoming in the near future.

CONCLUSION

Adolescence is a critically vulnerable time for the development of risky drinking habits that may lead to permanent neurobiological changes with significant consequences including the development of addiction. Environmental risk–resilience factors have been well documented and have so far been the main focus for preventive measures. However, recent studies indicate that genetic vulnerability in combination with environmental factors may affect the risk–resilience balance. Thus it is likely that a complex mix of gene(s)–environment(s) interactions are likely to underlie addiction vulnerability and development. This fact should be taken into account when planning future measures to prevent harmful drinking in adolescence.

REFERENCES

1. Johnston, L.D., P.M. O'Malley, J.G. Bachman, *et al.* 2005. Monitoring the Future. National Results on Adolescent Drug Use: Overview of Key Findings, 2004. (NIH Publication No. 05-5726). National Institute on Drug Abuse. Bethesda, MD.
2. Harford, T.C., B.F. Grant, H.Y. Yi, *et al.* 2005. Patterns of DSM-IV alcohol abuse and dependence criteria among adolescents and adults: results from the 2001 National Household Survey on Drug Abuse. Alcohol. Clin. Exp. Res. **29:** 810–828.
3. Kessler, R.C., P. Berglund, O. Demler, *et al.* 2005. Lifetime prevalence and age-of-onset distributions of DSM-IV disorders in the National Comorbidity Survey Replication. Arch. Gen. Psychiatry **62:** 593–602.
4. Koob, G.F. 2003. Alcoholism: allostasis and beyond. Alcohol. Clin. Exp. Res. **27:** 232–243.
5. Goldman, D., G. Oroszi & F. Ducci. 2005. The genetics of addictions: uncovering the genes. Nat. Rev. Genet. **6:** 521–532.

6. ENOCH, M.-A. 2003. Pharmacogenomics of alcohol response and addiction. Am. J. PharmacoGenomics **3:** 217–232.
7. ENOCH, M.-A. 2006. Genetics, stress and the risk for addiction. *In* Stress and Addiction: Biological and Psychological Mechanisms. M. al'Absi, Ed.: 127–146. Elsevier Neuroscience. New York. In Press.
8. BONOMO, Y.A., G. BOWES, C. COFFEY, *et al.* 2004. Teenage drinking and the onset of alcohol dependence: a cohort study over seven years. Addiction **99:** 1520–1528.
9. GRANT, B.F. & D.A. DAWSON. 1998. Age of onset of drug use and its association with DSM-IV drug abuse and dependence: results from the National Longitudinal Alcohol Epidemiologic Survey. J. Subst. Abuse **10:** 163–173.
10. DE BELLIS, M.D., D.B. CLARK & S.R. BEERS. 2000. Hippocampal volume in adolescent-onset alcohol use disorders. Am. J. Psychiatry **157:** 737–744.
11. HILLER-STURMHOFEL, S. & H.S. SWARTZWELDER. 2004/2005. Alcohol's effects on the adolescent brain. Alcohol Res. Health **28:** 213–221.
12. CREWS, F.T. & K. NIXON. 2005. Adolescent binge drinking causes life-long changes in brain. *In* Monti P.M., Miranda R. Jr., Nixon K. *et al.* Adolescence: booze, brains, and behavior. Alcohol. Clin. Exp. Res. **29:** 207–220.
13. SCHUCKIT, M.A. 1994. Low level of response to alcohol as a predictor of future alcoholism. Am. J. Psychiatry **151:** 184–189.
14. WILSNACK, S.C., N.D. VOGELTANZ, A.D. KLASSEN, *et al.* 1997. Childhood sexual abuse and women's substance abuse: national survey findings. J. Stud. Alcohol **58:** 264–271.
15. NATIONAL INSTITUTE ON DRUG ABUSE (NIDA). 1994. Capsules, Women Drug Abuse **6:** 2.
16. KOSS, M.P., N.P. YUAN, D. DIGHTMAN, *et al.* 2003. Adverse childhood exposures and alcohol dependence among seven Native American tribes. Am. J. Prev. Med. **25:** 238–244.
17. KIM-COHEN, J., T.E. MOFFITT, A. TAYLOR, *et al.* 2005. Maternal depression and children's antisocial behavior: nature and nurture effects. Arch. Gen. Psychiatry **62:** 173–181.
18. NIEMELA, S., A. SOURANDER, K. POIKOLAINEN, *et al.* 2006. Childhood predictors of drunkenness in late adolescence among males: a 10-year population-based follow-up study. Addiction **101:** 512–521.
19. WEAVER, I.C., N. CERVONI, F.A. CHAMPAGNE, *et al.* 2004. Epigenetic programming by maternal behavior. Nat. Neurosci. **7:** 847–854.
20. NEUMARK, Y.D., Y. FRIEDLANDER, R. DURST, *et al.* 2004. Alcohol dehydrogenase polymorphisms influence alcohol-elimination rates in a male Jewish population. Alcohol Clin. Exp. Res. **28:** 10–14.
21. THOMASSON, H.R., H.J. EDENBURG, D.W. CRABB, *et al* 1991. Alcohol and aldehyde dehydrogenase genotypes and alcoholism in Chinese men. Am. J. Hum. Genet. **48:** 677–681.
22. NEUMARK, Y.D., Y. FRIEDLANDER, H.R. THOMASSON, *et al.* 1998. Association of the ADH2*2 allele with reduced ethanol consumption in Jewish men in Israel: a pilot study. J. Stud. Alcohol **59:** 133–139.
23. MONTEIRO, M.G., J.L. KLEIN, M.A. SCHUCKIT. 1991. High levels of sensitivity to alcohol in young adult Jewish men: a pilot study. J. Stud. Alcohol **52:** 464–469.
24. TIET, Q.Q., H.R. BIRD, M. DAVIES, *et al.* 1998. Adverse life events and resilience. J. Am. Acad. Child. Adolesc. Psychiatry **37:** 1191–1200.
25. CASPI, A., J. MCCLAY, T.E. MOFFITT, *et al.* 2002. Role of genotype in the cycle of violence in maltreated children. Science **297:** 851–853.

26. FOLEY, D.L., L.J. EAVES, B. WORMLEY, *et al.* 2004. Childhood adversity, monoamine oxidase a genotype, and risk for conduct disorder. Arch. Gen. Psychiatry **61:** 738–744.
27. HARIRI, A.R., E.M. DRABANT, K.E. MUNOZ, *et al.* 2005. A susceptibility gene for affective disorders and the response of the human amygdala. Arch. Gen. Psychiatry **62:** 146–152.
28. HEINZ, A., D.F. BRAUS, M.N. SMOLKA, *et al.* 2005. Amygdala-prefrontal coupling depends on a genetic variation of the serotonin transporter. Nat. Neurosci. **8:** 20–21.
29. DREVETS, W.C. 2003. Neuroimaging abnormalities in the amygdala in mood disorders. Ann. N. Y. Acad. Sci. **985:** 420–444.
30. CASPI, A., K. SUGDEN, T.E. MOFFITT, *et al.* 2003. Influence of life stress on depression: moderation by a polymorphism in the 5-HTT gene. Science **301:** 386–389.
31. KENDLER, K.S., J.W. KUHN, J. VITTUM, *et al.* 2005. The interaction of stressful life events and a serotonin transporter polymorphism in the prediction of episodes of major depression: a replication. Arch. Gen. Psychiatry **62:** 529–535.
32. KAUFMAN, J., B.Z. YANG, H. DOUGLAS-PALUMBERI, *et al.* 2004. Social supports and serotonin transporter gene moderate depression in maltreated children. Proc. Natl. Acad. Sci. USA **101:** 17316–17321.
33. BARR, C.S., T.K. NEWMAN, S. LINDELL, *et al.* 2004. Interaction between serotonin transporter gene variation and rearing condition in alcohol preference and consumption in female primates. Arch. Gen. Psychiatry **61:** 1146–1152.
34. SMOLKA, M.N., G. SCHUMANN, J. WRASE, *et al.* 2005. Catechol-O-methyltransferase val158met genotype affects processing of emotional stimuli in the amygdala and prefrontal cortex. J. Neurosci. **25:** 836–842.
35. ENOCH, M.A., K. XU, E. FERRO, *et al.* 2003. Genetic origins of anxiety in women: a role for a functional catechol-O-methyltransferase polymorphism. Psychiatr. Genet. **13:** 33–41.
36. OLSSON, C.A., R.J. ANNEY, M. LOTFI-MIRI, *et al.* 2005. Association between the COMT Val158Met polymorphism and propensity to anxiety in an Australian population-based longitudinal study of adolescent health. Psychiatr. Genet. **15:** 109–115.
37. ZUBIETA, J.K., M.M. HEITZEG, Y.R. SMITH, *et al.* 2003. COMT val158met genotype affects mu-opioid neurotransmitter responses to a pain stressor. Science **299:** 1240–1243.
38. KAUHANEN, J., T. HALLIKAINEN, T.P. TUOMAINEN, *et al.* 2000. Association between the functional polymorphism of catechol-O-methyltransferase gene and alcohol consumption among social drinkers. Alcohol. Clin. Exp. Res. **24:** 135–139.
39. HALLIKAINEN, T., H. LACHMAN, T. SAITO, *et al.* 2000. Lack of association between the functional variant of the catechol-o-methyltransferase (COMT) gene and early-onset alcoholism associated with severe antisocial behavior. Am. J. Med. Genet. **96:** 348–352.
40. TIIHONEN, J., T. HALLIKAINEN, H. LACHMAN, *et al.* 1999. Association between the functional variant of the catechol-o-methyltransferase (COMT) gene and type 1 alcoholism. Mol. Psychiatry **4:** 286–289.
41. ENOCH, M.-A., J. WAHEED, C.R. HARRIS, *et al.* 2006. Sex differences in the influence of COMT Val158Met on alcoholism and smoking in Plains American Indians. Alcohol. Clin. Exp. Res. **30:** 399–406.

Stress and the Adolescent Brain

RUSSELL D. ROMEO AND BRUCE S. McEWEN

Laboratory of Neuroendocrinology, Rockefeller University, New York, New York, USA

ABSTRACT: During adolescence the brain shows remarkable changes in both structure and function. The plasticity exhibited by the brain during this pubertal period may make individuals more vulnerable to perturbations, such as stress. Although much is known about how exposure to stress and stress hormones during perinatal development and adulthood affect the structure and function of the brain, relatively little is known about how the pubertal brain responds to stress. Furthermore, it is not clear whether stressors experienced during adolescence lead to altered physiological and behavioral potentials in adulthood, as has been shown for perinatal development. The purpose of this review is to present what is currently known about the pubertal maturation of the hypothalamic-pituitary-adrenal (HPA) axis, the neuroendocrine axis that mediates the stress response, and discuss what is currently known about how stressors affect the adolescent brain. Our dearth of knowledge regarding the effects of stress on the pubertal brain will be discussed in the context of our accumulating knowledge regarding stress-induced neuronal remodeling in the adult. Finally, as the adolescent brain is capable of such profound plasticity during this developmental stage, we will also explore the possibility of adolescence as a period of interventions and opportunities to mitigate negative consequences from earlier developmental insults.

KEYWORDS: adolescence; adrenocorticotropic hormone (ACTH); *amygdale;* hippocampus; hypothalamic-pituitary-adrenal (HPA); axis neuroendocrine; stress

INTRODUCTION

Adolescence is increasingly being viewed as a significant period of developmental vulnerabilities.[5–7] For instance, puberty is marked by an increase in the morbidity and susceptibility to various psychological disorders, such as anxiety and depression.[8,9] However, it is presently unclear what central mechanisms may mediate the pubertal increase in these events. Interestingly, stressors in adulthood can lead to the onset and exacerbation of psychological disorders.[10] Furthermore, brain regions implicated in stress reactivity and

Address for correspondence: Russell D. Romeo, Laboratory of Neuroendocrinology, The Rockefeller University, Box 165, New York, NY 10021. Voice: +212-327-8623; fax: +212-327-8634.
e-mail: romeor@rockefeller.edu

Ann. N.Y. Acad. Sci. 1094: 202–214 (2006).
doi: 10.1196/annals.1376.022

emotionality, such as the hippocampus, medial prefrontal cortex (mPFC), and amygdala (AMY) undergo profound changes in both structure and function in response to stress.[4] Thus, stress-induced alterations in the pubertal nervous system may contribute to an individual's vulnerability to the onset of psychopathologies during adolescence. There is presently a paucity of knowledge regarding how stressors may affect the brain during adolescence. This is quite surprising for two reasons. First, stress reactivity changes dramatically depending on both the pubertal development and experience of an individual (see below). Second, brain regions that are highly sensitive to stress hormones play an important role in regulating emotionality and stress responsiveness (i.e., hippocampus, mPFC, AMY) continue to mature during the peripubertal period.[1–3,6,11–13] It is our hope that this review will provide a point of departure for future experiments elucidating the role of stress on the developing pubertal brain.

Pubertal Maturation of the Hypothalamic-Pituitary-Adrenal (HPA) Axis

The release of stress hormones by the HPA axis is driven by the release of corticotropin-releasing hormone (CRH) and vasopressin (AVP) from the medial parvocellular division of the paraventricular hypothalamic nucleus (PVN). CRH and AVP are released into the portal system of the pituitary, which in turn causes the release of adrenocorticotropic hormone (ACTH) from the anterior pituitary. ACTH then stimulates the secretion of the glucocorticoids (e.g., cortisol in primates and corticosterone in most rodent species) from the adrenal cortex. The stress hormones secreted by the HPA axis indirectly control their own secretion through a classic neuroendocrine negative feedback loop. That is, the glucocorticoids feedback on the PVN and many other extrahypothalamic sites, in particular, the hippocampus and mPFC, to inhibit further release of CRH[14] (FIG. 1). In addition to extrahypothalamic sites of negative feedback on the PVN, projections from the central nucleus of the amygdala (CeA) can activate the PVN and modulate stress reactive behaviors[14] (FIG. 1).

Studies that have examined stress responsiveness in juvenile animals have demonstrated that although basal and stress-induced ACTH and corticosterone secretion are similar in prepubertal and adult animals, prepubertal animals have a much more prolonged ACTH and corticosterone stress response compared to adults. For example, in males exposed to either intermittent foot shock,[15] ether vapors,[16] or restraint,[17] corticosterone levels of prepubertal males take at least 45 to 60 min longer to return to baseline compared to adults (FIG. 2). It is important to note that this extended response exhibited by prepubertal animals is to both total and free corticosterone,[18] indicating that corticotropin-binding globulin (CBG) is not upregulated to "buffer" the prepubertal animal from this prolonged exposure to corticosterone.

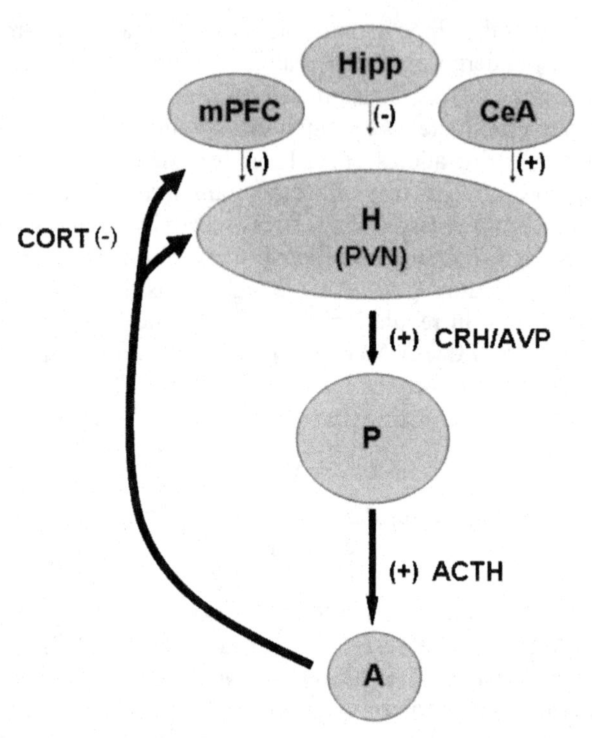

FIGURE 1. A diagram of the HPA axis and various extrahypothalamic sites that play a role in modulating stress hormone secretion. Abbreviations, A = adrenal; ACTH = adrenocorticotropic hormone; AVP = vasopressin; CeA = central nucleus of the amygdala; CORT = corticosterone; CRH = corticotropin-releasing hormone; Hipp = hippocampus; H = hypothalamus; mPFC = medial prefrontal cortex; P = pituitary; PVN = paraventricular nucleus; (+), positive drive; and (−), negative feedback.

The above-mentioned studies examined the hormonal stress response in prepubertal and adult animals only in the context of a single, acute stressor. However, it is well documented that experience with a stressor can also influence stress reactivity. For instance, in adults, repeated exposure to a stressor leads to habituation of the stress response, such that peak stress hormone levels are blunted.[19–22] Interestingly, we found that experience and pubertal maturation interact to affect HPA axis plasticity.[18] Specifically, we showed that, in contrast to the extended response observed after acute stress, chronic stress resulted in prepubertal males exhibiting a higher peak ACTH and corticosterone (free and total) response immediately following the stressor, but a faster return to baseline, compared to adults (FIG. 3).

In addition to these endocrine differences in stress reactivity, we have also found that this differential response to acute and chronic stress is associated with differential neuronal activation in the PVN of prepubertal and adult

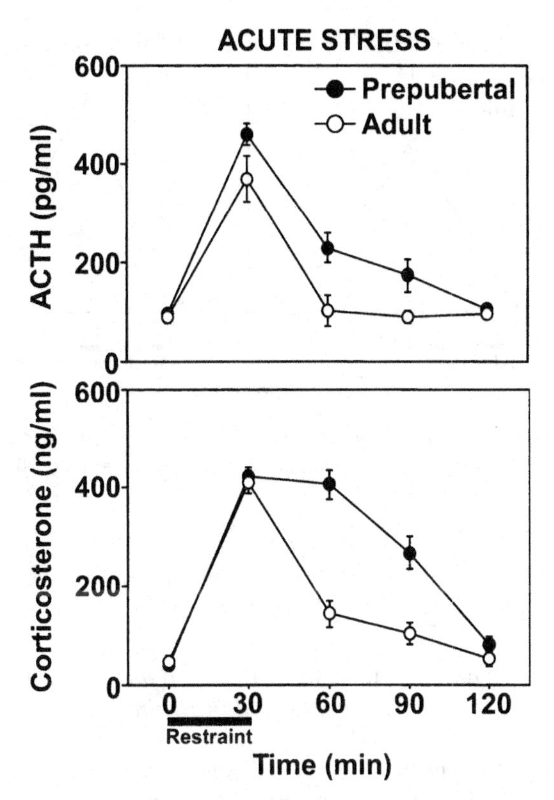

FIGURE 2. Plasma ACTH and corticosterone concentrations in prepubertal and adult males before and after a 30-min session of restraint stress.[17]

animals.[18] Moreover, we have established that a significantly larger proportion of CRH, but not AVP, cells are activated in the PVN in response to both acute and chronic stress in prepubertal compared to adult animals.[18] Together, these data indicate that experience-dependent plasticity of the HPA axis is markedly influenced by pubertal development, and that CRH neurons of the PVN are at least one neural locus involved in these changes.

The physiological and behavioral implications of these differential stress responses in prepubertal compared to adult animals are currently unknown. However, two factors may render the prepubertal brain especially vulnerable to stress. First, the prepubertal brain may be more sensitive to corticosterone, as a recent study showed an equivalent dose of corticosterone increased hippocampal N-methyl-D-aspartate (NMDA) receptor subunit expression (e.g., NR2A and NR2B) to a greater degree in prepubertal than adult males.[23] Second, brain regions that continue to mature during adolescence, such as hippocampus,[24–26] PFC,[1,11,27] and AMY,[12,28] are also the most sensitive to corticosterone.[4] Thus, upon encountering a similar stressor, the immature, and possibly more

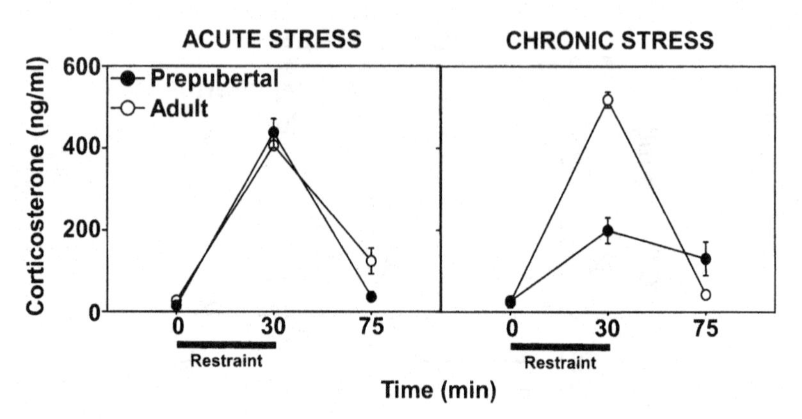

FIGURE 3. Plasma corticosterone concentrations in prepubertal and adult males exposed to a single 30-min session of restraint (acute stress) or a daily 30-min session of restraint for 1 week (chronic stress).[18]

sensitive, prepubertal brain experiences differential exposure to corticosterone compared to the more fully developed adult brain.

Stress and the Adolescent Brain: What We Can Learn from the Adult Brain

Though few experiments have examined the effects of stress on the structure of the pubertal brain, it is widely recognized that stressors experienced during adolescence can have long-lasting and profound consequences for the future behavioral and psychological function of an individual. For instance, human studies clearly demonstrate that stress burden during adolescence is strongly correlated with the subsequent onset of depressive and/or anxiety disorders in adulthood.[29] Similarly, studies in rodents indicate that animals exposed to stress during puberty show increases in basal and stress-induced anxiety-like behaviors upon reaching adulthood.[30,31] The neural correlates associated with these long-lasting changes in emotionality and behavior remain unknown. However, the effects of stress on the structural remodeling of the adult brain have been relatively well studied.[4] Thus, we will next discuss stress and structural remodeling of the adult brain, namely in the hippocampus, PFC, and AMY, to highlight current and future directions regarding the influence of stress on the adolescent brain.

Hippocampus

The hippocampus is critically important in learning and memory,[32] and continues to develop well into adolescence.[24,33] In adult male rats, chronic restraint (6-h per day of restraint stress for 3 weeks) or social stress significantly

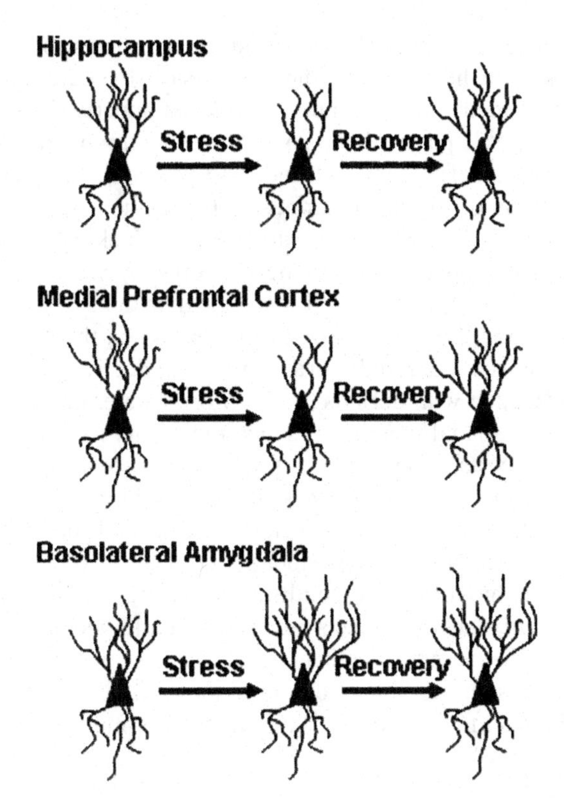

FIGURE 4. Schematic diagrams of dendritic remodeling in the adult hippocampus (*top*), mPFC (*middle*), and basolateral amygdala (*bottom*). Note that the dendritic remodeling of both the hippocampus and mPFC are reversible, while basolateral amygdala dendritic hypertrophy is longer lasting.

reduces branching of the apical dendrites of the CA3 region of hippocampus[34–36] (FIG. 4). The apical dendrites of CA3 neurons receive inputs from the granule neurons of the dentate gyrus.[37] The stress-induced remodeling in the hippocampus is dependent on corticosterone as cyanoketone, a corticosterone synthesis inhibitor, blocks the stress-induced atrophy of the CA3 dendrites,[19] while chronic injections of corticosterone mimic the stress-induced atrophy.[38] Interestingly, these effects of stress on hippocampal structure are reversible such that 10 days after the last stress session dendritic branching reverts to prestress levels[39] (FIG. 4).

Parallel to these morphological studies, it was found that chronic stress results in spatial memory impairment.[40] Furthermore, chronically stressed animals pretreated with tianeptine, an antidepressant that blocks stress-induced CA3 dendritic atrophy,[41] showed spatial abilities similar to nonstressed control animals.[40] Together, these data indicated that stress potently affects the adult hippocampus and suggests that the stress-induced dendritic atrophy demonstrated by the CA3 pyramidal cells adversely affects spatial cognition. It is important to note, however, that these effects of stress are reversible.

A recent study aimed at understanding stress and puberty showed that male rats exposed to variable physical and social stressors throughout adolescence exhibited volumetric deficits in CA1 and CA3 pyramidal cell layers as well as the dentate gyrus of the hippocampus.[25] The authors suggested that the reduction in hippocampal volume was due to stress blocking the normal maturational increase in hippocampal volume.[25] Interestingly, these effects on the hippocampus were not observed until 3 weeks after the stress sessions were terminated, indicating these effects of chronic stress on the developing adolescent hippocampus are delayed. Furthermore, the decrease in hippocampal volume was associated with deficits on the Morris water maze, a commonly used task to assess spatial memory.[25] Thus, these data indicate that, similar to the adult, the pubertal hippocampus is sensitive to stress. However, unlike the reversibility of the effect of stressors on the adult hippocampus, it appears that the effects of pubertal stress may be long-lasting, and perhaps permanent. Future studies will need to assess whether pubertal stress affects the structure and function of the hippocampus months after the stressors have been terminated, and whether behavioral effects persist into adulthood and aging. It will also be interesting to examine whether various pharmacological interventions shown to block stress-induced remodeling of the adult hippocampus, such as tianeptine,[41] phenytoin,[42] or lithium,[43] mitigate stress-induced changes in the pubertal hippocampus.

Prefrontal Cortex

The PFC is a key brain region involved in the regulation of emotional behaviors, executive function, and fear extinction.[44] In adults, chronic restraint stress (6-h per day of restraint stress for 3 weeks) results in reductions in both apical dendritic branching and spine density of medial prefrontal cortical pyramidal neurons in layer II/III of the anterior cingulate cortex and prelimbic area[45,46] (FIG. 4). As chronic injections of corticosterone mimic the effects of chronic stress on the prefrontal cortex it appears that stress-induced release of corticosterone is involved in the mechanism for these morphological changes.[47] The remodeling of the mPFC in response to stress is reversible such that animals allowed to recover for 3 weeks after exposure to chronic stress show dendritic branching similar to nonstress controls[48] (FIG. 4). The stress-induced remodeling in the PFC is associated with impairment of attention set-shifting,[49] an adaptive behavior that is also impaired by lesions of the mPFC.[50] Moreover, whereas mPFC neurons show atrophy with chronic stress, neurons in the orbitofrontal cortex show growth as a result of repeated stress.[49] These data indicate the structure of the prefrontal cortex is sensitive to the remodeling effects of stress and these morphological changes may mediate, at least in part, the changes in emotionality after prolonged exposure to stress.[4]

Similar to the hippocampus, the prefrontal cortex continues to mature throughout adolescence.[1,11] However, it is presently unknown whether exposure to stress during puberty affects the structure and function of the prefrontal cortex. Given that the pubertal mPFC expresses glucocorticoid receptors (R. D. Romeo, unpublished observation), it seems likely that this brain area would be sensitive to stress. Based on the accumulating evidence that exposure to stressors during adolescence can lead to an increased propensity to develop emotional and psychological disorders (i.e., depression and anxiety),[29] it is imperative to understand the influence of stress and stress hormones on such an important node in the neuronal circuitry of emotional regulation.

Amygdala

The AMY plays a central role in emotional memory and fear conditioning.[51] Unlike the stress-induced dendritic atrophy exhibited by the adult hippocampus and mPFC, adults show dendritic hypertrophy in the basolateral, but not central nucleus, of the amygdala after chronic immobilization stress (2-h per day of immobilization stress for 10 days; FIG. 4).[52,53] This chronic immobilization stress paradigm also results in elevated anxiety-like behaviors, suggesting that the dendritic hypertrophy influences anxiety levels.[54] Dissimilar to the reversibility of dendritic atrophy of the hippocampus[39] and mPFC,[48] stress-induced dendritic hypertrophy in the amygdala and increased levels of anxiety-like behaviors remain even after 3 weeks of stress-free recovery[55] (FIG. 4). It is presently unknown whether these effects of stress on amygdalar morphology are dependent upon stress-induced release of corticosterone. However, as glucocorticoid receptors are expressed in the amygdala,[56] it would appear likely that the effects of stress on the amygdala are, at least in part, due to the actions of corticosterone.

Pubertal development is marked by changes in the structure and function of the AMY.[28,33] However, the effects of stress on AMY during pubertal development remain unknown. Like the mPFC, the adolescent amygdala expresses abundant glucocorticoid receptors (R. D. Romeo, unpublished observation), indicating corticosterone sensitivity in this area. Future studies will need to examine the impact of stress on the developing AMY during puberty, and whether any effects on the structure and function of this brain region are transient or permanent.

Adolescence as a Period of Interventions and Opportunities

Puberty is marked by profound changes in an individual's nervous system, physiology, and behavior.[12,57,58] Although this may render an individual especially vulnerable to harm during this period, it may also allow for interventions to mitigate earlier or concurrent emotional and/or physical trauma.[5]

A stunning example of puberty as a period of opportunity to diminish the impact of an earlier, negative trauma comes from a classic paper by Twiggs, Popolow, and Gerall.[59] In this study, prepubertal males were housed alone (solitary) or in groups (social) and then given lesions of the medial preoptic nucleus of the anterior hypothalamus (MPN), an area of the brain critical for the display of male reproductive behavior.[60] Although MPN lesions in adulthood lead to irreversible deficits in male mating, males receiving a lesion prior to puberty were able to show copulatory behaviors upon reaching adulthood.[59] Interestingly, however, only the animals raised in the social groups during adolescence demonstrated substantial behavioral reversal of the effects of MPN lesions.[59] These data indicate that pubertal development and the social environment can interact to diminish or even reverse prior brain damage.

Recent studies have also explored the ability of environmental enrichment during adolescence to offset the negative influences of perinatal stress. For instance, animals derived from stressful pregnancies show increases in anxiety-related behaviors and HPA reactivity and depressed play behavior later in life.[61,62] However, animals raised in an enriched environment (larger housing, toys, running wheel) during puberty do not show these negative physiological and behavioral effects of prenatal stress compared to prenatally stressed offspring raised under normal laboratory conditions.[61,62] In addition to prenatal stress, postnatal stress in the form of suboptimal maternal care and maternal separation leads to increased HPA reactivity and emotionality and reduced cognitive function in adulthood.[63,64] Similar to the studies mentioned above, animals exposed to postnatal stress, but raised in enriched environments during puberty, show less HPA reactivity and emotionality and greater cognitive abilities compared to their postnatally stressed counterparts that were raised in standard laboratory environments.[65–67] Taken together, these studies clearly demonstrate that the pubertal period of development can serve as a time of interventions and opportunities to reduce or reverse the adverse effects accumulated from earlier insults.

CONCLUSIONS

The literature reviewed above indicates that stress reactivity is markedly influenced by both the pubertal maturation and the experience of the individual. Furthermore, although stress affects key regulatory nuclei related to stress responsiveness, emotional behavior, and cognitive function in adulthood, scant information exist about the effects of stress on the pubertal nervous system. Finally, it is important to note that despite the possible vulnerabilities of the pubertal brain to stress, adolescence may also provide opportunities to alleviate adverse effects of stress experienced earlier in development. Although much research remains to be done regarding the effects of stress on the structure and function of the adolescent brain, the vast body of stress research on adults may aid in honing our potential hypothesis and provide a point of departure for future experiments.

REFERENCES

1. GIEDD, J.N. 2004. Structural magnetic resonance imaging of the adolescent brain. Ann. N.Y. Acad. Sci. **1021:** 77–85.
2. BLAKEMORE, S.-J. & S. CHOUDHURY. 2006. Development of the adolescent brain: implications for executive function and social cognition. J. Child Psychol. Psychiatry **47:** 296–312.
3. MACCARI, S. *et al.* 2003. Prenatal stress and long-term consequences: implications of glucocorticoid hormones. Neurosci. Biobehav. Rev. **27:** 119–127.
4. MCEWEN, B.S. 2005. Glucocorticoids, depression, and mood disorders: structural remodeling in the brain. Metabolism **54:** 20–23.
5. ANDERSEN, S.L. 2003. Trajectories of brain development: point of vulnerability or window of opportunity. Neurosci. Biobehav. Rev. **27:** 3–18.
6. SPEAR, L.P. 2000. The adolescent brain and age-related behavioral manifestations. Neurosci. Biobehav. Rev. **24:** 417–463.
7. DAHL, R.E. 2004. Adolescent brain development: a period of vulnerabilities and opportunities. Ann. N.Y. Acad. Sci. **1021:** 1–22.
8. CONGER, J. & A. PETERSEN. 1984. Adolescence and Youth: Psychological Development in a Changing World. Harper and Row. New York.
9. MASTEN, A. 1987. Toward a developmental psychopathology of early adolescence. *In* Early Adolescent Transitions. M. Levin & E. McArnarny, Eds.: 261–278. Heath. Lexington, KY.
10. MCEWEN, B.S. 2003. Mood disorders and allostatic load. Biol. Psychiatry. **54:** 200–207.
11. GOGTAY, N. *et al.* 2004. Dynamic mapping of human cortical development during childhood through early adulthood. Proc. Natl. Acad. Sci. USA **101:** 8174–8179.
12. ROMEO, R.D. 2003. Puberty: a period of both organizational and activational effects of steroid hormones on neurobehavioral development. J. Neuroendocrinol. **15:** 1185–1192.
13. SUZUKI, M. *et al.* 2005. Male-specific volume expansion of the human hippocampus during adolescence. Cerebral Cortex **15:** 187–193.
14. HERMAN, J.P. *et al.* 2003. Central mechanisms of stress integration: hierarchical circuitry controlling hypothalamic-pituitary-adrenocortical responsiveness. Front Neuroendocrinol. **24:** 151–180.
15. GOLDMAN, L. *et al.* 1973. Postweaning development of negative feedback in the pituitary-adrenal system of the rat. Neuroendocrinology **12:** 199–211.
16. VAZQUEZ, D.M. & H. AKIL. 1993. Pituitary-adrenal response to ether vapor in the weanling animal: characterization of the inhibitory effect of glucocorticoids on adrenocorticotropin secretion. Pediatric Res. **34:** 646–653.
17. ROMEO, R.D. *et al.* 2004. Testosterone cannot activate an adult-like stress response in prepubertal male rats. Neuroendocrinology **79:** 125–132.
18. ROMEO, R.D. *et al.* 2006. Stress history and pubertal development interact to shape hypothalamic pituitary adrenal axis plasticity. Endocrinology **147:** 1664–1674.
19. MAGARINOS, A.M. & B.S. MCEWEN. 1995. Stress-induced atrophy of apical dendrites of hippocampal CA3c neurons: involvement of glucocorticoid secretion and excitatory amino acid receptors. Neuroscience **69:** 89–98.

20. MARTI, O. & A. ARMARIO. 1997. Influence of regularity of exposure to chronic stress on the pattern of habituation of pituitary-adrenal hormones, prolactin and glucose. Stress **1:** 179–189.
21. HELMREICH, D.L. *et al.* 1997. Correlation between changes in stress-induced corticosterone secretion and GR mRNA levels. Stress **2:** 101–112.
22. HARRIS, R.B.S. *et al.* 2004. Increased glucocorticoid response to a novel stress in rats that have been restrained. Physiol. Behav. **81:** 557–568.
23. LEE, P.R., D. BRANDY & J.I. KOENIG. 2003. Corticosterone alters N-methyl-D-aspartate receptor subunit mRNA expression before puberty. Mol. Brain Res. **115:** 55–62.
24. MEYER, G., R. FERRES-TORRES & M. MAS. 1978. The effects of puberty and castration on hippocampal dendritic spines of mice. A Golgi study. Brain Res. **155:** 108–112.
25. ISGOR, C. *et al.* 2004. Delayed effects of chronic variable stress during peripubertal-juvenile period of hippocampal morphology and on cognitive and stress axis function in rats. Hippocampus **14:** 636–648.
26. ANDERSEN, S.L. & M.H. TEICHER. 2004. Delayed effects of early stress on hippocampal development. Neuropsychopharmacol **29:** 1988–1993.
27. GIEDD, J.N. *et al.* 1999. Brain development during childhood and adolescence: a longitudinal MRI study. Nat. Neurosci. **2:** 861–863.
28. ROMEO, R.D. & C.L. SISK. 2001. Pubertal and seasonal plasticity in the amygdala. Brain Res. **889:** 71–77.
29. TURNER, R.J. & D.A. LLOYD. 2004. Stress burden and the lifetime incidence of psychiatric disorder in young adults. Arch. Gen. Psychiatry **61:** 481–488.
30. AVITAL, A. *et al.* 2006. Effects of early-life stress on behavior and neurosteroid levels in the rat hypothalamus and entorhinal cortex. Brain Res. Bull. **68:** 419–424.
31. AVITAL, A. & G. RICHTER-LEVIN. 2004. Exposure of juvenile stress exacerbates the behavioural consequences of exposure to stress in the adult rat. Int. J. Neuropsychopharmacol. **8:** 1–11.
32. EICHENBAUM, H. 1997. Declarative memory: insights from cognitive neurobiology. Ann. Rev. Neurosci. **48:** 547–572.
33. GIEDD, J.N. *et al.* 1996. Quantitative MRI of the temporal lobe, amygdala, and hippocampus in normal human development: ages 4–18 years. J. Comp. Neurol. **366:** 223–230.
34. WATANABE, Y., E. GOULD & B.S. MCEWEN. 1992. Stress induces atrophy of apical dendrites of hippocampal CA3 pyramidal neurons. Brain Res. **588:** 341–345.
35. MCEWEN, B.S. 1999. Stress and hippocampal synaptic plasticity. Ann. Rev. Neurosci. **22:** 105–122.
36. MCKITTRICK, C.R. *et al.* 2000. Chronic social stress reduces dendritic arbors in CA3 hippocampus and decreases binding to serotonin transporter sites. Synapse **36:** 85–94.
37. BLACKSTAD, T.W. & A. KJAERHEIM. 1961. Special axo-dendritic synapses in the hippocampal cortex: electron and light microscopic studies on the layer of mossy fibers. J. Comp. Neurol. **117:** 133–159.
38. WOOLLEY, C.S., E. GOULD & B.S. MCEWEN. 1990. Exposure to excess glucocorticoids alters dendritic morphology of adult hippocampal pyramidal neurons. Brain Res. **531:** 225–231.

39. CONRAD, C.D. *et al.* 1999. Repeated restraint stress facilitates fear conditioning independently of causing hippocampal CA3 dendritic atrophy. Behav. Neurosci. **113:** 902–913.
40. CONRAD, C.D. *et al.* 1996. Chronic stress impairs rat spatial memory on the Y maze, and this effect is blocked by tianeptine pretreatment. Behav. Neurosci. **110:** 1321–1334.
41. WATANABE, Y. *et al.* 1992. Tianeptine attenuates stress-induced morphological changes in the hippocampus. Eur. J. Pharmacol. **222:** 157–162.
42. WATANABE, Y. *et al.* 1992. Phenytoin prevents stress- and corticosterone-induced atrophy of CA3 pyramidal neurons. Hippocampus **2:** 431–435.
43. WOOD, G.E. *et al.* 2004. Stress-induced structural remodeling in hippocampus: prevention by lithium treatment. Proc. Natl. Acad. Sci. USA **101:** 3973–3978.
44. SOTRES-BAYON, F., C.K. CAIN & J.E. LEDOUX. 2006. Brain mechanisms of fear extinction: historical perspectives on the contribution of prefrontal cortex. Biol. Psychiatry. **60:** 329–336.
45. RADLEY, J.J. *et al.* 2006. Repeated stress induces dendritic spine loss in the rat medial prefrontal cortex. Cerebral Cortex **16:** 313–320.
46. RADLEY, J.J. *et al.* 2004. Chronic behavioral stress induces apical dendritic reorganization of pyramidal neurons of the medial prefrontal cortex. Neuroscience **125:** 1–6.
47. WELLMAN, C.L. 2001. Dendritic reorganization in pyramidal neurons in medial prefrontal cortex after chronic corticosterone administration. J. Neurobiol. **49:** 245–253.
48. RADLEY, J.J. *et al.* 2005. Reversibility of apical dendritic retraction in the rat medial prefrontal cortex following repeated stress. Exp. Neurol. **196:** 199–203.
49. LISTON, C. *et al.* 2006. In review. Stress-induced alterations in prefrontal cortical dendritic morphology predict selective impairments in perceptual attentional set-shifting. J. Neurosci. **26:** 7870–7874.
50. BIRRELL, J.M. & V.J. BROWN. 2000. Medial frontal cortex mediates perceptual attentional set shifting in the rat. J. Neurosci. **20:** 4320–4324.
51. LEDOUX, J.E. 2000. Emotion circuits in the brain. Ann. Rev. Neurosci. **23:** 155–184.
52. VYAS, A. *et al.* 2002. Chronic stress induces contrasting patterns of dendritic remodeling in hippocampus and amygdala neurons. J. Neurosci. **22:** 6810–6818.
53. VYAS, A., S. BERNAL & S. CHATTARJI. 2003. Effects of chronic stress on dendritic arborization in the central and extended amygdala. Brain Res. **965:** 290–294.
54. VYAS, A. & S. CHATTARJI. 2004. Modulation of different states of anxiety-like behavior by chronic stress. Behav. Neurosci. **118:** 1450–1454.
55. VYAS, A., A.G. PILLAI & S. CHATTARJI. 2004. Recovery after chronic stress fails to reverse amygdaloid neuronal hypertrophy and enhanced anxiety-like behavior. Neuroscience **128:** 667–673.
56. VAN EEKELEN, J.A., M.C. BOHN & E. R. DE KLOET. 1991. Postnatal ontogeny of mineralocorticoid and glucocorticoid receptor gene expression in regions of the rat tel- and diencephalon. Dev. Brain Res. **61:** 33–43.
57. ROMEO, R.D. 2005. Neuroendocrine and behavioral development during puberty: a tale of two axes. Vitam. Horm. **71:** 1–25.
58. ROMEO, R.D., H.N. RICHARDSON & C.L. SISK. 2002. Puberty and the maturation of the male brain and sexual behavior: recasting a behavioral potential. Neurosci. Biobehav. Rev. **26:** 379–389.

59. TWIGGS, D.G., H.B. POPOLOW & A.A. GERALL. 1978. Medial preoptic lesions and male sexual behavior: age and environmental interactions. Science **200:** 1414–1415.
60. HEIMER, L. & K. LARSSON. 1966/1967. Impairment of mating behavior on male rats following lesions of the preoptic-anterior hypothalamic continuum. Brain Res. **3:** 248–263.
61. MORLEY-FLETCHER, S. *et al.* 2003. Environmental enrichment during adolescence reverses the effects of prenatal stress on play behaviour and HPA axis reactivity in rats. Eur. J. Neurosci. **18:** 3367–3374.
62. LAVIOLA, G. *et al.* 2004. Beneficial effects of enriched environment on adolescent rats from stressed pregnancies. Eur. J. Neurosci. **20:** 1655–1664.
63. MEANEY, M.J. 2001. Maternal care, gene expression, and the transmission of individual differences in stress reactivity across generations. Ann. Rev. Neurosci. **24:** 1161–1192.
64. PRYCE, C.R. *et al.* 2005. Long-term effects of early-life environmental manipulations in rodents and primates: potential animal models in depression research. Neurosci. Biobehav. Rev. **29:** 649–674.
65. BREDY, T.W. *et al.* 2004. Peripubertal environmental enrichment reverses the effects of maternal care on hippocampal development and glutamate receptor subunit expression. Eur. J. Neurosci. **20:** 1355–1362.
66. BREDY, T.W. *et al.* 2003. Partial reversal of the effect of maternal care on cognitive function through environmental enrichment. Neuroscience **118:** 571–576.
67. FRANCIS, D.D. *et al.* 2002. Environmental enrichment reverses the effects of maternal separation on stress reactivity. J. Neurosci. **22:** 7840–7843.

Effects of Therapeutic Interventions for Foster Children on Behavioral Problems, Caregiver Attachment, and Stress Regulatory Neural Systems

PHILIP A. FISHER,[a,b] MEGAN R. GUNNAR,[c] MARY DOZIER,[d]
JACQUELINE BRUCE,[a] AND KATHERINE C. PEARS[a]

[a]*Oregon Social Learning Center, Eugene, Oregon, USA*

[b]*Center for Research to Practice, Eugene, Oregon, USA*

[c]*University of Minnesota, Minneapolis, Minnesota, USA*

[d]*University of Delaware, Newark, Delaware, USA*

ABSTRACT: Young children in foster care are exposed to high levels of stress. These experiences place foster children at risk for poor social, academic, and mental heath outcomes. The role of adverse events in stimulating neurobiological stress responses presumably plays a role in shaping neural systems that contribute to these problems. Systematic and developmentally well-timed interventions might have the potential to change developmental trajectories and promote resilience. Moreover, understanding how specific dimensions of early adversity affect underlying stress response systems and how alterations in these systems are related to later psychosocial outcomes might facilitate more precise and targeted interventions. Data are drawn from two ongoing randomized trials involving foster infants/toddlers and preschoolers. Consistent with prior animal models of early adversity, these studies have shown that early adversity—particularly neglect, younger age at first foster placement, and higher number of placements—is associated with altered hypothalamic-pituitary-adrenal (HPA) axis function. The interventions under investigation have produced evidence that it is possible to impact many areas that have been negatively affected by early stress, including HPA axis activity, behavior, and attachment to caregivers.

KEYWORDS: adrenocorticotropic hormone (ACTH); cortisol; hypothalamic-pituitary-adrenal (HPA) axis; stress; stress hyporesponsive period (SHRP)

Address for correspondence: Dr. Philip A. Fisher, Oregon Social Learning Center, 10 Shelton McMurphey Blvd., Eugene, OR 97401-4928. Voice: 541-485-2711; fax: 541-485-7087.
e-mail: philf@oslc.org

Ann. N.Y. Acad. Sci. 1094: 215–225 (2006).
doi: 10.1196/annals.1376.023

INTRODUCTION

In a society in which approximately 900,000 children are reported to be maltreated every year,[1] foster care is a necessary societal institution. It is also a much-maligned institution in which shortcomings and failures often garner considerable negative public scrutiny and successes frequently go unnoticed. The tasks with which the U.S. foster care system and the larger national child welfare system are charged are monumental: to investigate alleged child maltreatment and protect children from further maltreatment; to ensure that physical and psychological needs of children in care are met; and to provide services to parents necessary to achieve permanent and stable living circumstances. Numerous studies comparing foster children to nonmaltreated children have found elevated rates of psychopathology, developmental delays, substance abuse, and mortality among individuals placed in foster care.[2–4] There is also an apparent intergenerational transmission of risk for foster care involvement: individuals placed in care as children are more likely to have their own children placed in care.[5]

Although many foster children fare poorly, others appear to emerge relatively unscathed. Little scientific knowledge exists about which variables direct life course trajectories toward poor versus healthy adjustment in these children. In the context of two ongoing studies of foster children, involving infants and toddlers[6] and preschoolers,[7] we have worked to address these issues. This research, guided by a network of basic and applied scientists,[8] has had two primary emphases. First, we have synthesized prior animal and human research on the neurobiology of early adversity into a model that specifies underlying neural mechanisms hypothesized to mediate the association between stress and later outcomes. Second, we have applied this model to research on caregiver-based interventions foster care. In this article we describe elements of the model and show how ongoing randomized trials to evaluate the efficacy of the interventions are being employed to test the validity of the model.

THE NEUROBIOLOGY OF STRESS AND EARLY ADVERSITY

More than half a century of research on rodents and nonhuman primates has demonstrated that disruption in early parental care exerts a profound and lasting impact on brain development, gene expression, and vulnerability to later stress, anxiety, and affective disorders.[9] These studies have applicability to the foster care population and might indicate a window into basic mechanisms of risk in foster children. Although requiring cross-species translation and caution in drawing conclusions that are applicable to human experience, these studies have the potential to guide research toward far more precise linkages than have been established between specific dimensions of adverse early experience and later outcomes among foster children.

One neurobiological pathway that has been the focus of much of this preclinical research is the hypothalamic-pituitary-adrenal (HPA) axis. The HPA axis is activated in response to physical and psychological stressors. HPA axis activation involves a hormonal cascade in which corticotrophin-releasing hormone (CRH), secreted in the paraventricular nucleus (PVN) of the hypothalamus, stimulates the release of adrenocorticotropic hormone (ACTH) in the anterior pituitary, which enters the bloodstream and ultimately stimulates the release of glucocorticoids (cortisol in humans and nonhuman primates; corticosterone in rodents) in the adrenal cortex. Glucocorticoids in turn exert negative feedback on the upstream structures, slowing the release of ACTH and CRH.[10]

Glucocorticoids have numerous additional effects throughout the body, including stimulation of the immune system and metabolism of stored energy. In the brain, glucocorticoids act through two types of receptors—mineralocorticoid (MR) and glucocorticoid (GR). MRs primarily maintain a homeostatic balance of neurotransmitters to neurons; in contrast, GRs are involved in stress responding, limiting the impact of other biological stress responses and facilitating return to prestress functioning following exposure to stress. Although GR actions are critical to stress regulation, this system operates optimally only in response to acute, short-term stressors. Exposure to chronic, long-term stress has been shown to have a negative impact on the HPA axis and other neural and bodily systems.[11]

The HPA axis functions in concert with a number of other neural pathways in the regulation of stress responses. These include a second CRH pathway, emanating from the central nucleus of the amgydala (CeA), which is involved in threat detection and response. The CeA–CRH pathway has indirect connections to the HPA axis via the bed nucleus of the stria terminalis (BNST) and direct connections to the norepinephrine (NE) system via the locus coeruleus. NE is critical in supporting anxiety and fear responding. In addition, bidirectional linkages exist between the amygdala and areas of the medial prefrontal cortex (mPFC), which is involved in executive cognitive functioning, particularly the modulation of emotions and stress hormones (cortisol and adrenaline). Elsewhere,[8] we describe the interrelationships among these stress regulatory neural pathways, and their implications for understanding early adversity effects in humans. For this article, we concentrate on the HPA axis.

Studies of rodents, using experimental paradigms in which pups are separated from their mothers at varying time points and for varying intervals postparturition, have documented long-term effects of disrupted caregiving on HPA axis function. Gunnar *et al.*[8] have synopsized the results of these studies into three areas. First, the timing of the disruption to maternal care is likely to be of key importance. In particular, maternal separation during the first 1 to 2 weeks of life often appears to have the greatest impact on the development of the HPA axis. One explanation that has been offered for this is that there is extensive GR gene methylation during this developmental period in rodents that is clearly associated with maternal licking and grooming.[12] Methylation of the GR gene results in it being inactivated and unavailable for stress modulation. In the absence of maternal care, or at lower levels of such care, there is more methylation and consequently less GR gene transcription (and fewer GRs). As is noted above, GRs play a central role in the regulation of neural stress responses; thus lowered potential for GRs would be expected to produce problematic outcomes. (It is interesting to note that the 1- to 2-week postparturition period in rodents corresponds roughly to the final trimester of pregnancy and early postnatal period in humans, suggesting that the effects of prenatal stress should be an emphasis in human studies of early adversity.)

Second, permanent alterations in HPA axis function are most likely to stem from events that occur during the stress hyporesponsive period (SHRP) of development. The SHRP in rodents occurs during the first 2 postnatal weeks and is believed to be critical in the development of neural circuitry involved in learning, memory, and stress responsivity. The presence of this period is marked by an absence of HPA axis activation in response to external stress.[11] Notably, studies of humans responding to laboratory and everyday stressors suggest that a much longer SHRP might exist, emerging in infancy and persisting until the onset of adolescence;[8] however, this is an area of emerging knowledge in which cross-species translation of results is quite challenging. Additional research on normative and at-risk human populations will help to specify time points across this broad developmental span in which disruptions in care have more or less impact.

Third, the buffering from stress that occurs during the SHRP is caregiver mediated.[13] Thus, disruptions in care during the SHRP appear to have the most pervasive effect on HPA axis function. A similar buffering role of supportive caregiving has been obtained in children. When children are in out-of-home care, cortisol levels tend to rise over the day, and this rise is sharper for younger children (toddlers) and children who receive less supportive care from their child care provider(s).[14] Similarly, children in insecure attachment relationships are more likely than those in secure relationships to show elevations in cortisol when they encounter mildly threatening events (e.g., getting their childhood inoculations or being confronted by an intrusive stranger).[14,15] In sum, the availability of a sensitive, responsive, and supportive caregiver during human infancy and childhood appears to be required to buffer the individual and the developing HPA axis from the negative effects of mild everyday threats and stressors.

IMPLICATIONS FOR CHILDREN IN FOSTER CARE

The implications of these studies for foster children run counter to some prevalent beliefs about this population. To summarize, in the rodent SHRP, the pup is unable to regulate competent physiological response to stressors independently and is therefore dependent on maternal care for stress modulation.

The absence of such a parental regulator during this time period renders the pup vulnerable to environmental adversity in ways that have the potential to permanently affect neurobiology and behavior. Although in the rat SHRP appears to extend from the postnatal into the late prenatal period in humans, the SHRP in humans appears to have a wider window, perhaps due to evolutionary influences that allow human children to use relationships with parents and other supportive adults to modulate stress for much longer in brain and behavioral development. Thus, in humans, the unavailability of a caregiver to serve as a stress regulator until a child is able to competently manage stressors more independently could have similar negative effects.

In the case of foster children, physical abuse and sexual abuse are often the focus of treatment efforts, as these events are deeply traumatic and can interfere with subsequent functioning in a number of ways. However, the above summary suggests that *the absence of a responsive, supportive caregiver to serve an external extension of the child's stress regulatory system* might have the most pervasive long-term effects on the child. There are a number of circumstances common in the lives of foster children in which a sufficient caregiving regulatory system might not be present. These include being severely neglected in the family of origin, being placed in foster care with a nonresponsive caregiver, and experiencing multiple brief foster placements with unexpected moves. Given this, we hypothesize that it is among children who have had these experiences that we will see the greatest impact on HPA axis functioning and the least resiliency in the face of subsequent stressful events.

If the absence of a caregiver to modulate responses to adversity has significant negative effects during infancy and childhood, perhaps introducing an external source of stress regulation during this same period has the potential to reverse any of these early adversity effects. There is some evidence from rodent studies that remediation of early adversity effects on neural development is possible.[16] However, in the context of foster care, this is not a simple task. Simply placing children in foster care might not be a sufficient intervention, as not all foster parents can provide responsive, supportive care. This might not be due solely to foster parent limitations but also to the foster child's ability to communicate distress and more generally to accept the caregiver as a source of external regulation.[17]

Although placement in foster care might not prove a sufficient remedy to the effects of early adversity in the absence of an adequate caregiving regulatory system, it represents an opportunity. If foster parents are able to develop a relationship with the child that allows adequate stress regulation to occur, progress might be possible. Inasmuch as parenting is malleable, it might be possible to develop systematic interventions to help facilitate these processes. Our work has been based on the supposition that foster caregiver–based interventions might help to provide foster children with the necessary caregiver–child regulatory system to protect children from deleterious consequences of adversity and to support the development of the child's internal stress and emotion regulatory capacity; as this capability develops, we hypothesize that changes in other domains will also be observable.

In the remainder of this article, we present relevant evidence from our ongoing research. First, we show that rates of atypical HPA axis activity are higher in foster children than in the general population. We then show that neglect and other experiences associated with lack of a caregiver who can serve as stress regulator are associated with alterations in HPA axis activity. Finally, we present evidence suggesting that foster children who show altered HPA axis activity show improvements in neurobehavioral functioning in the context of therapeutic caregiver-based interventions designed to address these underlying deficits.

One clarification is necessary: to date, we have focused on the daytime diurnal activity of the HPA axis, in particular on a blunting of the daily rhythm in cortisol levels in toddlers and preschoolers due to atypically low morning cortisol. Such blunting, which has been suggested to be a consequence of exposure to chronic as opposed to acute stress,[18] is likely the result of downregulation of hypothalamic CRH in response to frequent HPA axis activation[19] and downregulation of pituitary CRH receptors.[20] Such blunting has also been observed among young children living in institutional orphanages in Russia and Romania[21] and in toddlers within a month following their adoption from Russian and Chinese orphanages.[22] It is important to acknowledge that this sort of blunting in response to chronic stress does not presuppose that low levels of cortisol will also be observed in the same individuals in response to acute stressors. For example, Kaufman *et al.*[23] observed hyperresponding during a CRH challenge among depressed, abused children who were subject to ongoing emotional maltreatment. Given the ages of the children in our studies and the vulnerability of this population, examination of responses to laboratory stressors has not yet been possible.

CORTISOL LEVELS IN FOSTER INFANTS, TODDLERS, AND PRESCHOOLERS

As is noted above, the work described here occurred within the context of two ongoing longitudinal studies of children in foster care. Research by Fisher and colleagues[7] included a sample of 117 foster children (FC) who were in the age range of 3 to 5 years and entering a new foster placement at entry into their study and a low-income, same-aged comparison sample of 60 community children (CC). Research by Dozier and colleagues[6] included a sample of 60 foster infants and toddlers (less than 20 months old when first placed in care and 20–60 months old at entry into the study) and a comparison sample of 110 same-aged, nonmaltreated community children. Both investigators evaluated the impact of therapeutic caregiver-based interventions. The work by Fisher involved dividing the foster children roughly in half at entry into the study, assigning them to foster care intervention (FCI) or regular foster care

(RFC) conditions. Dozier's work involved a second foster care sample (n = 60) randomly assigned to one of two intervention groups at intake.

LOW MORNING CORTISOL LEVELS AMONG FOSTER CHILDREN

Analyses of baseline data from both studies have revealed atypical diurnal patterns of cortisol production in foster children. Most notable is the higher proportion of FC with low cortisol values. Bruce *et al.*[24] classified children into high (>0.60 μg/dL), average (0.30–0.60 μg/dL), or low (<0.30 μg/dL) morning cortisol groups based on upper and lower quartile values for the overall sample. In total, 32% of the FC were classified as having low morning cortisol, whereas 14% of the CC had low morning cortisol. In contrast, 61% of the CC had average morning cortisol, whereas 42% of the FC had average morning cortisol. There was a significant group difference in cortisol classification, Pearson $\chi^2(2, 176) = 8.00$, $P < 0.05$, with FC being more likely to have low morning cortisol than CC, Pearson $\chi^2(1, 176) = 6.73$, $P < 0.01$, and CC more likely to have average morning cortisol, Pearson $\chi^2(1, 176) = 5.75$, $P < 0.05$. The percentage of children classified as high did not differ across the two groups, Pearson $\chi^2(1, 176) = 0.02$, *ns*.

Very similar results were obtained by Dozier *et al.*,[25] who classified children into high, average, and low cortisol groups based on extreme values at morning, afternoon, or bedtime cortisol collections (>2 SD above the CC group M for high; <1 SD below the CC group M for low). Differences between groups were observed, Pearson χ^2 (159) = 16.06, $P < 0.001$, $\phi = 0.32$, $P < 0.001$. In total, 38% and 18% of FC showed low and high patterns of cortisol production, respectively, compared with only 14% and 11% of CC.

ASSOCIATIONS BETWEEN EARLY ADVERSITY AND LOW CORTISOL

As is discussed above, one component of the conceptual model is that alterations in HPA axis functioning occur in the context of disruptions in care. These can arise due to a caregiver who is unattentive to the child's needs or to frequent transitions in caregivers. Bruce *et al.*[24] used the maltreatment classification system (MCS)[26] and child welfare placement records to test these hypotheses. The MCS allows for categorization of incidents of maltreatment according to type and severity. Types of maltreatment defined in the MCS include physical abuse, sexual abuse, failure to provide, lack of supervision, and emotional maltreatment. Consistent with the conceptual model, one-way analyses of variance (ANOVAs) indicated that morning cortisol classification (low, average, or high) was significantly related to the severity of failure to provide, $F(2, 114) = 4.01$, $P < 0.05$. Children with low morning cortisol levels had significantly more severe failure to provide instances than children with average or high cortisol levels, $t(84) = 2.15$, $P < 0.05$, and $t(66) = 2.68$, $P < 0.01$. In contrast, there were no main effects for morning cortisol classification on the number of maltreatment incidents, $F(2, 114) = 0.23$, *ns*, the number of different types of maltreatment experienced, $F(2, 114) = 0.03$, *ns*, the mean severity of physical abuse, $F(2, 114) = 0.29$, *ns*, the mean severity of sexual abuse, $F(2, 114) = 0.10$, *ns*, or lack of supervision, $F(2, 114) = 0.04$, *ns*. Also consistent with the conceptual model, separate analyses found that FC who had four or more prior foster placements, $F(2, 173) = 3.44$, $P < 0.05$, and FC first placed in care before the age of 2 years, $F(2, 173) = 3.23$, $P < 0.05$, had significantly lower morning cortisol than other FC or CC. It is notable that, when the maltreatment and placement variables were included in the analysis, failure to provide emerged as the significant predictor of low morning cortisol, whereas the placement variables did not.

EFFECTS OF FOSTER CARE INTERVENTIONS ON PROMOTING RESILIENCY

The interventions that have been the focus of the research described here focus on distinct age groups. Dozier's Attachment and Biobehavioral Catch-Up study is designed for infants and toddlers, whereas Fisher's Multidimensional Treatment Foster Care for Preschoolers (MTFC-P) study is designed for 3- to 5-year-olds. Although the treatment techniques and theoretical frameworks for these approaches differ, the interventions are strongly linked in targeting developmental issues that prevent foster caregivers from becoming a reliable resource for modulating stress and arousal. Dozier's study focuses on improving the caregivers' ability to detect signals of distress from the child—even when these signals are ambiguous or unclear—and to respond sensitively and to follow the child's lead. Fisher's study emphasizes supporting caregivers to respond consistently and contingently to positive and negative behavior. In both cases, an underlying assumption of the conceptual model is that, by supporting the foster parent–child relationship, adverse effects of early stress on the HPA axis and related neural systems will be reversed and that this will in turn increase the potential for improvements in psychosocial functioning.

Evidence from the randomized trials evaluating these interventions provides support for these assertions. Among FCI children with low morning cortisol, there was a significant Condition × Time interaction for change in morning cortisol levels measured at entry into the study and at 8–9 months postentry, $F(2, 32) = 3.91$, $P < 0.05$. *Post hoc* analyses revealed that the cortisol levels of the FCI, RFC, and CC groups of children did not differ at entry, $F(2, 42) = 0.01$, *ns*. However, by 8–9 months postentry, the FCI and CC groups had significantly higher cortisol levels than the RFC group, $F(2, 32) = 3.92$, $P < 0.05$. Furthermore, among those with low morning cortisol, only FCI had a significant increase in cortisol from entry into the study to 8–9 months postentry.[24] In addition to these group differences, parallel effects were observed in two related domains. Fisher and Kim[27] reported improvements in attachment security and decreases in avoidant attachment as (assessed by Dozier's Attachment Diary) for FCI children but not for RFC children. FCI children also had significantly fewer permanent placement failures than RFC following their time in foster care.[7] Dozier *et al.*[6] also noted intervention effects on cortisol. In her study, children in regular foster care showed diurnal cortisol patterns (as assessed by morning and bedtime salivary cortisol measures) that were significantly different from the intervention and community comparison groups postintervention. Fewer behavior problems were also observed on a caregiver-report measure for toddlers than for infants in the intervention group postintervention, but no age differences in behavior problems were observed for the regular foster care group.

SUMMARY AND CONCLUSIONS

Taken together, these studies provide evidence that caregiver-based interventions can help normalize HPA axis function, and that such changes co-occur with improved behavioral functioning. This is noteworthy, first, because it represents preliminary validation of a translational model derived largely from rodent studies of early stress. This model, as is discussed above, emphasizes the importance of the caregiver as an extension of the infant's regulatory system whose actions buffer or protect the infant from potentially deleterious effects of external stressors, thus promoting resiliency. In the absence of such caregiving, alterations in HPA axis activity appear likely to occur. Second, these studies show that, by supporting more responsive, competent caregiving in the context of foster care, some of these early adversity effects might be reversible.

In spite of the progress that this research represents, extensive work remains. First, the HPA axis is just one system known to be affected by early stress. Understanding whether similar results are possible in related structures, such as the amygdala and the medial prefrontal cortex, will be critical to the validation of a more comprehensive translational model of early adversity. Second, although changes in behavioral and biological systems have been documented in our studies, little is known about the temporal sequence of change in these domains. It will be important to develop a knowledge base about whether changes in stress regulatory neural systems occur prior to, simultaneously with, or after changes in behavior. Third, this research we have summarized here does not incorporate molecular genetics. Identifying genes that increase or decrease the stress vulnerability of neurobiological systems will increase the precision of our explanatory models. Finally, although we have emphasized children who show disturbances in HPA axis and/or behavioral functioning in foster care, many children do not show such disturbances. Our understanding of resiliency will be further enhanced by studying children who, despite early maltreatment and out-of-home placement, seem to function adequately without additional support. In sum, this research represents only the initial iteration of a translational process. Additional iterations will be required to clarify associations between the effects of early stress on neurobiology, and subsequent outcomes.

ACKNOWLEDGMENT

The support for this research was provided by the following grants: MH59780, NIMH, U.S. PHS; MH65046, NIMH, U.S. PHS; and MH52135, NIMH, U.S. PHS.

REFERENCES

1. National Clearinghouse on Child Abuse and Neglect Information. 2005. Child maltreatment 2003: summary of key findings. Retrieved February 22, 2006, from http://nccanch.acf.hhs.gov/pubs/factsheets/canstats.cfm.
2. Burns, B.J. *et al.* 2004. Mental health need and access to mental health services by youth involved with child welfare: a national survey. J. Am. Acad. Child Adolesc. Psychiatry **43:** 960–970.
3. Juon, H.S., M.E. Ensminger & M. Feehan. 2003. Childhood adversity and later mortality in an urban African American cohort. Am. J. Public Health **93:** 2044–2046.
4. Leslie, L.K. *et al.* 2004. Outpatient mental health services for children in foster care: a national sample. Child Abuse Negl. **28:** 699–714.
5. Roman, N. & P. Wolfe. 1997. The relationship between foster care and homelessness. Public Welfare **55:** 4–9.
6. Dozier, M. *et al.* 2006. Developing evidence-based interventions for foster children: an example of a randomized clinical trial with infants and toddlers. J. Soc. Iss. **62:** 767–786.
7. Fisher, P.A., B. Burraston & K. Pears. 2005. The early intervention foster care program: permanent placement outcomes from a randomized trial. Child Maltr. **10:** 61–71.
8. Gunnar, M.R., P.A. Fisher & The Early Experience, Stress, and Prevention Science Network. 2006. Bringing basic research on early experience and stress neurobiology to bear on preventive intervention research on neglected and maltreated children. Dev. Psychopathol.: **18:** 651–677.
9. Levine, S. 2005. Stress: an historical perspective. *In* Handbook on Stress, Immunology and Behavior. T. Steckler, N. Kalin & J.M.H.M. Reul, Eds.: 1–30. Elsevier Press. Amsterdam, the Netherlands.
10. Herman, J.P. & W.E. Cullinan. 1997. Neurocircuitry of stress: central control of the hypothalamo-pituitary-adrenocortical axis. Trends Neurosci. **20:** 78–84.
11. Sapolsky, R.M. & M.J. Meaney. 1986. Maturation of the adrenocortical stress response: neuroendocrine control mechanisms and the stress hyporesponsive period. Brain Res. Rev. **11:** 65–76.
12. Meaney, M. & M. Szyf. 2005. Environmental programming of stress responses through DNA methylation: life at the interface between a dynamic environment and a fixed genome. Dialogues Clin. Neurosci. **7:** 103–123.
13. Rosenfeld, P., D. Suchecki & S. Levine. 1992. Multifactorial regulation of the hypothalamic-pituitary-adrenal axis during development. Neurosci. Biobeh. Rev. **16:** 553–568.

14. GUNNAR, M. & B. DONZELLA. 2002. Social regulation of the cortisol levels in early human development. Psychoneuroendocrinology **27:** 199–220.
15. NACHMIAS, M. *et al.* 1996. Behavioral inhibition and stress reactivity: moderating role of attachment security. Child Dev. **67:** 508–522.
16. FRANCIS, D. *et al.* 2002. Environmental enrichment reverses the effects of maternal separation on stress reactivity. J. Neurosci. **22:** 7840–7843.
17. DOZIER, M., K.C. STOVALL & K.E. ALBUS. 1999. Attachment and psychopathology in adulthood. *In* Handbook of Attachment: Theory, Research, and Clinical Applications. J. Cassidy & P.R. Shaver, Eds.: 497–519. Guilford. New York.
18. FRIESE, E. *et al.* 2005. A new view on hypocortisolism. Psychoneuoendocrinology **30:** 1010–1016.
19. MAKINO, S., P.W. GOLD & J. SCHULKIN. 1994. Corticosterone effects on corticotropin-releasing hormone mRNA in the central nucleus of the amygdala and the parvocellular region of the paraventricular nucleus of the hypothalamus. Brain Res. **640:** 105–112.
20. HEIM, C., P. PLOTSKY & C.B. NEMEROFF. 2004. The importance of studying the contributions of early adverse experiences to the neurobiological findings in depression. Neuropsychopharmacology **29:** 641–648.
21. GUNNAR, M. & D.M. VAZQUEZ. 2001. Low cortisol and a flattening of expected daytime rhythm: potential indices of risk in human development. Dev. Psychopathol. **13:** 515–538.
22. BRUCE, J. *et al.* 2000. The relationships between cortisol patterns, growth retardation, and developmental delays in post-institutionalized children. Presented at the International Conference on Infant Studies. Brighton, UK, July.
23. KAUFMAN, J. *et al.* 1997. The corticotropin-releasing hormone challenge in depressed abused, depressed nonabused, and normal control children. Biol. Psychiatry **42:** 669–679.
24. BRUCE, J. *et al.* 2006. Morning cortisol levels in preschool-aged foster children: Differential effects of maltreatment type. Manuscript submitted for publication.
25. DOZIER, M. *et al.* 2006. Foster children's diurnal production of cortisol: an exploratory study. Child Maltr.: **11:** 189–197.
26. BARNETT, D., J.T. MANLY & D. CICCHETTI. 1993. Defining child maltreatment: the interface between policy and research. *In* Child Abuse, Child Development, and Social Policy. D. Cicchetti, S.L. Toth & I.E. Sigel, Eds.: 7–73. Ablex. Westport, CT.
27. FISHER, P.A. & H.K. KIM. 2006. Intervention effects on foster preschoolers' attachment-related behaviors from a randomized trial. *Prevention Sci.*: In press.

Psychobiological Processes of Stress and Coping

Implications for Resilience in Children and Adolescents—Comments on the Papers of Romeo & McEwen and Fisher *et al.*

BRUCE E. COMPAS

Department of Psychology & Human Development, Vanderbilt University, Nashville, Tennessee, USA

ABSTRACT: The significance of psychosocial stress and ways of coping with stress for understanding resilience in childhood and adolescence are reviewed. Psychological and biological processes of reactivity to and recovery from stress are central in understanding the physical and emotional tolls that result from prolonged exposure to chronic stress. A central theme of this article is that stress exerts a double toll on physical and emotional health and well-being. First, as a consequence of allostatic load, stress contributes to disease and disorder. And second, because of effects on specific brain regions, chronic stress takes a second toll by disrupting function in those regions primarily responsible for coping and self-regulation. Implications for future research on resilience and the development of interventions to promote resilience are highlighted.

KEYWORDS: allostatic load; amygdale; coping theory; sympathetic-adrenal-medullary (SAM) axis; hypothalamic-pituitary-adrenal (HPA) axis; resilience; stress

Psychosocial stress plays a central role in models of resilience in children and adolescents.[1–4] Exposure to major and minor stressful events and chronic conditions of adversity are primary sources of risk for mental and physical health problems in development. Resilience is defined, in part, as the ability to sustain adaptive functioning and positive growth and development in the face of significant stress and adversity. Therefore, understanding biological and

Address for correspondence: Bruce E. Compas, Department of Psychology & Human Development, Vanderbilt University, Peabody 512, 230 Appleton Place, Nashville, TN 37203. Voice: 615-322-8306; fax: 615-343-9494.

e-mail: bruce.compas@vanderbilt.edu

**Ann. N.Y. Acad. Sci. 1094: 226–234 (2006). © 2006 New York Academy of Sciences.
doi: 10.1196/annals.1376.024**

psychological processes that are involved in stress and responses to stress can provide important clues to distinguishing resilient from vulnerable individuals.

Substantial evidence suggests that stress takes a double toll on the ability of children and adolescents to sustain resilience in the face of prolonged stress and adversity. First, psychosocial stress initiates a series of biological and psychological processes captured by the concept of *allostatic load*.[5] Allostatic load, or the cost of wear and tear on the body produced by repeated activation of biological stress response systems, contributes to physical disease and emotional and behavioral disorder.[6] The effects of allostatic load include a second, less well-recognized but pernicious process that is reflected in the toll that stress takes on specific brain regions, including the hippocampus and the regions of the prefrontal cortex (PFC).[7] Furthermore, the brain regions most adversely affected by chronic stress are the very portions of the brain that are most responsible for effective coping and adaptation to stress.[8] Thus, the direct effects of chronic stress may be compounded by impairments in the ability to effectively cope with stress. Understanding these processes requires the integration of research on the biological and psychological processes through which stress affects individuals at multiple levels of analysis. Along this line, it has been 10 years since Taylor, Repetti, and Seeman [9] posed the question, "What is an unhealthy environment and how does it get under the skin?" With advances in research methods and technology and significant new findings from basic research, researchers are now poised to push this question further to ask, "What is an unhealthy (stressful) environment and how does it get under the skin, inside the brain, and inside of a cell?"

PSYCHOBIOLOGY OF STRESS

Psychological stress is the result of responses that are both within and outside of an individual's awareness. For example, animal and human research has highlighted the role of the amygdala in responding to threatening stimuli and fear conditioning.[10] These processes are rapid and can be triggered by emotionally threatening stimuli presented for very brief durations (e.g., 20 msec) and outside of the individual's awareness.[11] In addition to the rapid responses initiated by the amygdala, environmental events and conditions also activate psychological stress through conscious appraisal of threat and harm.[12] These conscious processes of stress appraisal are slower to transpire and are subject to substantial misinterpretation of the actual threat-value of the environment. Thus, consistent with the perspective of Taylor *et al.*,[9] stress "gets under the skin" by activating conscious and nonconscious processes in the brain that signal threat or harm to physical and/or psychological well-being.

A number of complex biological processes are set in motion in response to exposure to stress that form the basis for adaptation and survival in the face of adversity, threat, and challenge. The two primary mammalian neuroendocrine stress response systems are the sympathetic-adrenal-medullary (SAM) axis and the hypothalamic-pituitary-adrenal (HPA) axis.[13] Both of these systems are innervated by the amygdala and the hippocampus, and are partially modulated by activity in the regions of the PFC. Thus, both the rapid, automatic activation that occurs in the amygdala and the slower conscious processes of appraisal that occur in the PFC can activate and modulate the SAM and HPA axes. Activation of the SAM axis occurs rapidly in response to stress to prepare the body to make a sudden physical reaction of either approach (fight) or escape (flight). Epinephrine and norepinephrine (catecholamines) are released by the medulla of the adrenal gland and lead to increases in heart rate, respiration, blood flow, and blood pressure, and a concomitant decrease in activity in the digestive system. HPA axis activation occurs somewhat more slowly than in the SAM axis and involves a cascade of hormonal processes in which corticotrophin-releasing hormone (CRH), secreted in the paraventricular nucleus (PVN) of the hypothalamus, stimulates the release of adrenocorticotropic hormone (ACTH) in the anterior pituitary. ACTH then enters the bloodstream and ultimately leads to the release of glucocorticoids (cortisol in humans and nonhuman primates) in the adrenal cortex. Glucocorticoids in the bloodstream also exert negative feedback on the upstream structures, slowing the release of ACTH and CRH.[13]

Early descriptions of the mammalian stress response emphasized a broad, undifferentiated set of biological and behavioral reactions.[14] However, the HPA and SAM axes and other aspects of the human stress response show high levels of specificity in reactivity to and recovery from stress. With regard to *activation* of the stress systems, for example, decades of laboratory research with humans has shown that the HPA axis shows the greatest level of activation in response and the longest time to recovery in response to stressors that involve motivated performance, present a threat to self-evaluation, and are uncontrollable to the individual.[15] The prototype of a laboratory stressor that leads to HPA activation is the Trier Social Stress Test (TSST) in which the individual is required to engage in a hypothetical task that involves being evaluated by others.[16] There also appears to be specificity in the process of biological *recovery* from stress. For example, the HPA and SAM axes appear to follow different patterns of habituation to repeated stress. Schommer *et al.*[17] found that more than three administrations of the TSST, the HPA axis became nonresponsive while the SAM axis continued to show a classic pattern of stress activation. Thus, to determine the role of stress biology in processes of resilience (and vulnerability), careful attention must be given to the type and duration of stress that an individual encounters.

As noted above, these systems have evolved to allow for feedback and self-regulation. The PFC, hippocampus, and amygdala all are densely populated with receptors that, when stimulated, downregulate the hypothalamus and decrease production of CRH. Although glucocorticoids act on the brain through both mineralocorticoid receptors and glucocorticoid receptors, glucocorticoid receptors are most centrally involved in the regulation of stress responses, as they modulate other biological stress responses and facilitate recovery from stress through return to baseline (prestress) functioning. The HPA and SAM axes operate optimally only in response to acute, short-term stressors. Chronic stress, or prolonged allostatic load, however, takes a significant toll on these systems.[5]

At least two aspects of stress exposure lead to adverse effects on the brain and components of the stress response system. First, HPA activity is affected by early stress and adversity. Work by Fisher and colleagues has provided important evidence that early adversity, especially disruptions to the primary caregiving environment, can lead to long-term disregulation of HPA responses to stress.[18,19] For example, Dozier *et al.*[20] examined daytime patterns of cortisol production among young children placed into foster care as contrasted with children not in foster care. Saliva samples were taken at wake-up, afternoon, and bedtime for 2 days and average salivary cortisol values for each time of day were computed. These researchers found that children who had been in foster care had higher incidences of atypical patterns of cortisol production than children who had not. These differences suggest that conditions associated with foster care interfere with children's ability to regulate neuroendocrine functioning. Specifically, it is hypothesized that unstable caretaking environments fail to provide the level of environmental support that is needed for the development of regulated responding by the HPA axis.

Second, prolonged exposure to stress, and concomitantly, prolonged activation of the stress axes, is linked to neural degeneration in specific brain regions, most notably areas of the PFC and the hippocampus. The seminal work of McEwen and colleagues has shown that prolonged exposure to stress leads to atrophy and impaired neuronal function in the hippocampus and the medial PFC.[7,21,23] For example, Radley *et al.*[23] showed that repeated restraint stress in rats led to significant loss of dendritic spine density and length in pyramidal neurons in the medial PFC. Similarly, Isgor *et al.*[21] found that chronic variable stress led to decreased hippocampal volume in peripubertal rats. Both of these regions contain high levels of glucocorticoid receptors and when stimulated these receptors lead to downregulation of the HPA. However, these studies suggest that if the system remains activated by repeated and prolonged exposure to stress, the system breaks down leading to neuronal atrophy and cell death. Perhaps even more importantly, the effects of prolonged stress on the brain are not random, as most pronounced effects occur in brain regions that are responsible for higher order executive functions that are central in successful adaptation to stress.

PSYCHOBIOLOGY OF COPING

Individuals are not passive victims of stress and adversity. Upon exposure to stress, complex cognitive, behavioral, emotional, and biological processes are set in motion that serve the purpose of adaptation through either avoiding/withdrawing from the source of stress, acting on the source of stress to reduce its effects, or adjusting to the source of stress when neither escape nor confrontation are possible. These processes have been most often studied within the general rubric of *coping*. Research on coping with stress has a long and rich history.[24] However, much of this work has been undermined by several limitations in research methodology and in the conceptualization of the coping process. Problems with coping research include overreliance on a single methodology, self-report checklists, to assess the construct; failure to clearly specify the context in which coping efforts are enacted; and failure to distinguish coping from other processes of responses to stress, most importantly automatic stress responses that are typically referred to within the construct of stress reactivity.

Building on previous coping theory and research, we have proposed a dual-process model of responses to stress.[8,25] Two fundamental processes are involved in self-regulation in response to stress. First, there is a set of automatic processes that are activated in response to stress that are related to but distinct from coping. As noted above, automatic responses to stress may be triggered by activation of the amygdala in response to threat in the environment. Examples of automatic responses to stress include physiological and emotional arousal, intrusive thoughts, impulsive action, emotional numbing, and some forms of escape behavior.[25] Second, individuals initiate a set of controlled, volitional responses to stress. It is these voluntary responses to stress that are included in the concept of coping. We define coping as "conscious volitional efforts to regulate emotion, cognition, behavior, physiology, and the environment in response to stressful events or circumstances" (Compas *et al.*,[25] p. 89). These regulatory processes both draw on and are constrained by the biological, cognitive, social, and emotional development of the individual. An individual's developmental level both contributes to the resources that are available for coping, and limits the types of coping responses the individual can enact. Coping is a subset of broader self-regulatory processes, with coping referring to regulatory efforts that are volitionally and intentionally enacted specifically in response to stress. Recent confirmatory factor analytic studies have supported a model of coping that includes three primary subtypes: primary control coping, or efforts to directly act on the source of stress or one's emotions (problem solving, emotional expression, emotion modulation); secondary control coping, or efforts to adapt to the source of stress (acceptance, distraction, cognitive restructuring, positive thinking); and disengagement coping, or efforts to withdraw from the source of stress and one's emotions (avoidance, denial, wishful thinking).[26–28]

Advances in methods to examine brain and central nervous system structure and function have now provided the tools to study both the neurobiological structure and processes that underlie coping and adaptation to stress. Evidence is accumulating that coping is a part of the overall set of executive functions that are regulated by the PFC. For example, in a study of adolescents, Copeland and Compas [29] found that both primary control (e.g., problem solving) and secondary control (e.g., cognitive restructuring, acceptance) engagement coping strategies were related to neuropsychological measures of inhibitory control, whereas disengagement coping (e.g., avoidance) was related to poorer performance on measures of inhibition. Furthermore, mediation analyses found that primary and secondary control coping mediated the association between inhibition and externalizing behavior problems. These findings suggest that inhibitory control may be an important cognitive mechanism for understanding self-regulatory strategies under stressful situations.[29] Using a free-vision task to measure left and right hemispheric activation (based on orientation to the left vs. right visual field), Flynn and Rudolph [30] found that secondary control coping and involuntary disengagement stress responses (e.g., emotional numbing, cognitive interference) mediated the association between reduced posterior right hemispheric bias and depressive symptoms in adolescents. These studies provide some of the first evidence for the link between coping and executive functions of the PFC.

If coping is indeed an executive function that is regulated by the PFC and related brain regions, then research showing the adverse effects of prolonged and chronic stress on these brain regions suggests that chronic stress would lead to impairments in the ability to cope. Consistent with this hypothesis, several studies using parents' and adolescents' reports of adolescents' coping suggest that coping becomes less effective under conditions of greater stress.[27–29] Specifically, all of these studies have found that as the level of stress increases, the use of primary control and secondary control coping decreases.[31,32]

Pediatric Oncology: Moving from the Exception to the Rule

A more dramatic example of the relation between executive function and coping can be found in research on survivors of childhood cancer. Although cancer remains a relatively rare disease in children, affecting approximately 15 in 100,000 children and 12,400 new diagnoses each year in the United States,[33] findings from studies of neurocognitive function and coping in these children may help inform a broader understanding of the neurobiology of coping. Survival rates of childhood cancer, especially acute lymphocytic leukemia (ALL) have increased dramatically in the last 15 years, due in part to the administration of high doses of intrathecal chemotherapy delivered directly into the cerebral spinal fluid to prevent metastases in the brain. In spite of the remarkable improvement in survival, these treatments are not without some costs. Chemotherapeutic agents (e.g., anthracyclines) are designed to identify fast growing cells (such as cancer cells) and either preventing them from dividing out of control or by promoting cell death. However, other fast growing cells may be adversely affected. The effects of intrathecal chemotherapy (including dexamethazone, a synthetic glucocorticoid) include neurocognitive impairment, including deficits in working memory.[34] Thus, the negative side effects of chemotherapy may mimic the effects of chronic stress on the developing brain and offer an opportunity to examine the consequences of such damage on the ability to cope with stress. Recent work has shown that working memory function in childhood ALL survivors is significantly correlated with their ability to cope with stress.[35] Specifically, working memory was negatively correlated with children's use of secondary control coping ($r = -0.56$, $P < 0.01$) and positively related to the use of disengagement coping ($r = 0.46$, $P < 0.01$), suggesting that impairments in working memory were associated with impairments in coping.[35]

IMPLICATIONS FOR INTERVENTION

Interventions that are designed to enhance resilience in children and adolescents are informed by the research described above on the effects of stress on HPA reactivity and the effects of chronic stress and HPA activity on the PFC. First, early interventions to address deficits in the caretaking environment of young children can potentially ameliorate the impact of early adversity and deprivation. Fisher *et al.*[36] reported on a pilot study of the effectiveness of the Early Intervention Foster Care (EIFC) program in the period immediately following a preschool child's placement in a new foster home. Data were collected from an EIFC group (mean age 5.35 years), a regular foster care group, and a community comparison group via salivary cortisol sampling. EIFC children's behavioral adjustment improved and changes occurred in several salivary cortisol measures. Moreover, regular foster care children exhibited decrements in functioning in several areas over the same time period. And second, interventions that can simultaneously reduce children's exposure to significant sources of stress and adversity while simultaneously enhancing children's skills for coping and adaptation in the face of stress may have two pathways to enhance resilience.[37] The integration of research on social contextual and biological processes of stress and coping shows great promise to inform and enhance interventions to promote resilience in children and adolescents.

REFERENCES

1. LUTHAR, S.S., Ed. 2003. Resilience and Vulnerability: Adaptation in the Context of Childhood Adversities. Cambridge University Press. New York.
2. LUTHAR, S.S. 2006. Resilience in development: a synthesis of research across five decades. *In* Developmental Psychopathology, Vol. 3: Risk, Disorder and Adaptation (2nd ed.). D. Cecchetti & D.J. Cohen, Eds.: 739–795. John Wiley. Hoboken, NJ.
3. MASTEN, A.S. 2001. Ordinary magic: resilience processes in development. Am. Psych. **56:** 227–238.

4. WRIGHT, M.O. & A.S. MASTEN. 2005. Resilience processes in development: fostering positive adaptation in the context of adversity. *In* Handbook of Resilience in Children. S. Goldstein & R.B. Brooks, Eds.: 17–37. Kluwer Academic/Plenum Publishers. New York.
5. MCEWEN, B.S. 1998. Protective and damaging effects of stress mediators. N. Eng. J. Med. **338:** 171–179.
6. MCEWEN, B.S. 2003. Early life influences on life-long patterns and behavior and health. Ment. Retard. Dev. Disabil. Res. Rev. **9:** 149–154.
7. MCEWEN, B.S. 2005. Glucocorticoids, depression, and mood disorders: structural remodeling in the brain. Metab. Clin. Exp. **54:** 20–23.
8. COMPAS, B.E. 2004. Processes of risk and resilience during adolescence: linking individuals and contexts. *In* Handbook of Adolescent Psychology, 2nd ed. R. Lerner & L. Steinberg, Eds.: 263–296. John Wiley. New York.
9. TAYLOR, S.E., R.L. REPETTI & T. SEEMAN. 1997. Health psychology: what is an unhealthy environment and how does it get under the skin? Ann. Rev. Psych. **48:** 411–447.
10. DAVIS, M. & P.J. WHALEN. 2001. The amygdala: vigilance and emotion. Mol. Psychia. **6:** 13–34.
11. WHALEN, P.J., J. KAGAN, R.G. COOK, *et al.* 2004. Human amygdala responsivity to masked fearful eye whites. Science **306**(no. 5704): 2061.
12. GAAB, J., N. ROHLEDER, U.M. NATER, *et al.* 2005. Psychological determinants of the cortisol stress response: the role of anticipatory cognitive appraisal. Psychoneuroendocrinology **30:** 599–610.
13. HERMAN, J.P. & W.E. CULLINAN. 1997. Neurocircuitry of stress: central control of the hypothalamo-pituitary-adrenocortical axis. Trends Neurosc. **20:** 78–84.
14. SELYE, H. & C. FORTIER. 1950. Adaptive reaction to stress. Psychosom. Med. **12:** 149–157.
15. DICKERSON, S.S. & M.E. KEMENY. 2004. Acute stressors and cortisol responses: a theoretical integration and synthesis of laboratory research. Psych. Bull. **130:** 355–391.
16. KIRSCHBAUM, C., S. WÜST & D.H. HELLHAMMER. 1992. Consistent sex differences in cortisol responses to psychological stress. Psychosom. Med. **54:** 648–657.
17. SCHOMMER, N.C., D.H. HELLHAMMER & C. KIRSCHBAUM. 2003. Dissociation between reactivity of the hypothalamus-pituitary-adrenal axis and the sympathetic-adrenal-medullary system to repeated psychosocial stress. Psychosom. Med. **65:** 450–460.
18. BRUCE, J., J.A. FISHER, K.C. PEARS, *et al.* 2006. Morning cortisol levels in preschool-aged foster children: differential effects of maltreatment type. Manuscript submitted for publication.
19. DOZIER, M., M. MANNI, M.K. GORDON, *et al.* 2006. Foster children's diurnal production of cortisol: an exploratory study. Child Maltreat: J. Am. Prof. Soc. Abuse Children. **11:** 189–197.
20. FISHER, P.A., M.R. GUNNAR, M. DOZIER, *et al.* 2006. Effects of therapeutic interventions for foster children on behavioral problems, caregiver attachment, and stress regulatory neural systems.
21. ISGOR, C., M. KABBAJ, H. AKIL, *et al.* 2004. Delayed effects of chronic variable stress during peripubertal juvenile period of hippocampal morphology and on cognitive and stress axis functions in rats. Hippocampus **24:** 636–648.

22. RADLEY, J.J., H.M. SISTI, J. HAO, *et al.* 2004. Chronic behavioral stress induces apical dendritic reorganization in pyramidal neurons of the medial prefrontal cortex. Neuroscience **125:** 1–6.
23. RADLEY, J.J., A.B. ROCHER, M. MILLER, *et al.* 2006. Repeated stress induces dendritic spine loss in the rat medial prefrontal cortex. Cereb. Cortex. **16:** 313–320.
24. SKINNER, E.A., K. EDGE, J. ALTMAN, *et al.* 2003. Searching for the structure of coping: a review and critique of category systems for classifying ways of coping. Psych. Bull. **129:** 216–269.
25. COMPAS, B.E., J.K. CONNOR-SMITH, H. SALTZMAN, *et al.* 2001. Coping with stress during childhood and adolescence: progress, problems, and potential in theory and research. Psych. Bull. **127:** 87–127.
26. COMPAS, B.E., M.C. BOYER, C. STANGER, *et al.* 2006. Latent variable analysis of coping, anxiety/depression, and somatic symptoms in adolescents with chronic pain. J. Cons. Clin. Psych. **74:** 1132–1142.
27. CONNOR-SMITH, J.K., B.E. COMPAS, A.H. THOMSEN, *et al.* 2000. Responses to stress: measurement of coping and reactivity in children and adolescents. J. Cons. Clin. Psych. **68:** 976–992.
28. WADSWORTH, M.E., T. REICKMANN, M. BENSON, *et al.* 2004. Coping and responses to stress in Navajo adolescents: psychometric properties of the Responses to Stress Questionnaire. J. Comm. Psych. **32:** 391–411.
29. COPELAND, W. & B.E. COMPAS. 2006. Neuropsychological correlates of coping: the role of executive inhibition. Manuscript submitted for publication.
30. FLYNN, M. & K.D. RUDOLPH. Perceptual asymmetry and youth's responses to stress: understanding vulnerability to stress. Cog. Emot. In press.
31. JASER, S.S., A.M. LANGROCK, G. KELLER, *et al.* 2005. Coping with the stress of parental depression ii: adolescent and parent reports of coping and adjustment. J. Clin. Child Adolesc. Psych. **34:** 193–205.
32. WADSWORTH, M.E. & B.E. COMPAS. 2002. Coping with family conflict and economic strain: the adolescent perspective. J. Res. Adolesc. **12:** 243–274.
33. NATIONAL CANCER INSTITUTE. 2002. Young people with cancer: a handbook for parents. Available from http://www.cancer.gov.
34. CAMPBELL, L.L., M. SCADUTO, W. SHARP, *et al.* A meta-analysis of the neurocognitive sequelae of treatment for childhood acute lymphocytic leukemia. Pediatr. Blood Cancer. In press.
35. CAMPBELL, L.K., M. SCADUTO, J.A. WHITLOCK & B.E. COMPAS. 2006. The role of working memory in coping with stress in survivors of childhood cancer. Paper presented at Psychosocial and Neurocognitive Consequences of Childhood Cancer Conference at St. Jude Children's Research Hospital, September13–15, Memphis, TN.
36. FISHER, P.A., M.R. GUNNAR, P. CHAMBERLAIN, & J.B. REID. 2000. Preventive intervention for maltreated preschool children: impact on children's behavior, neuroendocrine activity, and foster parent functioning. J. Am. Acad. Child Adolesc. Psychiatry **39:** 1356–1364.
37. COMPAS, B.E., A.M. LANGROCK, G. KELLER, *et al.* 2001. Children coping with parental depression: processes of adaptation to family stress. *In* Children of Depressed Parents: Alternative Pathways to Risk for Psychopathology. S. Goodman & I. Gotlib, Eds.: 227–252. American Psychological Association. Washington, DC.

Prevention of Pediatric Bipolar Disorder

Integration of Neurobiological and Psychosocial Processes

KIKI CHANG, MEGHAN HOWE, KIM GALLELLI, AND DAVID MIKLOWITZ

Pediatric Bipolar Disorders Program, Department of Psychiatry and Behavioral Sciences, Stanford University School of Medicine, Stanford, California, USA

ABSTRACT: Bipolar disorder (BD) is a prevalent condition in the United States that typically begins before the age of 18 years and is being increasingly recognized in children and adolescents. Despite great efforts in discovering more effective treatments for BD, it remains a difficult-to-treat condition with high morbidity and mortality. Therefore, it appears prudent to focus energies into developing interventions designed to *prevent* individuals from ever fully developing BD. Such interventions early in the development of the illness might prevent inappropriate interventions that may worsen or hasten development of BD, delay the onset of first manic episode, and/or prevent development of full BD. Studies of populations at high-risk for BD development have indicated that children with strong family histories of BD, who are themselves experiencing symptoms of attention-deficit/hyperactive disorder (ADHD) and/or depression or have early mood dysregulation, may be experiencing prodromal states of BD. Understanding the neurobiological and genetic underpinnings that create risk for BD development would help with more accurate identification of this prodromal population, which could then lead to suitable preventative interventions. Such interventions could be pharmacologic or psychosocial in nature. Reductions in stress and increases in coping abilities through psychosocial interventions could decrease the chance of a future manic episode. Similarly, psychotropic medications may decrease negative sequelae of stress and have potential for neuroprotective and neurogenic effects that may contribute to prevention of fully expressed BD. Further research into the biologic and environmental mechanisms of BD development as well as controlled early intervention studies are needed to ameliorate this significant public health problem.

Address for correspondence: Kiki D. Chang, M.D., Stanford University School of Medicine, Division of Child and Adolescent Psychiatry, 401 Quarry Road, Stanford, CA 94305-5540. Voice: 650-725-0956; fax: 650-723-5531.
e-mail: kchang88@stanford.edu

Ann. N.Y. Acad. Sci. 1094: 235–247 (2006).
doi: 10.1196/annals.1376.026

KEYWORDS: bipolar disorders; children; prevention; neurobiology; genetics

INTRODUCTION

Bipolar disorder (BD) affects up to 4% of the U.S. population[1] and leads to costs of more than $45 billion per year.[2] A total of 25–50% of individuals with BD attempt suicide at least once, and 8.6–18.9% die by suicide.[3] Suicidal risk appears highest in childhood-onset BD,[4] with nearly one-third of children and adolescents with BD already having had a suicide attempt.[5] Between 15% and 28% of bipolar adults experience illness onset before the age of 13 years, and between 50% and 66% before the age of 19 years.[6–8] The exact prevalence in children is unknown, but estimates range from 420,000–2,072,000 among U.S. children alone.[9] Onset of BD in childhood or adolescence confers a more severe, adverse, and continuously cycling course of illness than adult-onset, typically with more mixed episodes, psychosis, and comorbid disorders.[10] The complexity of early-onset BD, especially given high rates of comorbidity with attention-deficit/hyperactive disorder (ADHD), conduct disorder, anxiety disorders, and substance abuse, usually makes these patients more treatment-refractory than adults with BD.[8,11,12] Thus, pediatric-onset BD patients are often severely derailed in social, academic, and emotional development.

In the last decade, much research has gone into discovering effective pharmaco- and psychotherapies to treat BD in children and adults. However, despite these efforts, BD remains difficult to treat. Furthermore, morbidity and mortality have not appreciably improved over the last 20 years,[13,14] which likely reflects the chronic disabling nature of the disorder and the fact that other than lithium, medications used to treat this disorder have all originally been developed to treat other conditions. Therefore, it appears prudent to focus energies into developing interventions designed to *prevent* individuals from ever fully developing BD. Such interventions early in the development of the illness might prevent inappropriate interventions that may worsen or hasten development of BD, delay the onset of first manic episode, and/or prevent development of full BD.

IDENTIFICATION OF PRODROMAL PEDIATRIC BD

Before intervention studies can take place, methods for detecting a suitable high-risk population must be determined. It is clear that a family history of BD elevates risk for BD.[15] As twin and family studies report a 59-87% heritability of BD, first-degree relatives of probands with BD are at very high risk of BD themselves.[16] Therefore, these relatives are a good starting point for identifying children and adolescents at high-risk for BD development.

High-Risk Studies

Children of parents with BD (bipolar offspring) are a logical population in which to implement preventative interventions. A meta-analysis of studies conducted before 1997 found that offspring of parents with BD were at 2.7 times higher risk for development of any psychiatric disorder and 4 times higher risk for developing a mood disorder than children of parents without psychiatric illness.[17] Recent studies have found that 50–60% of such offspring have some type of psychiatric disorder,[18–20] especially mood, anxiety, and disruptive behavior disorders.[18–21] Rates of BD spectrum disorders in these offspring range from 14–50%, and rates of major depressive disorder (MDD) range from 7 to 43%.[22]

Putative Prodromal BD

Symptom complexes predating the first manic episode can be identified from studies of high-risk samples. The high rate of MDD in bipolar offspring raises the distinct possibility that those children are experiencing an initial bipolar depression, and will experience a manic episode in the near future. In fact, the most reliable symptom complex predating mania has been depression. In a cohort of 642 adults with BD onset before the age of 18 years, approximately 60% reported depression as their initial mood episode.[8] Prospective studies have found high rates (20–30%) of switching to mania in children who initially presented with prepubertal MDD.[23,24] The rate of conversion to BD in depressed children who are offspring of bipolar parents is even greater. In a 5-year prospective study of 129 children of bipolar parents, 12 of the 13 offspring who developed BD had an antecedent depressive episode.[25]

ADHD in bipolar offspring also may be a harbinger of later BD development.[8,18,22,26–28] In recent cross-sectional studies, approximately 27% of bipolar offspring have met criteria for ADHD or significant behavioral or attention problems.[22] This finding, combined with the high comorbidity of ADHD and BD in childhood,[29] family studies,[29,30] and retrospective histories of ADHD predating BD onset,[18,31] supports that ADHD in certain children with strong family histories of BD is a first sign of developing BD.

Given the above epidemiological and phenomenological data, it appears that children with ADHD and/or depression who have strong family histories of BD are at high risk for BD development. The few longitudinal studies published also have supported this hypothesis.[21,32,33] However, it is also likely that not all these children will develop full BD, and that some may never progress to this point. Therefore, diagnostic tools other than symptom complexes and family history would be helpful in diagnosing BD before mania onset. The most logical tools to pursue currently are neurobiological and genetic markers of the disorder.

NEUROBIOLOGICAL MARKERS

Despite this profile of BD prodromes in children, it is far from certain at what rates these children will develop full BD. Furthermore, by the time children present with such symptomatology, it may be relatively late in illness development for ideal intervention as a preventative measure. Therefore, other diagnostic tools, such as biological markers, would be helpful in identifying children at highest risk for BD. Neurobiological markers are a logical choice, but currently there are no neurobiological findings that are pathognomonic of BD. Identification of the brain characteristics most highly associated with BD development, along with the genetic factors that affect their development, could lead to early identification of those at highest risk for BD development and a better understanding of the pathophysiology of BD.

Neuroimaging studies in adults and children with BD have implicated numerous regions of the brain in the pathophysiology of BD, namely regions serving prefrontal-limbic circuitry.[34] Prefrontal areas include dorsolateral prefrontal cortex (DLPFC), medial prefrontal cortex (including anterior cingulate cortex), and ventrolateral (or orbitofrontal) cortex.[35] Subcortical areas include hippocampus, caudate, putamen, thalamus, and amygdala. The amygdala is particularly interesting due to its role in mood and emotion, and consistent findings of decreased amygdalar volume in children with BD.[36–39] However, this finding is not specific to BD[40] and currently cannot be used diagnostically. Nonetheless, prefrontal amygdalar circuits are good candidates for further study in this regard. Other potential tools for marker discovery include magnetic resonance spectroscopy (MRS),[41] fMRI,[42–44] and diffusion tensor imaging (DTI).[45]

GENETIC MARKERS

Genetic markers may also serve to help determine risk for BD as well as age at onset (AAO). It is becoming increasingly clear that BD is a polygenic disorder, with many genetic polymorphisms creating small risk for BD individually, presenting together to generate increased risk for BD.[46,47] These polymorphisms could be used to help quantify risk for BD development.

For example, two potential BD gene candidates code for the serotonin transporter (5-HTT) and for brain-derived neurotrophic growth factor (BDNF). Polymorphisms of these genes have been associated with depression and BD (including early-onset and rapid-cycling varieties).[48–53] However, because these polymorphisms are relatively common in the population, they likely have gross overarching effects on the brain (such as general changes in serotonergic transmission, or varied availability of BDNF), thus creating only small risk for BD by themselves. However, by a summation of various at-risk genes, it is possible that a certain level of quantification for genetic risk of BD can be achieved.

Nonetheless, it is the proteins coded by the genes, which then influence brain functioning, that are relevant to understanding how risk leads to disorder. Thus, it is useful to study the effect of genes on brain structure and function, both in "healthy" individuals as well as those with BD.[54] For example, subjects with compared to those without the short allele of the 5-HTT gene have been found to have increased amygdalar and orbitofrontal activation when watching fearful faces or aversive pictures.[55,56] This finding is interesting in light of the amygdalar abnormalities found in BD, including amygdalar overactivity,[44,57,58] and the association of the short allele with BD.[51]

Finally, AAO genes could also be used to determine risk for early-onset BD specifically. While there has been some progress in this direction,[59] more research is needed. One promising area of research remaining is the possibility of trinucleotide repeat expansion in AAO regions of the chromosome, leading to anticipation of the disorder.[60] Discovery of such phenomena would again help elucidate the degree of urgency needed for intervention in at-risk youth.

EARLY INTERVENTION/NEUROPROTECTION

First applied to seizure disorders, the theory of kindling in affective disorder holds that the combination of psychosocial stress and genetic vulnerability gradually leads to a full mood episode, after which it becomes progressively "easier" to trigger subsequent episodes, until they become spontaneous.[61] Interventions early in the course of kindling may reverse the illness course. For example, rats given repeated subseizure level electrical stimulation to their amygdalae will eventually develop seizures, leading to a spontaneous seizure disorder. However, if the same rat is administered valproate prior to the onset of electrical stimulation, no seizure disorder develops.[62] Thus, if similar interventions are performed early enough in bipolar illness development, it is possible that the full expression of BD could be completely averted.

Medications

Thus, medications have the potential to prevent BD due to antikindling effects. Another mechanism by which they might act is to stimulate healthy neurogenesis. For example, it is becoming clearer that areas in the prefrontal cortex, as well as other limbic areas, suffer neurodegeneration with prolonged bipolar illness.[63–66] Stress from repeated mood episodes has been postulated to be causal to this process.[67,68] leading to less prefrontal mood regulation and greater cycling and treatment resistance.[43] Thus, an intervention that prevents this process or restores healthy neuronal circuits in these regions could have a combined effect on preserving prefrontal function and neuronal integrity and thus prevent or delay future mood episodes.

Mood stabilizers, and to some degree antipsychotics, which are used to treat BD, have been found to have neuroprotective and neurogenic properties. Antikindling (seizure prophylaxis) properties have been described in animals with valproate[69–71] and lamotrigine.[72] Other animal studies have indicated that both valproate and lithium increase brain bcl2 (a neuroprotective protein), and activate protein kinases, which lead to increased neural dendritic growth.[73,74] In humans, lithium may increase gray matter volume,[75] and exposure to lithium or valproate may prevent decreased gray matter volumes in anterior cingulate[76] or amygdala.[36] Both lamotrigine and olanzapine have been reported to lead to increases in prefrontal N-acetylaspartate, a marker of neuronal density and viability.[77,78]

Because of these properties, mood stabilizers and antipsychotics may prove to be effective medications in early intervention/prevention schemas. In one[79] but not another[80] study, valproate was found effective in treating acute mood symptoms in children with subsyndromal BD, considered a group at high risk for BD development. Quetiapine was also effective in treating mood symptoms in a similar population, with some evidence of prefrontal N-acetyl aspartate (NAA) increase as well.[81] However, no longitudinal studies have been conducted to investigate *prevention* of the occurrence of full mania with these types of agents. Clearly, while difficult to conduct, this type of study is paramount for discovering valid options for BD prevention.

Psychotherapy

Psychosocial stressors such as dysfunctional family environments, stressful life events, and ineffective coping strategies interact with genetic predispositions to induce the full expression of BD.[82] The mechanisms by which environmental threats affect the course of BD may involve psychological vulnerability factors (e.g., negative cognitive styles[83,95] or activation of brain circuitry involved in emotional self-regulation.[43] Specific psychotherapeutic interventions targeted at psychosocial risk factors in high-risk individuals may help prevent or delay the onset of BD.

Although requiring more time and effort than psychopharmacology, psychotherapy can be a precise, targeted intervention with sustained effects even after it is completed. Furthermore, whereas treatment with medication may be accompanied by deleterious side effects and cannot specifically treat psychosocial stressors, psychotherapy is a safe modality that can address specific stressors and correct behaviors that lead to mood episodes, such as irregular sleep patterns or medication nonadherence.

Specific psychotherapeutic interventions for high-risk individuals should ameliorate psychosocial vulnerability factors and enhance the at-risk person's coping ability to prevent or delay the onset of BD. Recent research has suggested that family environments characterized by high expressed emotion (EE) attitudes[84] or low maternal warmth[85] are associated with poorer outcomes of pediatric BD over 2–4 year follow-ups. In a sample of children of mothers with BD, maternal negativity contributed to risk for offspring BD development through its association with impaired frontal lobe functioning as measured by the Wisconsin Card Sorting Task.[86] Thus, maternal relationships in the context of family environment is one area to target for BD prevention.

Other strategies for reducing the likelihood of developing full BD can be inferred from data supporting the efficacy of psychosocial interventions for the prevention of relapse of mood episodes in patients already with BD.[84] It is currently recommended that patients with BD receive both medication and adjunct psychotherapy.[87,88] Thus, although extensive advances have been made in the pharmacological treatment of BD, it has become apparent that medication alone is not enough for the management of this chronic, recurrent illness. Medication noncompliance, lack of ability to recognize symptom exacerbation, and the inability to cope with stressors that precipitate illness episodes are problematic for many individuals with BD and are often related to illness relapse.[89,90]

Thus, potential psychotherapeutic interventions geared toward prevention of worsening to full BD could be based on current techniques geared toward prevention of mood episode relapse in patients already with full BD. Family focused therapy (FFT) has been found effective for adolescents with BD,[91] and would be a good candidate for modification for a high-risk population. Other promising candidates would be cognitive behavioral therapy (CBT)-type therapies[92] or more behaviorally oriented therapies for younger children,[93] both found useful in pediatric BD. Due to the highly familial nature of the disorder, a unique factor of these therapies could be the treatment of family members with BD-spectrum disorders, thus decreasing EE and stress in the family and theoretically decreasing BD risk in the at-risk family member(s). Such controlled studies in at-risk populations are clearly warranted.

CONCLUSIONS

It is the hope that a combination of brain and genetic markers, symptom complexes, and family history can lead to more accurate diagnoses of prodromal BD. Then early intervention could occur in a population at clear, perhaps even quantifiable, risk for BD development. Promising areas for further exploration of brain markers for this purpose include prefrontal-limbic areas, especially the amygdala. However, more understanding about how alterations in the relevant circuitry lead to bipolar symptoms would likely reveal markers more specific to BD than morphometric or neurochemical abnormalities by themselves. Furthermore, the neurobiological underpinnings of circadian rhythm disruption, fairly specific to BD, are vastly understudied. The search for AAO genes as well as additional genes that are linked to BD will help the early identification/prevention cause. Early-onset cohorts particularly should be studied to generate these candidate genes for prevention purposes.[94]

Intervention studies should not wait until these markers are definitively established, as the burden of BD is too great.[9] The neuroprotective and neurogenic properties of psychotropic medications are exciting: in the future the grim sentence of lifelong medications for patients with BD may be lifted if intervention with these agents, along with appropriate psychotherapies, is instituted early enough in the disorder evolution to halt the kindling process. A short, corrective course of these medications at the "right" time could also prevent prolonged exposure to them later in life. Controlled, long-term intervention studies in high-risk populations should therefore include biological and genetic assessment to more precisely match intervention with underlying neurobiology and genetic predisposition and to study effects of these interventions on brain function. Implementing psychotherapeutic and psychopharmacologic interventions that are placed upon such a neurobiological and genetic framework would be a powerful step toward the eventual eradication of this disorder.

REFERENCES

1. KESSLER, R.C. *et al.* 2005. Lifetime prevalence and age-of-onset distributions of DSM-IV disorders in the National Comorbidity Survey Replication. Arch. Gen. Psychiatry **62:** 593–602.
2. KLEINMAN, L. *et al.* 2003. Costs of bipolar disorder. Pharmacoeconomics **21:** 601–622.
3. CHEN, Y.W. & S.C. DILSAVER. 1996. Lifetime rates of suicide attempts among subjects with bipolar and unipolar disorders relative to subjects with other Axis I disorders. Biol. Psychiatry **39:** 896–899.
4. CARTER, T.D. *et al.* 2003. Early age at onset as a risk factor for poor outcome of bipolar disorder. J. Psychiatr. Res. **37:** 297–303.
5. GOLDSTEIN, T.R. *et al.* 2005. History of suicide attempts in pediatric bipolar disorder: factors associated with increased risk. Bipolar Disord. **7:** 525–535.
6. LEVERICH, G.S. *et al.* 2003. Factors associated with suicide attempts in 648 patients with bipolar disorder in the Stanley Foundation Bipolar Network. J. Clin. Psychiatry **64:** 506–515.
7. LEVERICH, G.S. *et al.* 2002. Early physical and sexual abuse associated with an adverse course of bipolar illness. Biol. Psychiatry **51:** 288–297.
8. PERLIS, R.H. *et al.* 2004. Long-term implications of early onset in bipolar disorder: data from the first 1000 participants in the systematic treatment enhancement program for bipolar disorder (STEP-BD). Biol. Psychiatry **55:** 875–881.
9. POST, R.M. & R.A. KOWATCH. 2006. The health care crisis of childhood-onset bipolar illness: some recommendations for its amelioration. J. Clin. Psychiatry **67:** 115–125.
10. GELLER, B. *et al.* 2002. Two-year prospective follow-up of children with a prepubertal and early adolescent bipolar disorder phenotype. Am. J. Psychiatry **159:** 927–933.

11. BIEDERMAN, J. *et al.* 2003. Current concepts in the validity, diagnosis and treatment of paediatric bipolar disorder. Int. J. Neuropsychopharmacol. **6:** 293–300.
12. BIEDERMAN, J. *et al.* 2003. Can a subtype of conduct disorder linked to bipolar disorder be identified? Integration of findings from the Massachusetts General Hospital Pediatric Psychopharmacology Research Program. Biol. Psychiatry **53:** 952–960.
13. ANGST, J. *et al.* 2005. Suicide in 406 mood-disorder patients with and without long-term medication: a 40 to 44 years' follow-up. Arch. Suicide Res. **9:** 279–300.
14. KASPER, S.F. 2004. Living with bipolar disorder. Expert Rev. Neurother. **4:** S9–S15.
15. FARAONE, S.V. & M.T. TSUANG. 2003. Heterogeneity and the genetics of bipolar disorder. Am. J. Med. Genet. C Semin. Med. Genet. **123:** 1–9.
16. SMOLLER, J.W. & C.T. FINN. 2003. Family, twin, and adoption studies of bipolar disorder. Am. J. Med. Genet. C Semin. Med. Genet. **123:** 48–58.
17. LAPALME, M., S. HODGINS & C. LAROCHE. 1997. Children of parents with bipolar disorder: a metaanalysis of risk for mental disorders. Can. J. Psychiatry **42:** 623–631.
18. CHANG, K.D., H. STEINER & T.A. KETTER. 2000. Psychiatric phenomenology of child and adolescent bipolar offspring. J. Am. Acad. Child Adolesc. Psychiatry **39:** 453–460.
19. CHANG, K. *et al.* 2003. Bipolar offspring: a window into bipolar disorder evolution. Biol. Psychiatry **53:** 945–951.
20. WALS, M. *et al.* 2001. Prevalence of psychopathology in children of a bipolar parent. J. Am. Acad. Child Adolesc. Psychiatry **40:** 1094–1102.
21. CARLSON, G.A. & S. WEINTRAUB. 1993. Childhood behavior problems and bipolar disorder—relationship or coincidence? J. Affect. Disord. **28:** 143–153.
22. CHANG, K.D. & H. STEINER. 2003. Offspring studies in child and early adolescent bipolar disorder. *In* Bipolar Disorder in Childhood and Early Adolescence. B. Geller & M. DelBello, Eds.: 107–129. The Guilford Press. New York.
23. GELLER, B., L.W. FOX & K.A. CLARK. 1994. Rate and predictors of prepubertal bipolarity during follow-up of 6- to 12-year-old depressed children [see comments]. J. Am. Acad. Child Adolesc. Psychiatry **33:** 461–468.
24. GELLER, B. *et al.* 2001. Adult psychosocial outcome of prepubertal major depressive disorder. J. Am. Acad. Child Adolesc. Psychiatry **40:** 673–677.
25. HILLEGERS, M.H. *et al.* 2005. Five-year prospective outcome of psychopathology in the adolescent offspring of bipolar parents. Bipolar Disord. **7:** 344–350.
26. EGELAND, J.A. *et al.* 2000. Prodromal symptoms before onset of manic-depressive disorder suggested by first hospital admission histories. J. Am. Acad. Child Adolesc. Psychiatry **39:** 1245–1252.
27. FERGUS, E.L. *et al.* 2003. Is there progression from irritability/dyscontrol to major depressive and manic symptoms? A retrospective community survey of parents of bipolar children. J. Affect. Disord. **77:** 71–78.
28. LISH, J.D. *et al.* 1994. The National Depressive and Manic-depressive Association (DMDA) survey of bipolar members. J. Affect. Disord. **31:** 281–294.
29. FARAONE, S.V. *et al.* 1997. Is comorbidity with ADHD a marker for juvenile-onset mania? J. Am. Acad. Child Adolesc. Psychiatry **36:** 1046–1055.
30. FARAONE, S.V. *et al.* 1997. Attention-deficit hyperactivity disorder with bipolar disorder: a familial subtype? J. Am. Acad. Child Adolesc. Psychiatry **36:** 1378–1387; discussion 1387–1390.

31. SACHS, G.S. *et al.* 2000. Comorbidity of attention deficit hyperactivity disorder with early- and late-onset bipolar disorder. Am. J. Psychiatry **157:** 466–468.
32. EGELAND, J.A. *et al.* 2003. Prospective study of prodromal features for bipolarity in well Amish children. J. Am. Acad. Child Adolesc. Psychiatry **42:** 786–796.
33. HODGINS, S. *et al.* 2002. Children of parents with bipolar disorder: a population at high risk for major affective disorders. *In* Child and Adolescent Psychiatric Clinics of North America, Vol. 11. G.A. Carlson & J.H. Kashani, Eds.: 533–554. W.B. Saunders Co. Philadelphia, PA.
34. STRAKOWSKI, S.M. *et al.* 2000. Neuroimaging in bipolar disorder. Bipolar Disord. **2:** 148–164.
35. STRAKOWSKI, S.M., M.P. DELBELLO & C.M. ADLER. 2005. The functional neuroanatomy of bipolar disorder: a review of neuroimaging findings. Mol. Psychiatry **10:** 105–116.
36. CHANG, K. *et al.* 2005. Reduced amygdalar gray matter volume in familial pediatric bipolar disorder. J. Am. Acad. Child Adolesc. Psychiatry **44:** 565–573.
37. DELBELLO, M.P. *et al.* 2004. Magnetic resonance imaging analysis of amygdala and other subcortical brain regions in adolescents with bipolar disorder. Bipolar Disord. **6:** 43–52.
38. DICKSTEIN, D.P. *et al.* 2005. Frontotemporal alterations in pediatric bipolar disorder: results of a voxel-based morphometry study. Arch. Gen. Psychiatry **62:** 734–741.
39. CHEN, B.K. *et al.* 2004. Cross-sectional study of abnormal amygdala development in adolescents and young adults with bipolar disorder. Biol. Psychiatry **56:** 399–405.
40. DELBELLO, M. & K. CHANG. 2005. Bipolar disorder in children and adolescents—are we approaching the final frontier? Bipolar Disord. **7:** 479–482.
41. ADLEMAN, N.E., N. BARNEA-GORALY & K.D. CHANG. 2004. Review of magnetic resonance imaging and spectroscopy studies in children with bipolar disorder. Expert Rev. Neurother. **4:** 69–77.
42. BLUMBERG, H.P. *et al.* 2003. Frontostriatal abnormalities in adolescents with bipolar disorder: preliminary observations from functional MRI. Am. J. Psychiatry **160:** 1345–1347.
43. CHANG, K. *et al.* 2004. Anomalous prefrontal-subcortical activation in familial pediatric bipolar disorder: a functional magnetic resonance imaging investigation. Arch. Gen. Psychiatry **61:** 781–792.
44. RICH, B.A. *et al.* 2006. Limbic hyperactivation during processing of neutral facial expressions in children with bipolar disorder. Proc. Natl. Acad. Sci. USA **103:** 8900–8905.
45. ADLER, C.M. *et al.* 2006. Evidence of white matter pathology in bipolar disorder adolescents experiencing their first episode of mania: a diffusion tensor imaging study. Am. J. Psychiatry **163:** 322–324.
46. SCHULZE, T.G. & F.J. MCMAHON. 2003. Genetic linkage and association studies in bipolar affective disorder: a time for optimism. Am. J. Med. Genet. C Semin Med. Genet. **123:** 36–47.
47. TSUANG, M.T., L. TAYLOR & S.V. FARAONE. 2004. An overview of the genetics of psychotic mood disorders. J. Psychiatr. Res. **38:** 3–15.
48. CASPI, A. *et al.* 2003. Influence of life stress on depression: moderation by a polymorphism in the 5-HTT gene. Science **301:** 386–389.
49. GELLER, B. *et al.* 2004. Linkage disequilibrium of the brain-derived neurotrophic factor Val66Met polymorphism in children with a prepubertal and early adolescent bipolar disorder phenotype. Am. J. Psychiatry **161:** 1698–1700.

50. Neves-Pereira, M. *et al.* 2002. The brain-derived neurotrophic factor gene confers susceptibility to bipolar disorder: evidence from a family-based association study. Am. J. Hum. Genet. **71:** 651–655.
51. Lasky-Su, J.A. *et al.* 2004. Meta-analysis of the association between two polymorphisms in the serotonin transporter gene and affective disorders. Am. J. Med. Genet. B. Neuropsychiatr. Genet. **133:** 110–115.
52. Lohoff, F.W. *et al.* 2005. Confirmation of association between the Val66Met polymorphism in the brain-derived neurotrophic factor (BDNF) gene and bipolar I disorder. Am. J. Med. Genet. B Neuropsychiatr. Genet. **139:** 51–53.
53. Green, E.K. *et al.* 2006. Genetic variation of brain-derived neurotrophic factor (BDNF) in bipolar disorder: case-control study of over 3000 individuals from the UK. Br. J. Psychiatry **188:** 21–25.
54. Hariri, A.R. & D.R. Weinberger. 2003. Functional neuroimaging of genetic variation in serotonergic neurotransmission. Genes Brain. Behav. **2:** 341–349.
55. Hariri, A.R. *et al.* 2002. Serotonin transporter genetic variation and the response of the human amygdala. Science **297:** 400–403.
56. Heinz, A. *et al.* 2005. Amygdala-prefrontal coupling depends on a genetic variation of the serotonin transporter. Nat. Neurosci. **8:** 20–21.
57. Chen, C.H. *et al.* 2006. Explicit and implicit facial affect recognition in manic and depressed states of bipolar disorder: a functional magnetic resonance imaging study. Biol. Psychiatry **59:** 31–39.
58. Yurgelun-Todd, D.A. *et al.* 2000. fMRI during affect discrimination in bipolar affective disorder. Bipolar Disord. **2:** 237–248.
59. Faraone, S.V. *et al.* 2004. Three potential susceptibility loci shown by a genome-wide scan for regions influencing the age at onset of mania. Am. J. Psychiatry **161:** 625–630.
60. O'Donovan, M., I. Jones & N. Craddock. 2003. Anticipation and repeat expansion in bipolar disorder. Am. J. Med. Genet. C Semin. Med. Genet. **123:** 10–17.
61. Post, R.M. 1992. Transduction of psychosocial stress into the neurobiology of recurrent affective disorder. Am. J. Psychiatry **149:** 999–1010.
62. Post, R.M. 2002. Do the epilepsies, pain syndromes, and affective disorders share common kindling-like mechanisms? Epilepsy Res. **50;** 203–219.
63. Manji, H.K. & R.S. Duman. 2001. Impairments of neuroplasticity and cellular resilience in severe mood disorders: implications for the development of novel therapeutics. Psychopharmacol. Bull. **35:** 5–49.
64. Gallelli, K.A. *et al.* 2005. N-acetylaspartate levels in bipolar offspring with and at high-risk for bipolar disorder. Bipolar Disord. **7:** 589–597.
65. Rajkowska, G., A. Halaris & L.D. Selemon. 2001. Reductions in neuronal and glial density characterize the dorsolateral prefrontal cortex in bipolar disorder. Biol. Psychiatry **49:** 741–752.
66. Strakowski, S.M. *et al.* 2002. Ventricular and periventricular structural volumes in first- versus multiple-episode bipolar disorder. Am. J. Psychiatry **159:** 1841–1847.
67. Hashimoto, K., E. Shimizu & M. Iyo. 2004. Critical role of brain-derived neurotrophic factor in mood disorders. Brain Res. Brain Res. Rev. **45:** 104–114.
68. Rajkowska, G. 2000. Postmortem studies in mood disorders indicate altered numbers of neurons and glial cells. Biol. Psychiatry **48:** 766–777.
69. Loscher, W. *et al.* 1989. Valproic acid in amygdala-kindled rats: alterations in anticonvulsant efficacy, adverse effects and drug and metabolite levels in various brain regions during chronic treatment. J. Pharmacol. Exp. Ther. **250:** 1067–1078.

70. POST, R.M. & S.R. WEISS. 1996. A speculative model of affective illness cyclicity based on patterns of drug tolerance observed in amygdala-kindled seizures. Mol. Neurobiol. **13:** 33–60.
71. SILVER, J.M., C. SHIN & J.O. MCNAMARA. 1991. Antiepileptogenic effects of conventional anticonvulsants in the kindling model of epilespy. Ann. Neurol. **29:** 356–363.
72. STRATTON, S.C. *et al.* 2003. Effects of lamotrigine and levetiracetam on seizure development in a rat amygdala kindling model. Epilepsy Res. **53:** 95–106.
73. MANJI, H.K. & R.H. LENOX. 1999. Ziskind-Somerfeld Research Award. Protein kinase C signaling in the brain: molecular transduction of mood stabilization in the treatment of manic-depressive illness. Biol. Psychiatry **46:** 1328–1351.
74. MANJI, H.K., G.J. MOORE & G. CHEN. 2000. Clinical and preclinical evidence for the neurotrophic effects of mood stabilizers: implications for the pathophysiology and treatment of manic-depressive illness. Biol. Psychiatry **48:** 740–754.
75. MOORE, G.J. *et al.* 2000. Lithium-induced increase in human brain grey matter. Lancet **356:** 1241–1242.
76. DREVETS, W.C. *et al.* 1997. Subgenual prefrontal cortex abnormalities in mood disorders. Nature **386:** 824–827.
77. CHANG, K. *et al.* 2005. Prefrontal neurometabolite changes following lamotrigine treatment in adolescents with bipolar depression. 44th Annual Meeting of the American College of Neuropsychopharmacology, Dec 11–15, Waikoloa, HI, Poster.
78. DELBELLO, M.P. *et al.* 2006. Neurochemical effects of olanzapine in first-hospitalization manic adolescents: a proton magnetic resonance spectroscopy study. Neuropsychopharmacology **31:** 1264–1273.
79. CHANG, K.D. *et al.* 2003. Divalproex monotherapy in the treatment of bipolar offspring with mood and behavioral disorders and at least mild affective symptoms. J. Clin. Psychiatry **64:** 936–942.
80. FINDLING, R.L. *et al.* 2000. The rationale, design, and progress of two novel maintenance treatment studies in pediatric bipolarity. Acta. Neuropsychiatrica **12:** 136–138.
81. DELBELLO, M. 2006. Neuropharmacology of adolescents at risk for bipolar disorder. 5th Annual NIMH Pediatric Bipolar Disorder Conference. Chicago.
82. POST, R.M. *et al.* 2001. Developmental vulnerabilities to the onset and course of bipolar disorder. Dev. Psychopathol. **13:** 581–598.
83. ALLOY, L.B. *et al.* 1999. Depressogenic cognitive styles: predictive validity, information processing and personality characteristics, and developmental origins. Behav. Res. Ther. **37:** 503–531.
84. MIKLOWITZ, D. J. 2006. A review of evidence-based psychosocial interventions for bipolar disorder. J. Clin. Psychiatry **67**(Suppl. 11)**:** 28–33.
85. GELLER, B. *et al.* 2004. Four-year prospective outcome and natural history of mania in children with a prepubertal and early adolescent bipolar disorder phenotype. Arch. Gen. Psychiatry **61:** 459–467.
86. MEYER, S.E. *et al.* 2006. A prospective high-risk study of the association among maternal negativity, apparent frontal lobe dysfunction, and the development of bipolar disorder. Dev. Psychopathol. **18:** 573–589.
87. KELLER, M.B. 2004. Improving the course of illness and promoting continuation of treatment of bipolar disorder. J. Clin. Psychiatry **15**(Suppl. 65): 10–14.
88. KOWATCH, R.A. *et al.* 2005. Treatment guidelines for children and adolescents with bipolar disorder. J. Am. Acad. Child Adolesc. Psychiatry **44:** 213–235.

89. MIKLOWITZ, D.J. *et al.* 2000. Family-focused treatment of bipolar disorder: 1-year effects of a psychoeducational program in conjunction with pharmacotherapy. Biol. Psychiatry **48:** 582–592.
90. VIETA, E. & F. COLOM. 2004. Psychological interventions in bipolar disorder: from wishful thinking to an evidence-based approach. Acta. Psychiatr. Scand. Suppl. 34–38.
91. MIKLOWITZ, D.J. *et al.* 2004. Family-focused treatment for adolescents with bipolar disorder. J. Affect. Disord. **82**(Suppl. 1): S113–S128.
92. PAVULURI, M.N. *et al.* 2004. Child- and family-focused cognitive-behavioral therapy for pediatric bipolar disorder: development and preliminary results. J. Am. Acad. Child Adolesc. Psychiatry **43:** 528–537.
93. FRISTAD, M.A., S.M. GAVAZZI & B. MACKINAW-KOONS. 2003. Family psychoeducation: an adjunctive intervention for children with bipolar disorder. Biol. Psychiatry **53:** 1000–1008.
94. ALTHOFF, R.R. *et al.* 2005. Family, twin, adoption, and molecular genetic studies of juvenile bipolar disorder. Bipolar Disord. **7:** 598–609.
95. MIKLOWITZ, D.J. & S.L. JOHNSON. 2006. The psychopathology and treatment of bipolar disorder. Annual Review of Clinical Psychology **2:** 199–235.

A Multiple-Levels-of-Analysis Perspective on Resilience

Implications for the Developing Brain, Neural Plasticity, and Preventive Interventions

DANTE CICCHETTI[a] AND JENNIFER A. BLENDER[b]

[a]*Institute of Child Development and Department of Psychiatry, University of Minnesota, Minneapolis, Minnesota, USA*

[b]*Department of Clinical and Social Sciences in Psychology, University of Rochester, Rochester, New York, USA*

ABSTRACT: Resilient functioning, the attainment of unexpected competence despite significant adversity, is among the most intriguing and adaptive phenomena of human development. Although growing attention has been paid to discovering the processes through which individuals at high risk do not develop maladaptively, the empirical study of resilience has focused predominantly on detecting the psychosocial determinants of the phenomenon. For the field of resilience to grow in ways that are commensurate with the complexity inherent to the construct, efforts to understand underlying processes will be facilitated by the increased implementation of interdisciplinary research designed within a developmental psychopathology framework. Research of this nature would entail a consideration of psychological, biological, and environmental–contextual processes from which pathways to resilience might eventuate (known as equifinality), as well as those that result in diverse outcomes among individuals who have achieved resilient functioning (know as multifinality). The possible relation between the mechanisms of neural plasticity and resilience and specific suggestions concerning research questions needed to examine this association are discussed. Examples from developmental neuroscience and molecular genetics are provided to illustrate the potential of incorporating biology into the study of resilience. The importance of adopting a multiple-levels-of-analysis perspective for designing and evaluating interventions aimed at fostering resilient outcomes in persons facing significant adversity is emphasized.

KEYWORDS: resilience; multiple-levels-of-analysis; gene × environment interaction; resilience-promoting interventions

Address for correspondence: Dante Cicchetti, Ph.D., Institute of Child Development, University of Minnesota, 51 East River Road, Minneapolis, MN 55455. Voice: 612-625-4455; fax: 612-624-6373. e-mail: cicchett@umn.edu

Ann. N.Y. Acad. Sci. 1094: 248–258 (2006). © 2006 New York Academy of Sciences.
doi: 10.1196/annals.1376.029

INTRODUCTION

Child maltreatment sets in motion a probabilistic path of epigenesis for abused and neglected children characterized by an increased likelihood of failure and disruption in the successful resolution of salient developmental tasks, resulting in a profile of relatively enduring vulnerability factors that increase the probability of the emergence of maladaptation and psychopathology.[1] Because the vast majority of children are adversely affected by their maltreatment experiences, child abuse and neglect may represent the greatest failure of the caregiving environment to provide opportunities for normal development. However, not all maltreated children develop maladaptively. Indeed, some abused and neglected youngsters function in a competent fashion despite the pernicious experiences they have encountered.

The achievement of competent functioning in a subset of maltreated youngsters is but one example of how some individuals who have endured deleterious experiences nonetheless manage to develop adaptively. Understanding how individuals overcome significant adversity and function adaptively has captured the imagination and interest of humanity throughout the ages; however, it has been only a little more than three decades that the systematic empirical study of the phenomenon that is today known as resilience began.[2]

The roots of work on resilience can be traced back to prior research in diverse areas, including investigations of schizophrenia, poverty, and response to trauma.[2] Resilience is a dynamic developmental process that has been operationalized as an individual's attainment of positive adaptation and competent functioning despite having experienced chronic stress or detrimental circumstances, or following exposure to prolonged or severe trauma.[2] Resilience is multidimensional in nature, exemplified by findings that high-risk individuals may manifest competence in some domains and contexts, whereas they may exhibit problems in others.[2]

A large volume of research has examined the individual, family, interpersonal, and broader environmental–contextual correlates of, and contributors to, resilience. Despite the growing attention paid to discovering the processes through which individuals at high risk do not develop maladaptively, the empirical study of resilience has focused primarily on detecting the psychosocial determinants of the phenomenon.[2] Because self-righting, one of the basic mechanisms underlying resilience, has historical roots embedded in the fields of embryology and genetics,[3] it is unfortunate that researchers investigating the pathways to resilient adaptation have eschewed the inclusion of genetic and biological measures. For the field of resilience to grow in ways that are commensurate with the complexity inherent to the construct, efforts to understand underlying processes will be facilitated by the increased implementation of interdisciplinary research designed within a developmental psychopathology framework. Research of this nature would entail a consideration of psychological, biological, and environmental–contextual processes from which varied pathways to resilience might eventuate (known as equifinality), as well as those that result in diverse outcomes among individuals who have achieved resilient functioning (known as multifinality).[4]

The role of biological factors in resilience is suggested by evidence on neural and neuroendocrine system function in relation to stress reactivity,[5] and in behavior-genetic research on nonshared environment effects.[6] Similarly, molecular genetic research can reveal the genetic elements that may serve a protective function for individuals experiencing significant adversity, such as child maltreatment.[7] Furthermore, the map of human haplotypes recently has been completed, thereby providing valuable information about individual genetic variation, a powerful tool for identifying both vulnerability and protective genes, that, in interaction with specific environmental experiences, may eventuate in mental disorder or resilience, respectively.[8]

MULTIPLE-LEVELS-OF-ANALYSIS

We believe that a multiple-levels-of-analysis perspective, in which biological measures are incorporated into the predominantly psychosocial and environmental–contextual measurement batteries used in research on the determinants of resilience, is crucial for continued progress to take place in charting the pathways to competent functioning in the presence of significant adversity.[9] The concurrent examination of environmental–contextual, psychological, and biological processes and their interplay at varying developmental periods will provide a more integrative conceptualization of the developmental course.[10] Because levels of organization and processes of biological and psychological development are reciprocally interactive, it is difficult, if not impossible, to impute ultimate causation to one level of organization over another. The consideration of the totality of attributes, psychopathological conditions, and risk and protective processes in the context of each other rather than in isolation is crucial for understanding the course of development taken by individuals.

Although it would be impractical for most investigators to include all levels of analysis within the same experimental design, the growing movement toward collaborative interdisciplinary research within the disciplines of neuroscience and developmental psychopathology offers optimism that a multiple-levels approach will become increasingly prevalent.[11] The incorporation of such a perspective into the study of resilience will result in a more sophisticated and comprehensive portrayal of this phenomenon that will serve not only to advance the scientific knowledge of resilience, but also to inform efforts to translate research on positive adaptation in the face of adversity into the development of interventions to promote resilient functioning.

AVOIDING THE REDUCTIONIST PITFALL

In the context of resilience, we do not wish to convey or encourage the reduction of resilience to biological processes. Rather, we believe that biology is but one part of what should be an all-encompassing systems approach to understanding resilience, which needs to take into account all levels of analysis from the cellular to the cultural.[12,13] In fact, reducing psychological phenomena to components of genetic, neuroanatomical, neurochemical, and neurophysiological factors dismisses the great impact that experience has on these processes, and relegates psychology to the realm of an ephemeral behavioral marker of biological processes. This reductionism is the antithesis of a multiple-levels-of-analysis approach that emphasizes the primary importance of the interrelations of all factors. For example, just as gene expression alters social behavior, so, too, do social experiences, such as child maltreatment and institutional upbringing exert actions on the developing brain by feeding back upon it to modify gene expression,[14] and brain structure and functioning.[1,10] Furthermore, despite the fact that the molecular mechanisms whereby environmental factors exert long-term effects on gene expression in humans are not fully understood, alterations in gene expression induced by learning and by social and psychological experiences produce changes in patterns of neuronal and synaptic connections and, thus, in the function of nerve cells.[14] Such neuronal and synaptic modifications not only exert a prominent role in initiating and maintaining the behavioral changes that are provoked by experience, but also contribute to the biological bases of individuality, as well as to individuals being differentially affected by similar experiences, regardless of their valence.[14]

NEURAL PLASTICITY AND RESILIENCE

Recognizing that mechanisms of plasticity are integral to the very anatomical structures of cortical tissue and cause the formation of the brain to be an extended malleable process, developmental psychopathologists and neuroscientists are presented with new avenues for understanding the vulnerability and protective aspects of the brain as contributors to the etiology, course, and sequelae of maladaptation and resilience.[15] Now that it is evident that experience can impact the microstructure and biochemistry of the brain, a vital role for early and continuing neural plasticity throughout epigenesis in contributing to the development of, and recovery from, various forms of maladaption and psychopathology is suggested.

Children endowed with normal brains may encounter a number of experiences, including maltreatment, poverty, and parental mental disorder, that may exert a deleterious impact on the structure, function, and organization of the developing brain. The pathology induced in brain structure, functioning, and organization may distort the child's experience, with subsequent alterations in cognition or social interactions causing additional pathological experience and added brain pathology. Moreover, because some maltreated children function resiliently despite having experienced significant adversity,[1] it is likely that the experience of child abuse and neglect may exert different effects on the neurobiological structure, function, and organization in well-functioning maltreated children than in the typical maltreated child.[1]

More broadly, the artificial distinction among genetics, biology, and behavior within the human organism contradicts years of research indicating co-actions between all levels of analysis, from the environment broadly construed to the molecular.[16] The pathways to either psychopathology or resilience are influenced, in part, by a complex matrix of the individual's level of biological and psychological organization, experience, social context, timing of adverse event(s) and experiences, and developmental history.

The study of neural plasticity in modern neuroscience and associated disciplines has brought to bear a wide range of empirical methodologies to describe observed dynamic processes at the synaptic and cellular levels that appear to underlie neural plasticity.[17,18] Neural plasticity is viewed as a dynamic nervous system process that orchestrates nearly constant neurochemical, structural, and functional central nervous system (CNS) alterations in response to experience. Advances in the study of neural plasticity could be fruitfully employed as a model to begin to hypothesize about the genetic and biological underpinning of resilience. Several decades of empirical investigation have revealed that plasticity is an inherent property of the CNS, and that the manifestation of plasticity is part of a normative process in the mammalian CNS.[17,18] Indeed, it has been suggested that the plasticity of the human brain is one of the central defining mechanisms of the evolutionary success of the human species.[19]

MECHANISMS OF NEURAL PLASTICITY

Neural plasticity has predominantly been thought of as reorganization within systems of the CNS, evidenced by changes in anatomy, neurochemistry, or metabolism, and is most typically studied in the context of several types of events impinging on the CNS. The neuroplastic changes that take place are often dramatic, and can include observable changes in the neural substrate that are translated into changes observable at the behavioral level. Such changes that are hallmarks of plasticity can occur on one or more levels of analysis, including molecular, cellular, neurochemical, neuroanatomical, and at the level of brain systems.

The mechanisms of experience-based neural plasticity begin with the organism interfacing with its environment.[20] The fundamental processes undergirding neural plasticity at all levels of analysis are believed to be two mechanisms underlying the modulatory effects of neurotransmitters. One of these is protein phosphorylation and the other is the regulation of gene expression.

Protein phosphorylation appears to be the major molecular mechanism of neural plasticity, and is generally considered to be the mechanism by which the modulation of neuronal function is achieved through alterations in the functional state of many different types of neural proteins, such as ion channels, neurotransmitter receptors, and processes by which neurotransmitter storage and release is regulated.[20] Protein phosphorylation regulates both presynaptic and postsynaptic neurotransmitter receptors, with corroborative evidence suggesting that phosphorylation alters the functional activity of receptors. Additionally, protein phosphorylation plays a central role in cell growth and differentiation.

The second primary mechanism by which neurotransmitters can effect long-term changes in the function of target neurons is by regulating gene expression within those neurons. Such changes in gene expression produce quantitative and qualitative changes in the protein components of neurons, including, for example, alterations in the numbers and types of ion channels and receptors present on the cell membrane as well as levels of proteins that regulate the morphology of neurons and the numbers of synaptic connections that form. Further, neurotransmitters continually regulate neuronal gene expression as a way to fine-tune the functional state of neurons in response to many varied synaptic inputs.[20] Regulation of neural gene expression by neurotransmitters can in some cases produce long-lasting changes in virtually all aspects of neuronal functioning.

Generally, changes to the CNS mediated by protein phosphorylation do not involve changes in protein synthesis and therefore are likely to have a rapid onset, be more readily reversible, and have a shorter duration compared to neural plasticity mediated by gene expression. However, both of these processes serve to mediate the long-term effects of experience on the brain. The biochemical and molecular changes brought about through these two processes, through a cascade of intermediate neural processes, lead to changes in the function and efficacy of synapses, changes in the processing of information by individual neurons, and ultimately to changes in the way multicellular neural networks within the brain communicate with each other.[20]

The challenge of future research attempting to relate neural plasticity to particular behavioral phenomena is to find associations between specific alterations in neural processes, brought about by phosphorylation and gene expression, and behavior. Presently, we do not know if some of the difficulties displayed by persons who have experienced significant life adversity are irreversible, or whether there are particular sensitive periods when it is more likely that neural and behavioral plasticity will occur. Moreover, it is not known whether some neural or psychological systems may be more plastic than other neural or behavioral systems. Furthermore, it is not known whether particular neural or psychological systems may be more refractory to change or have a more time-limited window when neural plasticity can occur. Consequently, it is critical that research investigations on the correlates and determinants of resilient adaptation begin to incorporate molecular genetic and neurobiological methods into their predominantly psychological measurement armamentaria.

HOW PRINCIPLES OF NEURAL PLASTICITY MIGHT INFORM THEORY AND RESEARCH

Analogous to neural plasticity that takes place in response to brain injury, resilience can be viewed as the ability of an individual to recover after exposure to trauma or adversity. In this view, adversity is thought to exert a damaging effect on one or more neural substrates, and mechanisms of neural plasticity bring about recovery in an individual. This might lead to the conclusion that certain individuals, classified as resilient, may have some increased innate capacity (plasticity), above and beyond normative levels, to recover from environmental insults that exert an impact on the brain.

This view of resilience conceives of adversity in the environment as "bad" for the brain, with recovery as an innate property of the brain itself. This perspective, however, does not consider the impact of a positive environment, or of the individual's active attempts at coping, on such recovery.

Another conceptualization of resilience would be one of greater than normative resistance to the impact of environmental adversity on the brain, such that resilient individuals may not succumb to the potentially damaging effects that adversity may have on the brain and other biological systems. This view of brain–adversity interaction would not strictly be classified as involving neural plasticity. Thus, for these individuals, the term recovery of function may not apply, in that they did not "lose" function at all. The distinction between these two formulations of resilience also can generate important research questions concerning the relation of neural plasticity to resilience. Such questions underscore the importance of employing longitudinal research designs that can begin to examine the brain's capacity either to resist damage from adversity or to use its restorative capabilities.

For example, a number of questions about resilient adaptation could potentially be addressed using neuroimaging methodologies, including: (1) Do brain structure and function differ between resilient and nonresilient children matched on comparable experiences of adversity? (2) Are particular areas of the brain more or less likely to be activated in resilient than in nonresilient functioning during challenging or stressful tasks? (3) Are there changes over time in brain structure and/or functioning in individuals classified as resilient that may reflect processes of neural plasticity? (4) Are there differences in connectivity, assessed through diffusion tensor imaging, between regions of the cerebral cortex, possibly providing evidence of neural plasticity as one of the underlying mechanisms of resilient outcomes?

GENE × ENVIRONMENT INTERACTION AND RESILIENCE

Knowledge of genetic variation may help to identify which individuals are most vulnerable to adverse experiences. Through investigating gene ×

environment (G × E) interactions, protective functions of genes may also be discovered. Caspi *et al.*[7] examined how genetic factors contribute to why some maltreated children grow up to develop antisocial personality disorders, whereas other maltreated children do not. In this longitudinal study of males from birth to adulthood, it was found that a functional polymorphism in the promoter region of the gene encoding the neurotransmitter-metabolizing enzyme monoamine oxidase A (MAOA) moderates the effects of child maltreatment. The link between child maltreatment and antisocial behavior was far less pronounced among males with high MAOA activity than among those with low MAOA activity. Of relevance to the importance of including biological measures in research on resilience, it is conceivable that the gene for high MAOA activity may confer a protective function against the development of antisocial disorder in males who have experienced maltreatment.

The results of the Caspi *et al.*[7] investigation suggest that a G × E interaction helps to explain why some maltreated children, but not others, develop antisocial behavior via the effect that stressful experiences, such as child maltreatment, exert on neurotransmitter system development. Specifically, the probability that child maltreatment will eventuate in adult antisocial behavior is greatly increased among children whose MAOA is not sufficient to render maltreatment-induced changes on neurotransmitter systems inactive.

A second large-scale prospective investigation conducted by Caspi *et al.*[21] is another compelling example of how the incorporation of a multiple-levels perspective can elucidate the processes that contribute to pathological or resilient adaptation. These investigators found that adults with a functional polymorphism in the promoter region of the serotonin transporter (5-HTT) gene moderated the influence of stressful life events on depression. Specifically, individuals with one or two copies of the short (s) allele of the 5-HTT promoter polymorphism developed more depressive disorders, depressive symptoms, and suicidality than individuals homozygous for the long (l) allele when confronted with high stress. The s allele in the polymorphic region is associated with lower transcriptional efficiency of the promoter compared with the l allele.[9]

The Caspi *et al.*[21] study also provides evidence of a G × E interaction, in which an individual's response to environmental insults is moderated by his or her genetic makeup. Furthermore, Caspi *et al.* discovered that, congruent with a G × E interaction, adult depression was predicted by the interaction between the s allele in the 5-HTT gene-linked polymorphic region and child maltreatment that occurred during the first decade of life. The G × E interaction revealed that child maltreatment predicted adult depressive disorder only among individuals carrying an s allele (i.e., s/s or s/l), but not among l/l homozygotes. Thus, the l/l homozygous allele may prove to confer a protective function against the development of adult depression in individuals who have been maltreated.

As researchers increasingly integrate the tools of contemporary neuroscience and molecular genetics into behavioral science investigations that also precisely measure and define environmental and contextual variables, we believe that we are at the intersection of a new age of discovery for understanding pathways to maladaptive and resilient adaptation.

IMPLICATIONS OF A MULTIPLE-LEVELS-OF-ANALYSIS APPROACH FOR RESILIENCE-PROMOTING INTERVENTIONS

Luthar and Cicchetti[22] concluded that research on resilience "should target protective and vulnerability forces at multiple levels of influence" (p. 878). The incorporation of a neurobiological framework and the utilization of genetically sensitive designs into interventions seeking to promote resilient functioning or to repair positive adaptations gone awry may contribute to the ability to design individualized interventions that are based on knowledge gleaned from multiple biological and psychological levels of analysis. The inclusion of neurobiological assessments in the design and evaluation of interventions designed to foster resilience enables scientists to discover whether the various components of multifaceted interventions each exert a differential impact on separate brain systems. We think that successful resilience-promoting interventions may be conceptualized as examples of experience-dependent neural plasticity.[23] If assessments of biological systems are routinely incorporated into the measurement batteries employed in resilience-facilitating interventions, then we will be in a position to discover whether the nervous system has been modified by experience.

The incorporation of a neurobiological framework into the conceptualization of preventive intervention holds considerable promise for expansion of knowledge regarding complexity of the developmental process. By basing preventive trials on more comprehensive, integrative developmental theories of psychopathology, prevention research offers the opportunity to conduct developmental experiments that alter environment and experience in efforts to promote resilient functioning among individuals faced with significant adversity. Determining the multiple levels at which change is engendered through preventive trials will provide more insights into the mechanisms of change, the extent to which neural plasticity may be promoted, and the interrelations between biological and psychological processes in resilience and psychopathology.

CONCLUSION

A multiple-levels-of-analysis perspective on resilience should not be misinterpreted as equating resilience with biology. Moreover, the inclusion of biological measures in resilience research should not hearken scientists back to the time when some espoused the view that there were "invulnerable" children.

To the contrary, existing theories in developmental neuroscience are quite compatible with organizational and systems theories in the fields of developmental psychology and psychopathology.[24] The inclusion of biological measures into research on resilience still requires adherence to a dynamic transactional view that acknowledges the importance of context. Biological, psychological, and environmental–contextual domains are each essential to include in basic research on resilience and in resilience-promoting interventions. If we are to grasp resilience in its full complexity, then we must adopt a multiple-levels-of-analysis approach.

ACKNOWLEDGMENTS

The preparation of this manuscript was supported by a grant from the Spunk Fund, Inc.

REFERENCES

1. Cicchetti, D. 2002. The impact of social experience on neurobiological systems: illustration from a constructivist view of child maltreatment. Cog. Dev. **17:** 1407–1428.
2. Luthar, S.S., D. Cicchetti & B. Becker. 2000. The construct of resilience: a critical evaluation and guidelines for future work. Child Dev. **71:** 543–562.
3. Waddington, C.H. 1957. The Strategy of Genes. Allen & Unwin. London.
4. Cicchetti, D. & F.A. Rogosch. 1996. Equifinality and multifinality in developmental psychopathology. Dev. Psychopathol. **8:** 597–600.
5. Gunnar, M.R. & D.M. Vazquez. 2006. Stress neurobiology and developmental psychopathology. *In* Developmental Psychopathology. Second edition. Developmental Neuroscience. Vol. 2. D. Cicchetti & D. Cohen, Eds.: Wiley. New York.
6. Rende, R. & R. Plomin. 1993. Families at risk for psychopathology: who becomes affected and why? Dev. Psychopathol. **5:** 529–540.
7. Caspi, A., J. McClay, T. Moffitt, *et al.* 2002. Role of genotype in the cycle of violence in maltreated children. Science **297:** 851–854.
8. Insel, T. & R. Quirion. 2005. Psychiatry as a clinical neuroscience discipline. J. Am. Med. Assoc. **294:** 2221–2224.
9. Cicchetti, D. & J.A. Blender. 2004. A multiple-levels-of-analysis approach to the study of developmental processes in maltreated children. Proc. Natl. Acad. Sci. 101: 17325–17326.
10. Cicchetti, D. 2002. How a child builds a brain: insights from normality and psychopathology. *In* Minnesota Symposia on Child Psychology: Child Psychology in Retrospect and Prospect. W. Hartup & R. Weinberg, Eds.: Vol. 32. Lawrence Erlbaum Associates. Mahwah, NJ.
11. Grillner, S., A. Koslov & J.H. Kotaleski. 2005. Integrative neuroscience: linking level of analyses. Curr. Opin. Neurobiol. **15:** 614–621.
12. Kendler, K. 2005. Toward a philosophical structure for psychiatry. Am. J. Psychiatry **162:** 433–440.

13. SHONKOFF, J. & D. PHILLIPS, Eds.: 2000. From Neurons to Neighborhoods: The Science of Early Childhood Development. National Academy Press. Washington, DC.
14. KANDEL, E.R. 2005. Psychiatry, psychoanalysis, and the new biology of mind. American Psychiatric Association.
15. CICCHETTI, D. & D. TUCKER. 1994. Development and self-regulatory structures of the mind. Dev. Psychopathol. **6:** 533–549.
16. GOTTLIEB, G. & C.T. HALPERN. 2002. A relational view of causality in normal and abnormal development. Dev. Psychopathol. **14:** 421–436.
17. KEMPERMANN, G. 2006. Adult Neurogenesis. Oxford University Press. Oxford. UK.
18. HUTTENLOCHER, P. 2002. Neural plasticity. Harvard University Press. Cambridge, MA.
19. KEMPERMAN, G., H. VAN PRAGG & F.H. GAGE. Activity-dependent regulation of neuronal plasticity and self-repair. Prog. Brain Res. **127:** 35–48.
20. HYMAN, S.E. & E.J. NESTLER. 1993. The Molecular Foundations of Psychiatry. American Psychiatric Press, Inc. Washington, DC.
21. CASPI, A., K. SUGDEN, T. MOFFITT, *et al.* 2003. Influence of life stress on depression: moderation by a polymorphism in the 5-HTT gene. Science **301:** 386–389.
22. LUTHAR, S.S. & D. CICCHETTI. 2000. The construct of resilience: implications for intervention and social policy. Dev. Psychopathol. **12:** 857–885.
23. GREENOUGH, W., J. BLACK & C. WALLACE. 1987. Experience and brain development. Child Dev. **58:** 539–559.
24. CICCHETTI, D. & D. COHEN, Eds: Developmental Psychopathology. Second edition. Vol. 1: Theory and Method. Wiley. New York.

Evolutionary Basis of Adaptation in Resilience and Vulnerability

Response to Cicchetti and Blender

MYRON A. HOFER

New York State Psychiatric Institute, New York, New York, USA

ABSTRACT: This masterful and wide-ranging paper gives us a clear picture of the need for interdisciplinary studies of resilience and vulnerability. We need to go beyond the interacting events at the different levels to see clearly that multiple levels of analysis and concept do not themselves interact, but instead give us different aspects of a biological, psychological, or behavioral event. Thus, no levels are reducible to any of the others. In the rest of my discussion, I raise the likelihood that the multiple level responses of "resilience" are no more adaptive in their evolutionary history than the very different responses we call "vulnerability." Keeping in mind the evolved functions of these responses, and the circumstances of their selection during evolution, will provide us with new ideas and approaches for understanding and intervention.

KEYWORDS: adaptation; resilience; vulnerability

NYAS CONFERENCE ON RESILIENCE IN CHILDREN

Cicchetti and Blender have given us a wide-ranging description of the several levels on which the clinical concept of resilience operates. As they point out, much less is known about the biological processes that underlie the psychosocial observations and the language in which resilience has been defined. Two points that they make are particularly worthy of emphasis: first, that the cell–molecular and neural circuit mechanisms of the brain are as responsive and capable of change in the patterns of their functioning as the psychosocial measures and processes that we speak of as mediating resilience and vulnerability to adversity. Second, that the effects that the genetic endowment an individual has on his or her resilience is also strongly influenced by the prior history of the embryo, fetus, and child's active interactions with their environment

Address for correspondence: Myron A. Hofer, New York State Psychiatric Institute, 1051 Riverside Drive, Unit 40, New York, NY 10032. Voice: 212-543-5692; fax: 212-543-5467.
e-mail: mah6@columbia.edu

Ann. N.Y. Acad. Sci. 1094: 259–262 (2006).
doi: 10.1196/annals.1376.030

during early development and beyond, as well as by interactions between the expression patterns of one gene and those of other genes within the person's unique genome.

The "multiple levels" of the author's perspective are operating virtually simultaneously during an individual's exposure to adversity, so I would rather think of the neurochemical and genetic levels as "underlying" and "mediating" the behavioral and psychological events of the resilient individual, rather than thinking of an "interplay" between "reciprocally interactive" levels, as the authors describe. This distinction gets us out of the fallacy of thinking of neurochemical or genetic events as *causing* behavioral or psychological events, for example, if we were to speak of a "gene for resilience." Psychological constructs, such as "attachment," can often be understood better, to my mind, when we know the organization and dynamics of the underlying biological processes.[1] When we have this deeper level of understanding, then the psychological construct is more than a useful metaphor, for new properties of this construct are often revealed through knowing about attachment at multiple levels of biological organization. Thus, events occurring at one level can interact with events at another, but the levels of analysis themselves are different aspects of the same behavior or trait or concept. This may seem to be a small point, but making this distinction reveals the fallacy of the "reductionist position" and of genetic or environmental determinism. In addition, it provides the best way I know to bridge the conceptual gap between psychosocial processes and biological ones.

In the second part of my response to the authors' paper, I am going to do what discussants are always criticized for: focusing on what they are interested in, instead of the author's paper. But I suspect that this is why I was chosen to discuss this paper. Recent developments in evolutionary theory and animal research in the laboratory can add to the picture of resilience painted by the authors. First we should ask: What is the ultimate basis for the observations that have led to the concept of resilience—that is, what basic properties of humans, and other mammals, is resilience drawing upon? To answer this question, I will first give a little background that may be unfamiliar to some. The new field of evolutionary developmental biology, or "Evo-devo," has grown out of the recent discovery that genes play a key role in the organization and regulation of development as well as in their known role as agents of heredity.[2] Because all cells in the body have the same genes, developmental events and patterns are the result of organized patterns of gene regulation that are orchestrated by many interacting molecular signals originating from both endogenous and exogenous sources. This gives these developmental interactions a role in evolution as a major source of novel variation that functions in addition to the familiar mechanisms of mutation and natural selection. Thus, one of the evolutionary functions of development is the production of variation in the capacity of the next generation to adapt to environmental change—that is their capacity for "resilience" to a range of environmental conditions.

So it is the evolution of this function of development that has given us resilience. But why then does such a maladaptive thing as "vulnerability" exist? The answer comes from asking this question: Resilience in what circumstances? For it is likely that development evolved the capacity to generate different developmental courses that are particularly suited to a variety of conditions, including extremely adverse conditions—famine, social chaos, floods, volcanism, etc. Research in both rats and monkeys has revealed a pattern of developmental response to severe adversity that resembles the behavior and altered physiology of children raised in poverty and social upheaval.[3] In humans, these responses are often called "psychopathological" and regarded as evidence of vulnerability or failure of resilience. The transmission of these traits across generations in humans has been thought to be purely cultural. But there is now good experimental evidence of changed (less attentive) patterns of maternal behavior occurring in laboratory animals under adverse early environmental conditions (e.g., frequent separations) that are faithfully transmitted to the next generation (even when the adverse conditions no longer continue). In addition to maternal behavior differences, offspring grow up to be fearful, with highly reactive adrenocortical responses, increased appetite, a tendency to depressed behavior, certain cognitive differences ("deficits"), and rapid sexual maturation. These traits have one thing in common—they increase the chances that a greater number of offspring will survive under these particular conditions in subsequent generations. Offspring with "normal" and "healthy" patterns of behavior and physiology are less successful under such chaotic and persistently threatening conditions.

What we call "resilient" patterns are adaptive when adverse conditions are not so very severe and some resources are available. In these cases, standard psychosocial interventions can be beneficial, but what should be done when extremely adverse conditions have already occurred or cannot be changed significantly? This question is not going to be easy to answer, but if we do not recognize alternate pathways of development for what they are, we will never find the answers. One example of this sort of situation gives some insight. In offspring with nutritional deprivation *in utero* because of dietary or placental insufficiency, an increased incidence of type 2 diabetes (insulin resistance), hypertension, and anxiety are found in offspring reared in normal circumstances.[4] This outcome is now thought to be due to the overeating and obesity that occurs when there is a restoration of "more optimal" nurturing environment during the first year or two after birth. I am not saying we should not intervene in the case of children who appear to lack resilience. Quite the contrary, they may need more but different kinds of intervention. I will close with an observation told to me by Tiffany Field, who had just set up a special intervention clinic to supply increased tactile stimulation, holding and massage, to infants from deprived and abusive home circumstances. Not until the intervention was provided to the *mothers*, was the intervention successful.

REFERENCES

1. HOFER, M.A. 2005. The psychobiology of early attachment. Clin. Neurosci. Res. **4:** 291–300.
2. CARROLL, S.B. 2005. Endless Forms Most Beautiful: The New Science of Evo-Devo. W.W. Norton & Company. New York.
3. CAMERON, N.M., F.A. CHAMPAGNE, C. PARENT, *et al.* 2005. The programming of individual differences in defensive responses and reproductive strategies in the rat through variations in maternal care. Neurosci. Biobehav. Rev. **29:** 843–865.
4. OSMOND, C. & D.J. BARKER. 2000. Fetal, infant, and childhood growth are predictors of coronary heart disease, diabetes, and hypertension in adult men and women. Environ. Health Perspect. **108**(Suppl 3): 545–553.

Maternal Sensitivity Is Related to Hypothalamic-Pituitary-Adrenal Axis Stress Reactivity and Regulation in Response to Emotion Challenge in 6-Month-Old Infants

CLANCY BLAIR,[a] DOUGLAS GRANGER,[b] MICHAEL WILLOUGHBY,[c] KATIE KIVLIGHAN,[b] AND THE FAMILY LIFE PROJECT INVESTIGATORS[a,b,c,d]

[a]*Department of Human Development and Family Studies, Pennsylvania State University, University Park, Pennsylvania, USA*

[b]*Department of Biobehavioral Health, Pennsylvania State University, University Park, Pennsylvania, USA*

[c]*Frank Porter Graham Child Development Institute, University of North Carolina at Chapel Hill, Chapel Hill, North Carolina, USA*

[d]*Center for Developmental Science and Department of Psychology, University of North Carolina at Chapel Hill, Chapel Hill, North Carolina, USA*

ABSTRACT: This study examined relations between maternal sensitivity as observed in a free play interaction and changes in levels of the glucocorticoid hormone cortisol in response to procedures designed to elicit negative affect in 6-month old infants. The sample included 1,292 families in predominantly rural and low-income communities in Pennsylvania and North Carolina. Results indicated that infants of more sensitive mothers had lower levels of cortisol at baseline and increased cortisol reactivity and regulation in response to the emotion procedures. Maternal negativity was unrelated to infant cortisol. Findings highlight the need for further research on variation in early caregiving and the development of the stress response in young children.

KEYWORDS: stress; parenting; emotion

Studies with nonhuman animal models indicate normal variation in maternal behavior is associated with the development of the hypothalamic-pituitary-adrenal (HPA) axis response to stress and aspects of cognition and behavior

Address for correspondence: Clancy Blair, Human Development and Family Studies, Pennsylvania State University, 110 Henderson South, University Park, PA 16802-6504. Voice: 814-863-6423; fax: 814-863-6207.
e-mail: cbb11@psu.edu

Ann. N.Y. Acad. Sci. 1094: 263–267 (2006). © 2006 New York Academy of Sciences.
doi: 10.1196/annals.1376.031

dependent on effective stress regulation.[1,2] These studies suggest the need for further research examining the relation of caregiving in the normal range of care to the development of the HPA stress response and cognitive, emotional, and behavioral outcomes in human infants. Prior work with human infants and young children has shown that extreme neglect and maltreatment early in life are associated with disrupted HPA regulation and poor developmental outcomes.[3] A number of studies have also determined that maternal emotional unavailability is stressful for children and have indicated that developmental outcomes in children may to some extent be attributable to maternal effects on HPA regulation.[4] No prior studies, however, have examined relations among specific aspects of maternal behavior, the HPA stress response, and developmental outcomes for children in poverty. Given evidence for elevated levels of stress exposure and stress response in the context of poverty,[5] it may be that parenting and early life stress are important mediating mechanisms through which poverty influences child outcomes.

METHOD

Participants

Data for this analysis are provided by the Family Life Project (FLP), a longitudinal study examining multiple aspects of child and family functioning in predominantly low-income, nonurban communities. The FLP utilized complex sampling procedures to recruit a sample of 1,292 families beginning at child birth that are highly representative of families in nonurban counties in Pennsylvania and North Carolina from which the sample was drawn. Low-income families in both states and African American families in North Carolina were oversampled.

Procedure

As part of one of the two home visits conducted at child age 6 months, infants were presented with four procedures designed to elicit emotional reactivity.[6] The tasks included toy reach, mask presentation, barrier, and arm restraint tasks.

Three saliva samples were collected from infants: a baseline pretask sample and samples at 20- and 40-min post peak arousal in response to emotion challenge. All samples were assayed for cortisol using a highly sensitive enzyme immunoassay 510 k cleared for use as an *in vitro* diagnostic measure of adrenal function. The test used 25 μL of saliva (for singlet determinations), had a range of sensitivity from 0.007 to 1.8 μg/dL, and average intra- and interassay coefficients of variation of less than 10% and 15%. All samples were assayed in duplicate.

As a part of the second of two home visits, mothers and children were observed in a semistructured interaction for 15 min. The interaction was videotaped and later coded on a five-point scale using global ratings of behaviors indicative of sensitivity and negativity.[7]

RESULTS

We first examined change in the measures of salivary cortisol in response to the emotion challenge tasks. Paired t-tests indicated that on average infants reacted to the challenge with an increase in cortisol from baseline to the 20-min post peak arousal assessment, paired $t(987) = -3.55$, $P < 0.0001$, and then exhibited a significant decline from the 20- to the 40-min post peak arousal assessment, paired $t(884) = 5.74$, $P < 0.0001$. Baseline and 40-min post arousal levels were not significantly different from one another.

To test our primary hypotheses concerning relations of maternal behavior to variation in HPA reactivity and regulation, we used repeated measures analysis to examine the relation of parenting, family, and child variables to linear and quadratic change in cortisol in response to the emotion challenge. Results indicated a within subjects effect for maternal sensitivity $F(2,1674) = 3.60$, $P < 0.05$, and a significant quadratic within subjects contrast. Specifically, higher levels of maternal sensitivity were associated with lower baseline cortisol and a pattern of change characterized by an increase in cortisol between baseline and 20-min post peak arousal and a decrease in cortisol between 20- and 40-min post peak arousal. This relation is presented in FIGURE 1 and indicates that children of mothers exhibiting higher levels of sensitivity in the parent–child interaction task exhibited greater cortisol reactivity and regulation in response to the emotion challenge task. In contrast, children of mothers exhibiting lower levels of sensitivity were characterized by higher baseline cortisol and decreasing cortisol at 20- and 40-min post peak arousal. This effect was present when controlling for a within subjects effect for body temperature and between subjects effects for ethnicity and time of day. Maternal negativity was unrelated to cortisol at baseline or in response to emotion challenge.

DISCUSSION

Results indicated that normal variation in maternal sensitivity observed in a standard mother–child interaction was associated with child HPA reactivity and regulation in response to emotion challenge at age 6 months. Unlike previous studies that have called attention to the deleterious effects of abnormally

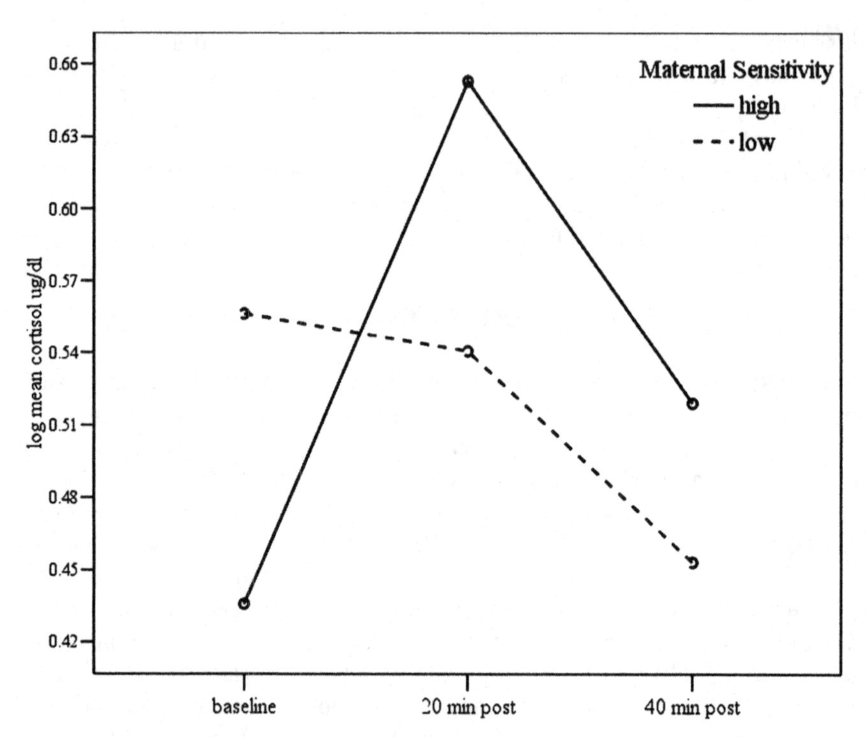

FIGURE 1. Children of mothers exhibiting higher levels of sensitivity in the parent–child interaction task exhibited cortisol reactivity and regulation in response to the emotion challenge task.

high or low mean levels of cortisol among children facing early psychosocial disadvantage, these results, as with our prior work with preschool children,[8] indicate the utility of a focus on physiological response to challenge. Specifically, findings indicated that higher level of maternal sensitivity was associated with lower baseline level of cortisol in children, with the mounting of a physiological response to challenge when needed, and with a down-regulation of this response once challenge had been met. In contrast, lower level of sensitivity, not negativity, was associated with higher baseline level of cortisol and the absence of cortisol reactivity and regulation in response to challenge.

REFERENCES

1. Liu, D., J. Diorio, B. Tannenbaum, *et al.* 1997. Maternal care, hippocampal glucocorticoid receptors, and hypothalamic-pituitary-adrenal responses to stress. Science **277:** 1659–1662.
2. Liu, D., J. Diorio, J. Day, *et al.* 2000. Maternal care, hippocampal neurogenesis, and cognitive development in rats. Nat. Neurosc. **3:** 799–806.

3. CICCHETTI, D. & F. ROGOSH. 2001. The impact of child maltreatment and psychopathology on neuroendocrine functioning. Dev. Psychopathol. **13:** 783–804.
4. GUNNAR, M.R. & B. DONZELLA. 2002. Social regulation of cortisol levels in early human development. Psychoneuroendocrinology **27:** 199–220.
5. EVANS, G. & K. ENGLISH. 2002. The environment of poverty: multiple stressor exposure, psychophysiological stress, and socioemotional adjustment. Child Dev. **73:** 1238–1248.
6. STIFTER, C., T. SPINRAD & J. BRAUNGART-RIEKER. 1995. Toward a developmental model of child compliance: the role of emotion regulation in infancy. Child Dev. **70:** 21–32.
7. NICHD EARLY CHILD CARE RESEARCH NETWORK. 1999. Child care and mother-child interaction in the first 3 years of life. Dev. Psychol. **35:** 1399–1413.
8. BLAIR, C., D. GRANGER & R.P. RAZZA. 2005. Cortisol reactivity is positively related to executive function in preschool children attending Head Start. Child Dev. **76:** 554–567.

Ultrasound Consultation to Reduce Risk and Increase Resilience in Pregnancy

ZACK BOUKYDIS

Erikson Institute, Chicago, Illinois, USA

ABSTRACT: Clinical evidence indicates the influence of viewing ultrasound on women's investment in health during pregnancy. Ongoing work on the effects of ultrasound consultation (UC) include: establishing a replicable UC and demonstrating validity of the UC by examining effects of UC on behavioral and physiological indicators of increased resilience in maternal health and pregnancy outcome. The study indicated that UC significantly increased maternal–fetal attachment, decreased maternal anxiety, and increased positive attitudes toward health during pregnancy. Ongoing research involves using UC in two protocols with pregnant women, for instance, those experiencing moderate-to-severe depression and those at risk for noncompliance in treatment for gestational diabetes.

KEYWORDS: ultrasound consultation; maternal health; maternal–fetal attachment

INTRODUCTION

Clinical evidence has indicated the influence of viewing ultrasound on women's investment in health during pregnancy.[1] Having an ultrasound as a routine screen is often enjoyed by women and can contribute to maternal "personification" of the fetus.[2] Prenatal interventions, especially ultrasound, in pregnancies where there is higher medical or psychosocial risk have the potential to increase maternal–fetal attachment and reduce the risk of behaviors that may harm the fetus and compromise the health status of the pregnancy.[3,4] In this way, prevention–intervention efforts aimed at higher risk populations in pregnancy are designed to reduce risk and produce a healthier base from which all children move forward in their ongoing transactions with the postnatal caregiving environment.[5]

There are two phases in the ongoing work on ultrasound consultation (UC) in second trimester pregnancy: establishing a replicable ultrasound consultation and demonstrating the validity and utility of the UC by using the UC to initiate

Address for correspondence: Zack Boukydis, Ph.D., Erikson Institute, 420 N. Wabash Ave., Chicago, IL 60611-5627. Voice: +312-893-7193; fax: +312-755-0928.
e-mail: zboukydis@erikson.edu

Ann. N.Y. Acad. Sci. 1094: 268–271 (2006).
doi: 10.1196/annals.1376.032

interventions to reduce risk factors and increase maternal–fetal health and pregnancy outcome.

DEVELOPMENT OF THE ULTRASOUND CONSULTATION

Two studies have contributed to the establishment of a replicable ultrasound. In the first study done at Women and Infants Hospital, Providence, RI, women observed an ultrasound during the second trimester of pregnancy.[6] A UC protocol was established that included: a screen of fetal anatomy; view of fetal facial features and physical characteristics; observation of fetal physical movement; and mother initiated interaction with the fetus. Eighty-five women consented to participate in the UC at an average of 24 weeks gestation. The UC was scheduled within 1 week of a screen done in the obstetric department. The UC lasted an average of 17 min. Pre- and post-UC questionnaires indicated that women significantly increased in maternal–fetal attachment and significantly decreased in trait anxiety following the ultrasound consultation. Sixty-six percent of the women indicated that seeing the baby, and seeing the baby moving, were the most helpful parts of the UC.

A second study was done at Hutzel Hospital, Detroit, MI.[7] The study consisted of two parts: an observation of routine ultrasounds in the sonography clinic, and a random assignment study of Ultrasound Consultation (UC) compared with Standard Care (SC). The observation component included 26 patients presenting for routine ultrasound screens. Average maternal age was 27 years; average gestational age was 19.7 weeks; average duration of ultrasound was 16.6 min (range 10–25); average length of time viewing the screen was 12.4 min (range 3–25). Women asked an average of 2.4 questions per session (range 1–7).

In the second part, low socioeconomic status women attending prenatal clinics were recruited to participate in a study examining the effects of UC on maternal–fetal attachment. Women attending the clinic for routine screens at 16–24 weeks g.a. were randomly assigned to either the UC ($N = 29$) or SC (routine screen following clinical protocol; $N = 26$) condition. Results indicated that UC significantly increased maternal–fetal attachment, decreased maternal anxiety, and increased positive attitudes toward maintaining health in pregnancy.

ULTRASOUND CONSULTATION TO INITIATE PREVENTION/ INTERVENTION IN AT-RISK PREGNANCIES

The second phase of the research using ultrasound to initiate intervention is currently being implemented. The use of the UC in two research protocols with pregnant women in second trimester: women with diabetes who are at risk for noncompliance in ongoing treatment and women experiencing moderate-to-severe depression—are being implemented in two different hospital research settings.

1. *Pregnant women with diabetes*. Having diabetes during pregnancy places mother and fetus at increased risk.[8] Depending on the ability to maintain diet, exercise, and medication requirements, morbidity and mortality factors can increase significantly.[9] The protocol in this research involves recruitment during ultrasound screens in the second trimester and random assignment to either SC or UC/Personal Coaching (UC–PC) groups. The UC–PC groups have an ultrasound consultation based on the established protocol and are assigned a personal counselor (nurse clinician) trained with principles from motivational interviewing, personal fitness training, infant mental health, and doula support. Mothers have weekly contact throughout pregnancy. Outcome data in the perinatal period involve comparing both groups on maternal health status, labor/delivery status, infant risk status, and infant neurobehavior.
2. *Pregnant women with significant depression*. Women having moderate-to-severe depression are at risk for poorer pregnancy outcomes and higher infant risk status.[10] Women are screened for depression during second trimester ultrasound screens. Women with moderate-to-severe depression are assigned to either SC or UC–PS groups. The UC–PS groups have an ultrasound consultation based on the established protocol and are assigned a personal support counselor who is trained with principles from infant mental health and has weekly contact with the women throughout pregnancy. Outcome data in the perinatal period include the same variables as those in the diabetes study.

REFERENCES

1. GRACE J.T. 1983. Prenatal ultrasound examinations and mother-infant bonding. N. Eng. J. Med. **309:** 561–562.
2. ZECHMEISTER I. 2001. Foetal images: the power of visual technology in antenatal care and the implications for women's reproductive freedom.. Hlth. Care Anal. **9:** 387–400.
3. POLLOCK P.H. & A. PERCY. 1999. Maternal antenatal attachment style and potential fetal abuse. Child Abuse Negl. **23:** 1345–1357.
4. VILLENEUVE C., C. LAROCHE, A. LIPPMAN & M. MARRACHE. 1998. Psychological aspects of ultrasound imaging during pregnancy. Can. J. Psychiatry **33:** 530–536.
5. SAMEROFF, A. 2004. Ports of entry and the dynamics of mother-infant interventions. *In* Treating Parent-Infant Relationship Problems. A. Sameroff, S.C. McDonough & K.L. Rosenblum, Eds: Guilford Press. New York.
6. BOUKYDIS, C.F.Z., L. LAGASSE, L. RUGGIERO, *et al.* 2006. Ultrasound consultation in pregnancy: incorporating psychological consultation into obstetric ultrasounds. Submitted to Ultrasound Ob. & Gyn.

7. BOUKYDIS, C.F.Z., M.C. TREADWELL, V. DELANEY-BLACK, *et al.* 2006. Women's response to viewing ultrasound during routine screens in an obstetric clinic. J. Ultrasound Med. **25:** 721–728.
8. SCHWARTZ, R. & K.A. TERAMO. 2000. Effects of pregnancy on the fetus and newborn. Semin. Perinatol. **24:** 120–135.
9. SILVERMAN, B.L., T.A. RIZZO, N.H. CHO & B.E. METZGER. 1998. Long-term effects of the intrauterine environment. The Northwestern University Diabetes in Pregnancy Center. Diabetes Care **21**(Suppl 2):B142–C149.
10. MARCUS, S.M., H.A. FLYNN, F.C. BLOW & K.L. BARRY. 2003. Depressive symptoms among pregnant women screened in obstetric settings. J. Women Hlth. **12:** 373–380.

Emotional Resilience in Early Childhood

Developmental Antecedents and Relations to Behavior Problems

ANNE M. CONWAY[a] AND SUSAN C. McDONOUGH[b]

[a]*University of Pittsburg, Pittsburg, PA, USA*

[b]*School of Social Work, University of Michigan, Ann Arbor, Michigan, USA*

ABSTRACT: To test whether the development of emotional resilience is a function of sensitive caregiving and child negative affect, we tested the joint contributions of 7-month maternal sensitivity and infant negative affect to the prediction of 33-month emotional resilience across the first 3 years of life. The aims of this study were to examine whether maternal sensitivity and infant negative affect predict long-term emotional resilience and whether this was associated with preschool behavior problems. Using a sample of 181 mother–infant dyads, we found that (*a*) maternal sensitivity at 7 months, but not infant negative affect, longitudinally predicted emotional resilience during preschool and (*b*) emotional resilience was negatively associated with anxiety/depression in preschool.

KEYWORDS: emotional resilience; behavior problems; early childhood

INTRODUCTION

The ability to generate positive emotions and recover quickly from negative emotional experiences is known as emotional resilience.[1] Theorists identify resilience as the ability to display positive adaptation despite stress and adversity[2] and this component reflects positive emotional adaptation.[1,3] Based on the Broaden and Build Theory of positive emotions,[4] positive emotions following challenge are expected to (*a*) undo the effects of negative emotions and speed cardiovascular recovery from challenge and (*b*) promote long-term resources. This may include protection from the development of behavior problems.

Studies with adults demonstrate that positive emotions following challenge are associated with faster cardiovascular recovery following challenge,[5,6] low levels of depression during crisis,[7] and positive adaptation following loss. [8]

Address for correspondence: Anne M. Conway, University of Pittsburg, Western Psychiatric, Detre Hall/Room E718, Pittsbrug, PA 15213. Voice: 412-246-5826; fax: 412-246-5880.
e-mail: conwayam@upmc.edu

**Ann. N.Y. Acad. Sci. 1094: 272–277 (2006). © 2006 New York Academy of Sciences.
doi: 10.1196/annals.1376.033**

However, few studies have examined relations between emotional resilience and children's behavior adaptation. This study seeks to address this gap by assessing relations between emotional resilience and behavior problems in childhood and examining the developmental antecedents.

Theories suggest that maternal sensitivity and infant negative reactivity predict the development of emotion regulation.[9] This may also extend to emotional resilience—ability to recover and express positive emotions following challenge. Indeed, sensitive and responsive maternal behaviors have been found to be concurrently associated with infants' ability to recover and express positive emotions following stressful interactions with parents (e.g., still-face paradigm).[10–12] Few studies, however, have examined these relations longitudinally.

The purpose of this study was to address this gap by (*a*) examining whether maternal sensitivity and infant negative affect longitudinally predict emotional resilience during preschool and (*b*) investigating whether emotional resilience predicts preschool behavior problems.

METHOD

One hundred eighty-one children and their mothers participated in a series of free play and problem-solving interactions in our laboratory.[13,14] Episodes were videotaped by research assistants behind a one-way mirror. The behavior and affect of mothers and infants were coded globally on a scale from 0

TABLE 1. Code Descriptions

Study measures	Description
Maternal sensitivity	Gentle, soothing, infant focused and responsive behaviors (e.g., attending to the infant's emotional state and exploration) were rated on a scale from 0 (no sensitivity) to 3 (high sensitivity) (Weighted kappa = 0.71)[15]
Infant negative affect	Fussing and crying were rated on a scale from 0 (no negative affect) to 3 (high negative affect) (Weighted kappa = 0.87)[15]
Child behavior problems	Maternal ratings of child internalizing (e.g., anxiety/depression, withdrawn), externalizing (e.g., aggression, destructive), sleep problems, somatic, and total problem 0 (none) to 3 (always) (Child Behavior Checklist 2–3; Achenbach, 1992)
Emotional resilience	Total number of seconds until children expressed joy following the anger tasks[a]

[a] Trained undergraduate research assistants coded children's emotional expression at 33 months during the four emotion induction tasks. Facial action and voice quality cues developed by Cole, Barrett, and Zahn-Waxler[20] were used to determine the presence of anger, sadness, and joy and were coded on a second by second basis and ranged from 0 to 3 (none, low, medium, and high). Angry tones consisted of harsh, insistent voices; sad voices included low, resigned voices and crying; joy was based on light-lifting voices or laughing and giggling. Percent agreements ranged from 0.71 to 0.99. Latencies to joy expression in the bubble and bunny tasks were summed and a log transformation was used to correct skewness. This transformed variable was also multiplied by –1 to put the dependent variable in the positive direction.

(none) to 3 (very high) for each task.[15] Codes included maternal sensitivity and infant negative affect (see TABLE 1). These were coded during (a) free play, (b) teaching task 1, and (3) high-chair free play of the still face. Infant negative affect was coded during the (1) teaching task 1, (2) teaching task 2, and (3) the still face.

When the children were 33 months old, they participated in four tasks used to induce joy or anger in children modified from the Preschool Laboratory Assessment Battery (Lab-TAB)[16]: (a) popping bubbles, (b) locked toy in container, and (3) draw a perfect circle. An additional task, "Tickle the Bunny," where children were asked to tickle a bunny puppet, was used to induce joy.[17] The anger–joy tasks were presented to children in pairs allowing for an assessment of individual differences in the latency to joy expressions following anger. Children were videotaped while participating in these tasks and tapes were subsequently coded by trained undergraduate research assistants. Results confirmed that the emotion tasks were successful in inducing the expected emotions for both boys and girls.[18] Groups were combined across gender and the total sample was used for all subsequent analyses.

RESULTS

Testing the Measurement Model

Structural equation modeling was used in the major analyses. Before testing the full-hypothesized model, the measurement model for the latent constructs—maternal sensitivity and infant negative affect—was tested using confirmatory factor analysis. Based on our conceptual model, a three-factor model was specified and tested. The two latent factors were: (*a*) maternal sensitivity, expressed during the free play, teaching, and high-chair tasks and (*b*) infant negative affect, expressed during teaching task 1 and 2, and the still face. The latent factors were allowed to correlate. The measurement model, which was evaluated with maximum-likelihood path estimation using AMOS,[19] was a good fit, χ^2 (8, $N = 181$) = 8.446, $P = 0.391$, with a TLI of 0.987, a CFI of 0.995, and a RMSEA measure of 0.018. All loadings for the indicators were significant.

Fit of the Models

Antecedents of Emotional Resilience

The model predicting to emotional resilience was a good fit, χ^2 (12, $N = 181$) = 9.012, $P = 0.702$, with a TLI of 1.00, a CFI of 1.00, and a RMSEA measure of 0.000 (see FIG. 1). In the model, the direct path from

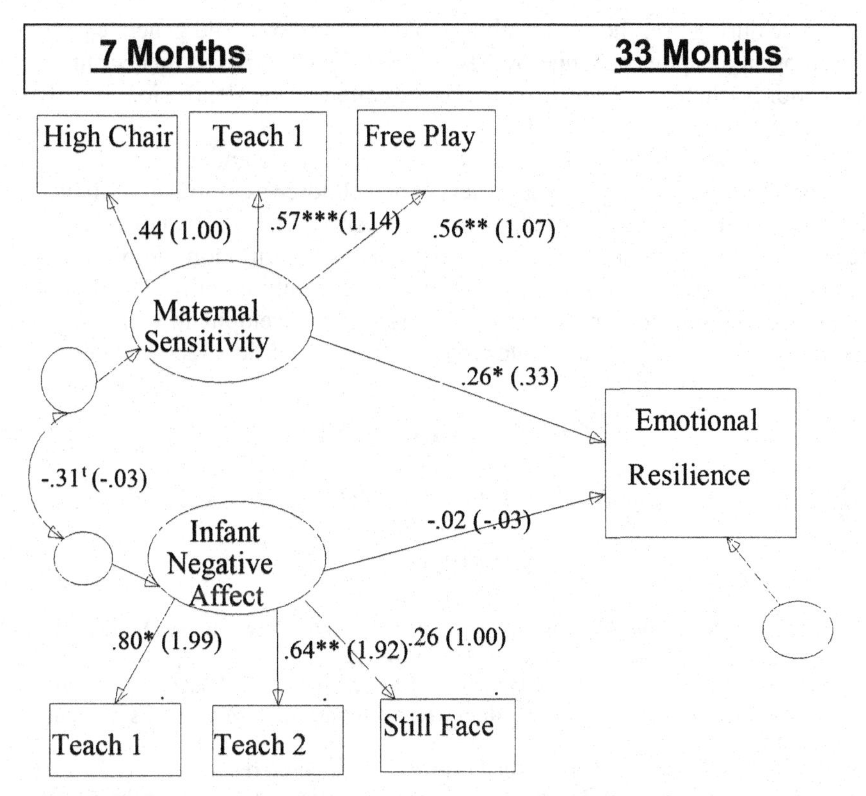

FIGURE 1. Relations of maternal sensitivity and infant negative affect to emotional resilience.

maternal sensitivity to emotional resilience was significant and positive, but infant negative affect was not.

Relations between Emotional Resilience and Behavior Problems

Correlational analyses were used to examine the relations between emotional resilience and child behavior problems. Results were that emotional resilience was not associated with children's aggressive and externalizing behavior, but was negatively correlated with low levels of parent-reported child anxiety-depression ($r = -0.16$, $P < 0.05$).

DISCUSSION

This study contributed to the literature by documenting that maternal sensitivity during infancy significantly predicted children's emotional resilience during preschool—the ability to quickly recover and generate positive emotions despite challenge. We also found that emotional resilience during preschool predicted low levels of concurrent anxiety and depression in early childhood.

Future research is needed to identify the mechanisms underlying the relations between early care giving experiences and children's emotional resilience to inform interventions designed to promote positive emotions in children. Indeed, the ability to quickly recover and express positive emotions despite challenge may also have long-term implications. Specifically, emotional resilience in early childhood may protect children from the development of affective disorders in later years or facilitate recovery from pediatric affective illness.

ACKNOWLEDGMENTS

This study was supported by NIMH Grant MH54322 to S.C.M.

REFERENCES

1. DAVIDSON, R.J. 2000. Affective style, psychopathology, and resilience: brain mechanisms and plasticity. Am. Psych. **55:** 1196–1214.
2. MASTEN, A.S., K.M. BEST & N. GARMEZY. 1990. Resilience and development: contributions from the study of children who overcome adversity. Dev. Psychopath. **2:** 425–444.
3. CURTIS, W.J. & D. CICCHETTI. 2003. Moving research on resilience into the 21st century: theoretical and methodological considerations in examining the biological contributors to resilience. Dev. Psychopath. **15:** 773–810.
4. FREDRICKSON, B.L. 2001. The role of positive emotions in positive psychology: the broaden and build theory of positive emotions. Am. Psych. **56:** 218–226.
5. FREDRICKSON, B.L. & R.W. LEVENSON. 1998. Positive emotions speed recovery from the cardiovascular sequelae of negative emotions. Cog. Emot. **12:** 191–220.
6. FREDRICKSON, B.L., R.A. MANCUSO, C. BRANIGAN & M.M. TUGADE. 2000. The undoing effect of positive emotions. Motiv. Emot. **24:** 237–258.
7. FREDRICKSON, B.L., M.M. TUGADE, C.E. WAUGH & G.R. LARKIN. 2003. What good are positive emotions in crisis? A prospective study of resilience and emotions following the terrorist attacks on the United States on September 11th, 2001. J. Person. Social Psych. **84:** 365–376.
8. BONANNO, G.A. & D. KELTNER. 1997. Facial expressions of emotion and the course of conjugal bereavement. J. Abnor. Psych. **106:** 126–137.
9. CALKINS, S.D. 1994. Origins and outcomes of individual differences in emotion regulation. *In* The Development of Emotion Regulation: Behavioral and Biological Considerations. N.A. Fox, Ed.: Vol. 59, 53–72. Chicago: University of Chicago.
10. BRAUNGART-RIEKER, J.M., M.M. GARWOOD, B.P. POWERS & P.C. NOTARO. 1998. Infant affect and affect-regulation during the still-face paradigm with mothers and fathers: the role of infant characteristics and parental sensitivity. Dev. Psych. **34:** 1428–1437.

11. KOGAN, N. & A.S. CARTER. 1996. Mother-infant reengagement following the still-face: the role of maternal emotional availability in infant affect regulation. Infant Behav. Dev. **19:** 359–370.
12. ROSENBLUM, K., S. MCDONOUGH, M. MUZIK, et al. 2002. Maternal representations of the infant: associations with infant response to the still face. Child Dev. **73:** 999–1015.
13. CROWELL, J.A. & S.S. FELDMAN. 1988. Mother's internal working models of relationships and children's behavioral and developmental status: a study of mother-child interaction. Child Dev. **59:** 1273–1285.
14. TRONICK, E.Z. & M.K. WEINBERG. 1992, November. Manual for the Face-to-Face Still-Face Paradigm. Boston Children's Hospital Harvard University Medical School.
15. MILLER, A., S. MCDONOUGH, K. ROSENBLUM & A. SAMEROFF. 2002. Emotion regulation in context: situational effects on infant and caregiver behavior. Infancy **3:** 403–433.
16. GOLDSMITH, H.H., J. REILLY, S. LEMERY, *et al.* 1999. The Laboratory Temperament Assessment Battery: Preschool Version. Unpublished manuscript.
17. CONWAY, A. 1999. Elicitors of Positive Emotions in Young Children: The tickle the bunny task. University of Michigan, Ann Arbor, Michigan.
18. CONWAY, A.M. 2005. The Development of Emotion Regulation: The role of effortful control and positive affect. Ph.D. thesis, University of Michigan, Ann Arbor, Michigan.
19. ARBUCKLE, J.L. 2003. Amos (Version 5.0). Small Waters Corporation, Chicago.
20. COLE, P.M., K.C. BARRETT & C. ZAHN-WAXLER. 1992. Emotion displays in two-year-olds during mishaps. Child Dev. **63:** 314–324.

The Role of Verbal Competence and Multiple Risk on the Internalizing Behavior Problems of Costa Rican Youth

FEYZA CORAPCI,[a] JULIA SMITH,[b] AND BETSY LOZOFF[c]

[a]*Center for Human Growth and Development, University of Michigan, Ann Arbor, Michigan, USA*

[b]*Educational Leadership, Oakland University, Rochester, Michigan, USA*

[c]*Center for Human Growth and Development, Department of Pediatrics and Communicable Diseases, University of Michigan, Ann Arbor, Michigan, USA*

ABSTRACT: This longitudinal study examined internalizing behavior problems (anxiety/depression) in early adolescence in relation to adversity in early childhood and child verbal competence. We hypothesized that verbal competence would act as a protective factor in the face of early adversity, that is, high verbal IQ would predict relatively lower internalizing problems in early adolescence primarily for those children who experienced the greatest adversity. The sample was based on 191 Costa Rican children and their mothers, who were recruited in infancy from an urban community and assessed again at 5 and 11–14 years. Families were generally lower-middle to working class. A total of 165 children (94 boys) participated in the early adolescent follow-up (mean age = 12.3 years). Internalizing problems were based on maternal report (Spanish Child Behavior Checklist). Our cumulative risk index (CRI) of adversity in early childhood consisted of home environment quality (HOME score), socioeconomic status, maternal depressed mood (CESD), and maternal IQ. Controlling for the effects of age, gender, internalizing problems at 5 years, and verbal IQ at 5 years, there was a significant interaction between early adversity and verbal IQ at age 11–14 years in predicting internalizing problems in early adolescence. Youth with high verbal IQ had comparable levels of internalizing problems regardless of high or low adversity in early childhood. In contrast, youth with low verbal IQ received higher internalizing problem ratings if they experienced high adversity early in life. The results raise the possibility that interventions to improve verbal competence might help lower the risk of internalizing problems in the face of early adversity.

Address for correspondence: Feyza Corapci, Ph.D., Psychology Department, Bogazici University, 34342 Bebek, Istanbul, Turkey. Voice: 90-212-359-7323; fax: 90-212-287-2472.
e-mail: feyza.corapci@boun.edu.tr

Ann. N.Y. Acad. Sci. 1094: 278–281 (2006).
doi: 10.1196/annals.1376.034

KEYWORDS: **internalizing behavior problems; multiple risk; verbal competence; protective factor; vulnerability; longitudinal design**

Internalizing behavior problems (IBP) in childhood such as symptoms of anxiety and depression are important markers for similar problems in adulthood.[1] However, there is still relatively little research on the operation of risk and protective factors to predict IBP. Risk factors for IBP include temperamental inhibition, exposure to stressful events and social adversity, parental anxiety, as well as parent–child interaction patterns such as insecure attachment and parental overcontrol.[2] Some factors have been associated with lower levels of IBP.[3] These include the child's emotion regulation and coping skills, verbal competence, maternal warmth, and kinship social support. There is a paucity of research on whether any of these factors moderate the impact of exposure to multiple risk factors in an early disadvantageous environment on later IBP.

The present study investigated the protective role of youth verbal competence on IBP using a longitudinal design. Based on research on IBP as well as theories of risk and resilience,[4] we tested two hypotheses. First, we expected that the cumulative combination of multiple risk factors early in life would predict IBP in early adolescence. Second, we expected that verbal competence would act as a protective factor and moderate the effects of multiple risk such that high verbal competence would reduce the risk of IBP, primarily for those youth who experienced greatest early adversity.

METHOD

Participants

This study used data from a longitudinal study of 191 Costa Rican children recruited in infancy and their mothers, from an urban community near San Jose as part of a community-based study of iron deficiency and child development.[5] Enrollment entailed door-to-door screening of the entire community and included all 12- to 23-month-old healthy infants. The community was predominantly lower-middle to working class. The average maternal education was 8.4 years. A total of 85% of the original cohort (n = 162; 87 boys) participated in the early childhood follow-up. The mean age of children was 60.3 months (SD = 1.1). At the early adolescence follow-up, data on 165 youth (94 boys) were available. The mean age of youth was 12.3 years with a range from 11 to 14 years.

Procedure and Measures

Our index of cumulative risk focused on aspects of the family environment at infancy. The quality of the family environment was assessed with the

Infancy-Toddler HOME. The socioeconomic status was measured by Hollingshead four-factor index. Mother's full scale IQ was assessed by the Wechsler Intelligence Scale for Adults-Revised. The Center for Epidemiologic Studies Depression Scale was used to assess maternal depressed mood. Following previous research,[6] each family environment variable was dichotomized to identify risk. The cumulative risk index (CRI) representing early adversity was computed by summing all binary risk factors for each family. In this sample, the mean number of risks was 1.2 (SD = 1.1). The Child Behavior Checklist (CBCL, parent report, Spanish version) was obtained at early childhood (age 5 years) and early adolescence (age 11–14 years) follow-ups to measure IBP. Verbal IQ scaled scores (Wechsler Scales; WPPSI-R and WISC-R) were the measure of verbal competence at both follow-ups.

RESULTS AND DISCUSSION

A hierarchical linear regression analysis was conducted to predict IBP at age 11–14 years from age, gender, CRI, IBP at age 5 years and verbal IQ at age 5 and 11–14 years. The overall model was significant, accounting for 25% of the variance. The CRI accounted for significant proportion of variance in IBP at 11–14 years ($\Delta r^2 = 0.03$, $P < 0.05$) after partialling out the effects of age, gender, IBP, and verbal IQ at age 5 years. This result suggests that the role of early adversity extends beyond the stability of IBP and child characteristics. There was also a significant interaction between the CRI and verbal IQ in early adolescence, $\Delta F(1, 118) = 7.83$, $P < 0.01$. The interaction accounted for 5% additional variance in IBP at age 11–14 years while controlling for the other main effects and the interaction of CRI by verbal IQ at age 5 years. The nature of the interaction was explored by estimating CBCL Internalizing scores at 1 SD above and below the mean on the CRI and verbal IQ predictors (see FIG. 1). Contrary to our expectations, high verbal IQ in early adolescence did not reduce the risk of IBP for youth who experienced greatest early adversity. Rather, youth with high verbal IQ had comparable levels of IBP under both adversity levels. On the other hand, youth with low verbal IQ received high IBP ratings if they experienced high adversity early in life.

This interaction suggests four conclusions. First, it appears that high verbal competence confers stability to youth's psychosocial adjustment regardless of the adversity level rather than acting as a protective factor to benefit primarily those children from high-risk families. Second, verbal IQ in early adolescence, but not in early childhood, moderated the role of early adversity on IBP, indicating that the same factor may act as either a protective or vulnerability factor in different periods of development. Third, the combination of early high adversity and low verbal IQ seems to render children most vulnerable to the highest level of IBP in early adolescence. This result appears to fit with the concept of "double jeopardy"—in this case worse outcome among children

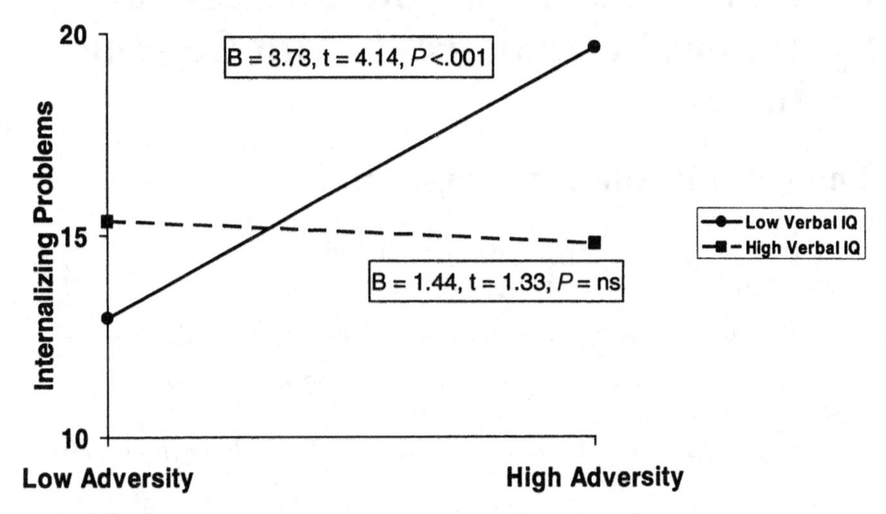

FIGURE 1. Interaction between early adversity level and verbal IQ at age 11–14 years predicting mother ratings of internalizing problems in early adolescence.

who experience both multiple risk and poor personal resources. Numerous processes could explain this pattern: youth with less verbal competence are likely to experience poor social and academic competence as well as poor problem solving and coping skills, which in turn may contribute to higher IBP. Finally, improving verbal competence might be a fruitful target for interventions to decrease anxiety and depression symptoms in at-risk youth.

REFERENCES

1. Hammen, C. & K.D. Rudolph. 2003. Childhood mood disorders. *In* Child Psychopathology. E.J. Mash & R.A. Barkley, Eds.: 233–278. Guilford. New York.
2. Zahn-Waxler, C., B. Klimes-Dougan & M. Slatterly. 2000. Internalizing problems of childhood and adolescence: prospects, pitfalls, and progress in understanding the development of anxiety and depression. Dev. Psychopathol. **12:** 443–466.
3. Spence, S.H. 2001. Prevention strategies. *In* The Developmental Psychopathology of Anxiety. M.W. Vasey & M.R. Dadds, Eds.: 325–354. University Press. Oxford, UK.
4. Masten, A.S. & J.L. Powell. 2003. A resilience framework for research, policy, and practice. *In* Resilience and Vulnerability: Adaptation in the Context of Childhood Adversities. S.S. Luthar, Ed.: 1–25. Cambridge University. New York.
5. Lozoff, B. *et al.* 1987. Iron deficiency anemia and iron therapy: effects on infant developmental test performance. Pediatrics **79:** 981–995.
6. Sameroff, A.J. *et al.* 1993. Stability of intelligence from preschool to adolescence: the influence of social and family risk factors. Child Dev. **64:** 80–97.

Preventing Co-Occurring Depression Symptoms in Adolescents with Conduct Problems

The Penn Resiliency Program

J.J. CUTULI,[a,b] TARA M. CHAPLIN,[a] JANE E. GILLHAM,[c]
KAREN J. REIVICH,[a] AND MARTIN E.P. SELIGMAN[a]

[a]*Psychology Department, University of Pennsylvania, Pennsylvania, USA*

[b]*Institute of Child Development, University of Minnesota, Minneapolis, Minnesota, USA*

[c]*Psychology Department, Swarthmore College, Swarthmore, Pennsylvania, USA*

ABSTRACT: Children who exhibit elevated levels of conduct problems are at increased risk for developing co-occurring depression symptoms, especially during adolescence. This study tests the effectiveness of a manualized after school intervention (the Penn Resiliency Program [PRP]) for the prevention of depression symptoms among a subset of middle-school-aged students who exhibited elevated levels of conduct problems, but not depression symptoms, at the start of the study. Longitudinal analyses demonstrate that the program successfully prevented elevations in depression symptoms across early- to mid-adolescence compared to no-intervention controls.

KEYWORDS: prevention; intervention; conduct problems; depression; adolescence

Conduct problems and depression symptoms often co-occur, especially in the adolescent years. Much attention has been paid to elaborating developmental pathways that result in this dual expression of symptoms. One explanation takes the form of a failure model of depression, whereby childhood disruptive behavior interferes with key domains of functioning, such as academic achievement and interactions with parents and peers.[1] Under this model, the child encounters more negative experiences and fewer positive ones, and the salience of these repeated failures intensifies in adolescence, a time when social and academic functioning have increased weight relative to childhood.

Address for correspondence: J.J. Cutuli, Institute of Child Development, University of Minnesota—TC, 51 East River Road, Minneapolis, MN, 55405. Fax: 612-624-6373.
e-mail: cutu0001@umn.edu

Ann. N.Y. Acad. Sci. 1094: 282–286 (2006).
doi: 10.1196/annals.1376.035

This preponderance of failures in important domains is associated with later depression symptoms, in addition to continued conduct problems.[1,2]

The present study attempts to elaborate on the mechanisms involved in the development of depression symptoms from earlier externalizing symptoms. The Penn Resiliency Program (PRP) is a 12-session after school intervention originally designed to prevent depression symptoms in middle-school-aged students. The sessions stress techniques in emotional regulation, cognitive abilities, and social skills. A key component of the intervention involves teaching the participants to cognitively challenge inaccurate, negative self-perceptions and interpretations of experiences, such as arguing with a friend or getting into trouble at school. Evidence suggests that the program is efficacious in preventing psychopathological symptoms.[3]

If children with elevated conduct problems have more negative experiences, then interventions like PRP that specifically target depressotypic interpretations of these experiences may be particularly efficacious in preventing depression symptoms in children who display higher levels of externalizing symptoms.

METHOD

All families enrolled in three suburban middle schools were invited to participate in a study of an intervention designed to teach coping and problem-solving skills to children. A total of 718 families consented to the study. Participants of consenting families were stratified by gender, grade, and depression symptom levels within each school and then randomly assigned to either the intervention or control conditions. A total of 231 students were assigned to a third condition where they received an alternative intervention, but this group is not considered here (for a full account of the project's methodology see Ref. 4). Of the remaining 466 families, 294 (63.1%) provided data on depressive symptoms and externalizing symptoms at baseline and data on depressive symptoms during at least one postintervention assessment, thereby allowing for their inclusion in the mixed models (MM) ANCOVA analyses described below. This was a primarily white (76.9%), middle-class sample. The mean age of the participants was 12.04 years (std. = 0.96 years). There were roughly equal numbers of male (170, 57.8%) and female participants, and 153 (52.0%) of the families had been randomly assigned to the intervention condition. Analyses were conducted to ensure that intervention and control participants who completed the follow-up assessments were similar on preintervention variables. ANOVA and chi-square analyses showed no significant differences among the conditions (PRP, control) on any preintervention demographic or outcome variable.

Participants and their parents completed questionnaire packets prior to the start of the intervention (baseline), at the conclusion of the 12-week intervention period, and again every 6 months through 3 years following the intervention. To gauge depression symptoms, participants completed the Children's

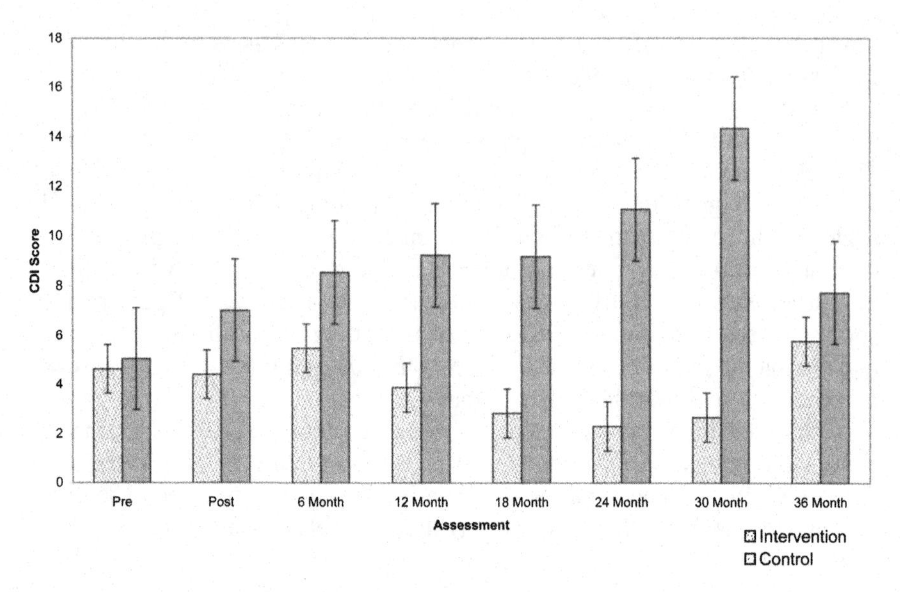

FIGURE 1. Depression symptoms among pure externalizers.

Depression Inventory (CDI).[5] Parents completed the Child Behavior Checklist (CBCL/4–18),[6] which provides externalizing scores that reflect each participant's level of conduct problems. All symptom score variables violated normality assumptions and were square root transformed. Untransformed means are presented in FIGURE 1 for ease of interpretation.

ANALYSES AND RESULTS

Participants were first divided into symptom groups based on their levels of symptom expression at baseline. Cut points were set at previously established cutoffs for each measure: 13 or above for the CDI to denote moderate to severe depression symptoms[4,5] and at or above the 80th percentile for the externalizing scale of the CBCL to indicate significant conduct problems.[6] This produced four groups: low symptom (low depression and externalizing, $n = 167$; 83 control, 84 intervention); pure externalizers (low depression, high externalizing $n = 56$; 24 control, 32 intervention); pure depression (moderate-high depression, low externalizing $n = 42$; 22 control, 20 intervention); and co-occurring (moderate-high depression, high internalizing $n = 29$; 12 control, 17 intervention). Chi-square analyses reveal that symptom groups significantly differed with respect to household income (χ^2 [15] $= 37.73$, $P < 0.01$). All analyses were rerun covarying income; this produced similar results. The composition of these groups did not significantly differ with respect to age, gender, condition assignment, and race. Also, symptom group assignment did not predict the number of sessions attended in the intervention condition, suggesting a comparable (if not equal) intervention dose between symptom groups. All analyses employed an intent-to-treat approach.

In line with failure models of depression, we anticipated that the program would be especially effective in preventing depression symptoms in the participants who exhibited high levels of externalizing symptoms at baseline, but have not yet developed depression symptoms. To test this hypothesis, we completed an MM ANCOVA predicting depression symptoms from intervention condition and symptom group assignments at baseline through the final assessment at 36 months postintervention, covarying initial depression scores. This MM ANCOVA yielded a significant result for the condition by symptom group interaction, suggesting that PRP's effect on depressive symptoms varied by symptom group, $F(3, 277) = 6.852, P < 0.001$. Follow-up MM ANCOVAs were run separately for each symptom group. In the pure externalizers group, a significant intervention effect was found, $F(1,52) = 8.563, P < 0.01$. No significant intervention effects were found in the other three symptom groups.

Finally, it is important to point out that many participants in the original study were excluded from these analyses as their parents did not provide CBCL data at baseline. An additional MM ANOVA with condition assignment predicting depression symptoms in these participants ($n = 142$) demonstrates that the program was efficacious for these participants as well, $F(1,130) = 13.447$, $P < 0.001$. This indicates that while the program seems to work particularly well for those assigned to the pure externalizers group, it also benefits most participants with regard to symptom expression, as has been shown in several studies.[3,7]

DISCUSSION

While the PRP intervention is generally beneficial to all participants, these findings suggest that it is especially efficacious in preventing depression symptoms in young adolescents who already express significant levels of conduct problems. Framed in terms of failure model theories on the development of depression, these results suggest that the intervention is buffering the negative impact of high levels of externalizing symptoms at the start of adolescence, possibly through the challenging and reframing of depressotypic beliefs about and interpretations of the increased number of negative experiences that accompany conduct problems.

ACKNOWLEDGMENTS AND DISCLOSURE

This study was supported through a grant from the NIMH (grant no. MH52270). The Penn Resiliency Program is owned by the University of

Pennsylvania. The University of Pennsylvania has licensed this program to Adaptiv Learning Systems. Drs. Reivich and Seligman own Adaptiv stock and could profit from the sale of this program. The other authors have no financial relationship with Adaptiv Learning Systems and have no financial interests to disclose. The Penn Resiliency Program is available for use in research. Requests for the curriculum should be made to Jane Gillham at jgillham@psych.upenn.edu.

REFERENCES

1. PATTERSON, G.R., J. REID & T. DISHION. 1992. A Social Interactional Approach: Antisocial Boys (Vol. 4). Castalia Publishing Company. Eugene, OR.
2. CAPALDI, D.M. 1992. Co-occurrence of conduct problems and depressive symptoms in early adolescent boys: II. A 2-year follow-up at Grade 8. Dev. Psychopathol. **4:** 125–144.
3. GILLHAM, J.E., K.J. REIVICH, L.J. JAYCOX & M.E.P. SELIGMAN. 1995. Prevention of depressive symptoms in schoolchildren: two year follow-up. Psychol. Sci. **6:** 343–351.
4. GILLHAM, J.E., K.J. REIVICH, D.R. FRERES, *et al.* School-based prevention of depressive symptoms: a randomized controlled study of the effectiveness and specificity of the Penn Resiliency Program. J. Consult. Clin. Psychol. In press.
5. KOVACS, M. 1992. Children's Depression Inventory Manual. Multi-Health Systems, Inc. North Tonawanda, NY.
6. ACHENBACH, T.M. 1991. Manual for the Child Behavior Checklist/4–18 and 1991 Profile. University of Vermont Department of Psychiatry. Burlington, VT.
7. QUAYLE, D., S. DZIURAWIEC, C. ROBERTS, *et al.* 2001. The effect of an optimism and lifeskills program on depressive symptoms in preadolescence. Behav. Change **18:** 194–203.

Maternal Depression and Psychotropic Medication Effects on the Human Fetus

EUGENE K. EMORY AND JOHN N.I. DIETER

Center for Prenatal Assessment and Human Development, Emory University, Atlanta, Georgia, USA

ABSTRACT: Ultrasound studies examined fetuses of depressed and nondepressed mothers. Fetuses of depressed mothers were more active during mid-gestation and exhibited lower baseline heart rate and moved less during late-term vibratory stimulation. Mid-gestation heightened activity and late-term diminished responsivity may be a prenatal manifestation of the "general adaptation syndrome." Color Doppler technology measured blood flow velocity in the middle cerebral artery of fetuses whose mothers were prescribed SSRIs or lithium. SSRIs were associated with velocity increases and lithium with velocity decreases. The effects of psychotropic medications on prenatal neurobehavioral development require further study to document potential benefits and adverse effects.

KEYWORDS: fetus; maternal depression; psychotropic medication

INTRODUCTION

Newborns of depressed mothers show "biobehavioral dysregulation" when compared to those of nondepressed mothers that includes poorer neurobehavioral organization, less responsivity to caregivers, lower vagal tone, higher cortisol, and greater right frontal EEG activity.[1,2] Such findings suggest that maternal depression has negative effects on the developing fetus. Two studies examined the effects of maternal depression on fetal behavior. Preliminary case studies of psychotropic medication effects on fetal cerebral blood flow are also presented.

STUDY 1: FETAL ACTIVITY ACROSS GESTATION

Participants

A cross-sectional design examined basal motor differences in fetuses of mothers who were (n = 45) or were not (n = 45) reporting symptoms

Address for correspondence: Eugene K. Emory, Ph.D., Department of Psychology, Emory University, 532 Kilgo Circle, Atlanta, GA30322. Voice: 404-727-7455; fax: 404-727-1284.

Ann. N.Y. Acad. Sci. 1094: 287–291 (2006). © 2006 New York Academy of Sciences.
doi: 10.1196/annals.1376.036

of depression during the second and third trimesters. Pregnancies were uncomplicated; none of the women were prescribed medications, smoked cigarettes, drank alcohol, or used illicit drugs. Women completed the Center for Epidemiological Studies-Depression Scale (CES-D) and the State Trait Anxiety Inventory (STAI) and were assigned to the Depressed Group if their CES-D score was 16 or more.[3]

Fetal Assessment

A lateral view of the fetus was obtained. Every 3 sec, a tape-recorded cue prompted the "blind" observer to record if the fetus was engaged in single limb, multiple limb, or gross body movement. The 5-min records were assigned to gestational month groups (i.e., 4th through 8th).

Results

Fetuses of depressed mothers spent a significantly greater % time being active (Depressed M = 44.04%, SD = 24.62; Nondepressed M = 28.25%, SD = 20.68), t (1, 88) = 3.28, $P < 0.01$ (two-tailed) across gestation and specifically during the 5th (F [1, 18] = 7.37, $P < 0.05$), 6th (F [1, 13] = 5.01, $P < 0.05$), and 7th (F [1, 13] = 6.22, $P < 0.05$) months (see FIG. 1). Stepwise regression suggested that 35% of the variance in activity was explained by maternal CES-D ($R^2 = 0.29$, $P < 0.01$ [two-tailed]) and STAI scores ($R^2 = 0.35$, $P < 0.05$ [two-tailed]).

STUDY 2: MATERNAL DEPRESSION AND ANXIETY EFFECTS ON VIBRATORY STIMULATION RESPONSE IN LATE-TERM FETUSES

Behavior and heart rate (HR) responsivity to vibratory stimulation was examined in late-term fetuses using a habituation paradigm to assess fetal CNS maturation and integrity.[4]

Participants

Women were assigned to either the Depressed (n = 17) or Nondepressed (n = 15) group based on their Beck Depression Inventory-II Score (>11). Women also completed the Beck Anxiety Scale. None of the pregnancies were complicated and none of the women smoked cigarettes, drank alcohol, used illicit drugs, or were prescribed medications. The mean gestational age at assessment was 33 weeks.

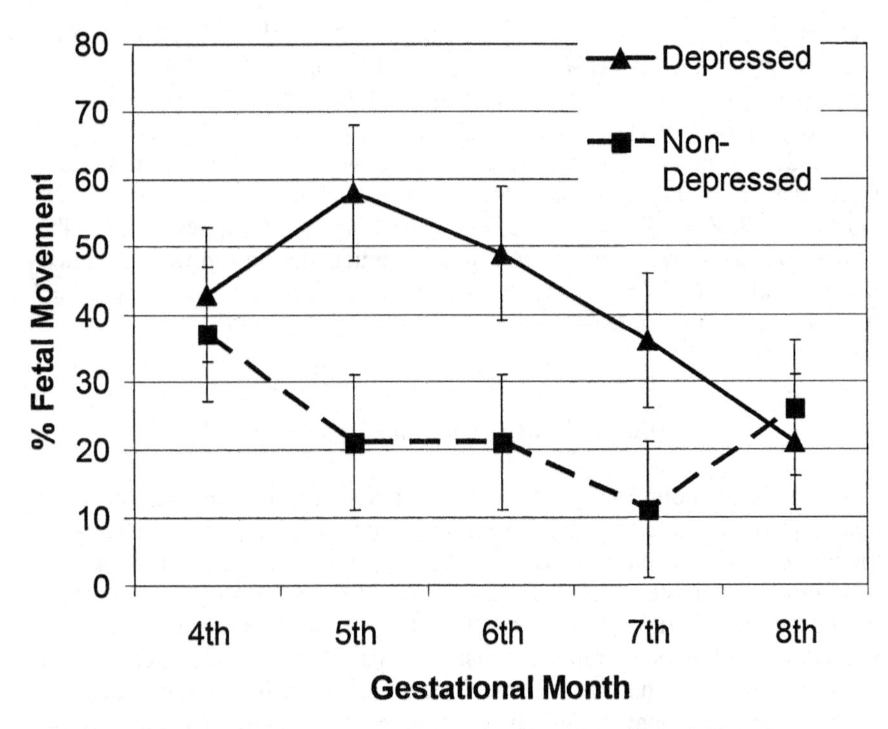

FIGURE 1. Movement in fetuses of "depressed" and "nondepressed" mothers across gestation.

Fetal Assessment

Actocardiographic monitoring provides quantitative measurement of fetal movement and HR. A computer program calculates summary variables for the biobehavioral measures. Fetal assessment consisted of three distinct phases: A 5-min baseline, stimulation trials whose number depended on if and when the fetus habituated (i.e., four consecutive trials without movement for 10 sec), and a 5-min poststimulation period.

Results

Repeated-measures multivariate analysis of variance (MANOVA) revealed a significant group effect on fetal movement and HR, F (2, 21) = 3.42, P = 0.05 (two-tailed). Fetuses of depressed mothers showed a significantly lower mean baseline HR (Depressed M = 133.87 BPM, SD = 13.30; Nondepressed M = 145.68 BPM, SD = 16.76, P = 0.04, one-tailed). During stimulation, the Depressed group showed less total movement (P = 0.03, one-tailed). A change score revealed that fetuses of depressed mothers showed a HR increase from baseline to the stimulation trials compared to a HR decrease in fetuses of Nondepressed mothers ($M = -3.10$, SD = 12.13), $t(22) = -1.83$, $P = 0.04$ (one-tailed). More of the Depressed group meet the criterion for habituation to vibratory stimulation (Depressed 52.94%; Nondepressed 26.67%), $U = 72.50$, $P = 0.02$, (two-tailed). The Depressed group showed fewer trials to habituation (Depressed $M = 12.18$, SD = 6.94; Nondepressed $M = 22.67$, SD = 7.57), $t(12) = 2.28$, $P = 0.04$, (two-tailed). Stepwise regression suggested that 34% of the variance in whether a fetus met the habituated criterion was explained by maternal BDI-II ($R^2 = 0.25$, $P < 0.01$ [two-tailed]) and BAI scores ($R^2 = 0.34$, $P < 0.01$ [two-tailed]).

Discussion of Study 1 and 2 Findings

These studies point to a possible neurobehavioral profile that reflects fetal reaction to maternal emotional distress and its possible biochemical effects on the intrauterine environment that may be analogous to the "general adaptation syndrome."[5] Heightened motor activity in mid-gestation may represent the fetus's "alarm reaction." While initially adaptive, the prolonged exposure to stress and the fetus's attempts at resistance, may diminish physiological and behavioral reserves that are reflected in the general decline in motor activity after the 5th gestational month. These adaptive efforts may then result in some degree of "exhaustion" during late gestation that manifests in a greater propensity toward receptor adaptation, effector fatigue, and diminished responsivity to vibratory stimulation.

STUDY 3: CASE STUDIES OF THE EFFECTS OF PSYCHOTROPIC MEDICATION ON FETAL CEREBRAL BLOOD FLOW

Investigations of cerebral blood flow in the human fetus (F-cbf) focus on the Circle of Willis (a polygon-shaped ring of cerebral vessels that include the middle cerebral artery [MCA], anterior cerebral artery [ACA], and posterior cerebral artery [PCA]).

Participants

Four psychiatric cases of women (two with major depression prescribed SSRIs and two with bipolar disorder prescribed lithium) underwent research F-cbf velocity measures. Obtained velocity values were compared to expected values based on clinical norms ($N = 600$).

Results

Women prescribed SSRIs showed overall increases in combined left (L)- and right (R)-MCA velocity ($M = +18.5\%$), with larger increases in the right than the left MCA. Women prescribed lithium showed minute increases, but mostly decreases ($M = -2.1\%$) in flow velocity in both L and R MCA.

Study 3 Interpretation

These case studies suggest that the human fetal brain is reactive to psychotropic medication. Moreover, the general direction of change in blood flow velocity mirrors what one would expect given the pharmacologic properties of these medications. It is entirely unknown if these effects persist into the neonatal period or if they materially affect cognitive or perceptual functioning.

Clinical Implications of These Studies

Findings highlight the importance of early clinical intervention for psychologically distressed pregnant women. A unique idea is that the negative effects of maternal stress and psychopathology on the developing fetus can be combated through interventions provided to the pregnant mother. Potential prenatal maternal interventions that require further research study include psychotropic medication, psychotherapy, and complimentary treatments, such as massage therapy, yoga, and relaxation therapy.

REFERENCES

1. FIELD, T. 1998. Maternal depression effects on infants and early interventions. Prev. Med. **27:** 200–203.
2. JONES, J.A., T. FIELD, N.A. FOX, *et al.* 1998. Newborns of mothers with depressive symptoms are physiologically less developed. Infant Behav. Dev. **21:** 537–541.
3. DIETER, J.N.I., T. FIELD, M. HERNANDEZ-REIF, *et al.* 2001. Maternal depression and increased fetal activity. J. Obstet. Gynaecol. **21:** 468.
4. DIETER, J.N.I., E.K. EMORY, K.C. JOHNSON, *et al.* Maternal depression and anxiety effects on the fetus: preliminary findings and clinical implications. Infant Mental Health J. In Press.
5. SELYE, H. 1998. A syndrome produced by diverse nocuous agents. 1936. J. Neuropsychiatry Clin Neurosci. **10:** 230–231.

More Than Maternal Sensitivity Shapes Attachment

Infant Coping and Temperament

MARINA FUERTES,[a,b] PEDRO LOPES DOS SANTOS,[b]
MARJORIE BEEGHLY,[a] AND EDWARD TRONICK[a]

[a]*Child Development Unit, Children's Hospital, Boston and Harvard Medical School, Boston, Massachusetts, USA*

[b]*Faculdade de Psicologia e de Ciências da Educação, University of Porto, Porto, Portugal*

ABSTRACT: The aim of this longitudinal study was to investigate the effect of a set of factors from multiple levels of influence: infant temperament, infant regulatory behavior, and maternal sensitivity on infant's attachment. Our sample consisted of 48 infants born prematurely and their mothers. At 1 and 3 months of age, mothers described their infants' behavior using the Escala de Temperamento do Bebé. At 3 months of age, infants' capacity to regulate stress was evaluated during Tronick's Face-to-Face Still-Face (FFSF) paradigm. At 9 months of age, mothers' sensitivity was evaluated during free play using the CARE-Index. At 12 months of age, infants' attachment security was assessed during Ainsworth's Strange Situation. A total of 16 infants were classified as securely attached, 17 as insecure-avoidant, and 15 as insecure-resistant. Mothers of securely attached infants were more likely than mothers of insecure infants to describe their infants as less difficult and to be more sensitive to their infants in free play. In turn, secure infants exhibited more positive responses during the Still-Face. Infants classified as insecure-avoidant were more likely to self-comfort during the Still-Face and had mothers who were more controlling during free play. Insecure-resistant exhibited higher levels of negative arousal during the Still-Face and had mothers who were more unresponsive in free play. These findings show that attachment quality is influenced by multiple factors, including infant temperament, coping behavior, and maternal sensitivity.

KEYWORDS: attachment; infants born prematurely; resilience; multidimensional approach

Address for correspondence: Marina Fuertes, Child Development Unit, Children's Hospital, 1295 Boylston Street, Suite 320, Boston, MA 02215. Voice: 617-355-3545; fax: 617-730-0074.
e-mail: marina.fuertes@childrens.harvard.edu

**Ann. N.Y. Acad. Sci. 1094: 292–296 (2006). © 2006 New York Academy of Sciences.
doi: 10.1196/annals.1376.037**

INTRODUCTION

Infants born prematurely are at risk for attachment problems.[1–3] Classical attachment theory postulates that maternal sensitivity is a primary factor in determining the quality of the attachment relationship.[4] However, modern attachment theorists argue for a transactional, multicontextual approach.[5,6] The aim of this longitudinal study is to investigate the effect of a set of factors from multiple levels of influence: infant temperament, infant regulatory behavior (coping), and maternal sensitivity on infant's attachment in a sample of infants born prematurely.

SAMPLE

The sample consisted of 48 Portuguese prematurely born infants (M gestational age at birth = 33.94; SD = 1.97; range: 31–36 weeks; M birth weight = 2.104 g.; SD = 0.495; range: 1.100–2.500 g.) and their mothers (M age = 27.98; SD = 5.69; range: 18 to 40 years). No infants had sensory or neuromotor disabilities or serious illnesses, and no parents had any known mental health or drug/alcohol addiction problems. Infants' age at each follow-up assessment was corrected for gestational age at delivery.

PROCEDURE

Infant Temperament

When infants were 1 and 3 months old, mothers described their infants' temperament using the Escala de Temperamento do Bebé.[7] This scale is statistically explained by a single factor and highly correlated with other parental ratings of infants' difficulty. Mothers rated infants' behavior (e.g., "My child calms down") on a 7-point Likert scale (1 = very easy, 7 = very difficult).

Infant Regulatory Behavior

At 3 months, infants' capacity to regulate stress was evaluated during Tronick's Face-to-Face Still-Face (FFSF) paradigm.[8] The infants' behavior was coded using the Infant Regulatory Scoring System (IRSS).[9] Following scoring, IRSS behaviors were grouped into three categories: positive expression, negative expression, and self-comfort.

Mother–Infant Play Interaction

At 9 months, mother–infant interactive behavior during free play was scored using the CARE-Index.[10] This scale assesses the mother's interactive behavior according to three qualifications (sensitive, controlling, and unresponsive), and the infant's interactive behavior according to four qualifications (cooperative, compulsive, difficult, and passive).

Attachment

At 12 months, the Strange Situation was administered and scored by trained and reliable coders. Infants were categorized as either secure, insecure-avoidant, or insecure-resistant using Ainsworth *et al.*[11] guidelines.

RESULTS

Distribution of Attachment Classifications

A total of 16 (33.3%) infants were classified as securely attached, 17 (35.4%) as insecure-avoidant, and 15 (31.3%) as insecure-resistant.

Infant Temperament and Infant Attachment

Compared to mothers of secure infants, mothers of avoidant infants were more likely to describe their infants as difficult at both 1 month (H-Kruskal-Wallis = 16.780; $P < 0.001$) and at 3 months of age (H-Kruskal-Wallis = 9.971; $P = 0.002$). Similarly, mothers of resistant infants were more likely than mothers of secure infants to rate their infants as difficult at both 1 month (H-Kruskal-Wallis = 16.924; $P < 0.001$) and 3 months of age (H-Kruskal-Wallis = 18.446; $P < 0.001$).

Infant Temperament and Maternal Interactive Behavior

Mothers who rated their infants' temperament as more difficult at 1 and 3 months interacted with them in a less sensitive and more passive manner during free play at 9 months (TABLE 1).

Infants' Regulatory Behavior and Attachment

Secure infants were more likely than avoidant infants (H-Kruskal-Wallis = 3.837; $P = 0.05$) or resistant infants (H-Kruskal-Wallis = 4.560; $P = 0.033$) to exhibit positive responses to their mother during the FFSF paradigm. Infants classified as avoidant used more self-comforting behaviors to regulate their

TABLE 1. Correlations (Spearman's ρ coefficients) between mothers' interactive behavior and their ratings of infants' difficult behavior at 1 month and at 3 months (corrected for the gestational age)

	Difficult temperament at 1 month	Difficult temperament at 3 months
Sensitivity	−0.752**	−0.684 **
Control	0.200	0.160
Passivity	0.326*	0.336*

*$P < 0.03$; **$P < 0.001$.

stress during the Still-Face than secure infants (H-Kruskal-Wallis = 3.982; $P = 0.05$) or resistant infants (H-Kruskal-Wallis = 12.233; $P < 0.001$). Finally, negative expression was significantly higher in ambivalent-resistant infants compared to avoidant-attached infants (H-Kruskal-Wallis = 4.948; $P = 0.026$), and marginally higher than in secure infants (H-Kruskal-Wallis = 2.9783; $P = 0.084$).

Maternal Interactive Behavior during Free Play and Attachment

Compared to mothers of insecure infants, mothers of secure infants were more sensitive with their infant during free play (H-Kruskal-Wallis = 26.884; $P < 0.001$). In turn, mothers of avoidant infants were more controlling (H-Kruskal-Wallis = 15.804; $P < 0.001$) and mothers of resistant infants were more unresponsive than mothers of secure infants (H-Kruskal-Wallis = 22.961; $P < 0.001$).

DISCUSSION

A relatively low incidence of secure attachment (33.3%) was found in this sample. These results corroborate findings from prior Portuguese studies that also reported a lower incidence of securely attached infants, compared with American and other Western samples.[12] The results are also consistent with findings from other attachment studies with infants born prematurely at high medical risk.[1–3]

In relation to coping and temperament, securely attached infants were more likely to be described by their mothers as less difficult and to exhibit more positive responses during the FFSF paradigm. Their mothers also were more sensitive in free play compared with insecure infants. Infants classified as insecure-avoidant were more likely to self-comfort during the FFSF paradigm and had mothers who were more controlling during free play. Insecure-resistant exhibited higher negative arousal during the FFSF paradigm and had mothers who were less responsive in free play. These findings are consistent with a transactional and multicontextual conceptual model of development rather than a single-factor causal model.

ACKNOWLEDGMENT

This work was supported with a fellowship from Fundação para a Ciência a e Tecnologia, Secretariado Nacional para a Reabilitação da Pessoa com Deficiência and Fundação Marquês de Pombal.

REFERENCES

1. Cox, S.M., J. Hopkins & S.L. Hans. 2000. Attachment in preterm infants and their mothers: neonatal risk status and maternal representations. Infant Ment. Health J. **21**(6)**:** 464–480.
2. Mangelsdorf, S.C. *et al.* 1996. Attachment security in very low birth weight infants. Dev. Psychol. **32:** 914–920.
3. Wille, D.E. 1991. Relation of preterm birth with quality of mother-infant attachment at one year. Infant Behav. Dev. **14:** 227–240.
4. Bowlby, J. 1969. Attachment and Loss. Penguin Books. London.
5. Sroufe, L.A. 1996. Emotional Development: The Organization of Emotional Life in the Early Years. Cambridge University Press. New York.
6. Cicchetti, D. & D. Barnett. 1991. Attachment organization in maltreated preschoolers. Dev. Psychopathol. **3:** 397–411.
7. Lopes dos Santos, P., M. Fuertes & M. Sanches-Ferreira. 2005. A percepção materna dos atributos temperamentais do bebé: características psicométricas de um questionário e seu valor prognóstico relativamente à qualidade da vinculação. *In* Desenvolvimento: Contextos Familiares e Educativos. J. Bairrao, Ed.: 142–170. Livpsic. Porto, Portugal.
8. Tronick, E.Z. *et al.* 1978. The infant's response to entrapment between contradictory messages in face-to-face interaction. J. Am. Acad. Child Adolesc. Psychiatry **17:** 1–13.
9. Tronick, E.Z. & K. Weinberg. 1990. The Infant Regulatory Scoring System (IRSS). Unpublished Manuscript. Children's Hospital and Harvard Medical School, Boston.
10. Crittenden, P.M. 2003. CARE-Index Manual. Unpublished Manuscript. Family Relations Institute, Miami, FL.
11. Ainsworth, M.D.S. *et al.* 1978. Patterns of Attachment: A Psychological Study of the Strange Situation. Lawrence Erlbaum Associates. Hillsdale, NJ.
12. Fuertes, M. 2005. Rotas da Vinculacao. Doctoral Thesis. Porto University. Porto, Portugal.

Infant Resilience to the Stress of the Still-Face

Infant and Maternal Psychophysiology Are Related

JACOB HAM[a] AND ED TRONICK

[a]*Beth Israel Medical Center, New York City, New York, USA*

[b]*Harvard Medical School, Boston, Massachusetts, USA*

ABSTRACT: Respiratory sinus arrhythmia (RSA) is related to infant emotion regulation and resilience. However, few studies have examined RSA of infants *and* mothers during a stressful experience. Even fewer studies have measured infant and mother skin conductance (SC), which in part reflects anxiety. This pilot study examined RSA, heart rate (HR), and SC patterns of 12 five-month-old infants and their mothers during normal interaction and a stressful perturbation of the interaction in which the mother does not respond to her infant—the Face-to-Face Still-Face (FFSF) paradigm. Dyads were grouped into four categories by two conditions: whether the infant protested to the Still-Face episode (SF) and whether they "recovered" from the SF by reducing protest when the mother resumed interaction in the Reunion (RE). Infants who recovered from the SF had the largest increase in RSA from SF to RE. Mothers of infants who recovered from the SF showed a decrease in RSA during the RE, suggesting mobilization of infant soothing behaviors. Mothers of infants who did not recover from the SF showed physiologic markers of anxiety in the form of continued increases in RSA and high levels of SC. Furthermore, these mothers behaved in a manner that was not responsive to their infant's disengagement cues. These pilot results demonstrate the feasibility of measuring infant SC, a measure long disregarded in infant research. The findings suggest that maternal psychophysiology may be related to infant resilience and suggest a bidirectional effect of maternal and infant reactivity.

KEYWORDS: mother-infant interaction; psychophysiology; respiratory sinus arrythmia; skin conductance

Address for correspondence: Jacob Ham, Ph.D., Beth Israel Medical Center, First Avenue at Sixteenth St. New York City, NY 10003. Voice: 212-420-4114; fax: 212-420-3936.
e-mail: jham@chpnet.org

**Ann. N.Y. Acad. Sci. 1094: 297–302 (2006). © 2006 New York Academy of Sciences.
doi: 10.1196/annals.1376.038**

INTRODUCTION

Resilience includes an ability to regulate one's emotions in the face of stress and challenge. In infancy, emotion regulation is thought to develop through interactions with primary caretakers.[1] This pilot study examines interactions between mothers and 5-month-old infants to explore whether physiologic measures of emotion regulation in both mothers and infants relate to interactive social behaviors.

The physiologic measures used in this study are heart rate (HR), respiratory sinus arrhythmia (RSA), and skin conductance (SC). RSA is an estimate of the parasympathetic influence on HR variability and has been found to be related to emotion regulation abilities. According to Porges' Polyvagal theory,[2] decreases in RSA indicate a decrease of parasympathetic activity in order to mobilize a sympathetic and behavioral response; whereas, increases in RSA indicate an increase of parasympathetic tone and is considered to indicate a recovery of response. SC is a direct measure of sympathetic arousal. Its measurement has never before been used in this type of infant research. This study is also unique in that both mother and infant physiologies are measured in the hopes of finding a relation between mother and infant physiologies as they relate to infant emotion regulation and resilience.

METHOD

Procedures

Clinically normal mother–infant dyads were recruited through a database of families who participated in a prior study at the Child Development Unit of Children's Hospital Boston.

Upon arrival to the lab, families were given the opportunity to settle into the waiting room and ensure that the infant was comfortable and alert. Study procedures were described to mothers and informed consent was obtained. Mother and infant were escorted into the observation room. Disposable, pre-gelled sensors for measurement of ECG and SC were placed on mother and infant. Physiologic data were collected and analyzed using the ADInstruments Powerlab 8SP modular instrument system connected to a notebook computer running Chart Software (v. 4.2) (Sydney, Australia). Video and physiologic recording were begun and manually synchronized.

Face-to-Face Still-Face Paradigm (FFSF)

The FFSF is a standard laboratory-based observational procedure for studying infant social capacities and capacity to cope with perturbations. The FFSF consists of three successive 2-minute episodes: an episode of ordinary mother–infant face-to-face interactive play (FF), an interactive perturbation episode called the Still-Face (SF), in which the mother looks at the infant and remains immobile, and a reunion play episode (RE) in which the mother reengages with her infant in her usual playful manner. The interactions are recorded using split-screen video techniques and coded using the Observer 5.0 software by Noldus Information Technology (Leesburg, VA). Mother and infant behaviors were coded using the Infant Caregiver Engagement Phases (ICEP),[3] which codes mothers and infants for facial expression (positive and negative affect), direction of gaze, and vocalizations on a second-by-second basis.

RESULTS

Sample

A total of 16 mother–infant dyads completed this pilot study. Four dyads were dropped for technical reasons. Dyads were first categorized into groups according to (i) whether or not the infant protested during the SF episode for more than 25% of the time and (ii) whether or not the infant "recovered" during the RE by reducing the percent time of protest behaviors. The 4 groups were: Recovered ($n = 4$) infants who protested during the SF for more than 25% of the time but then reduced percent time of Protest during the RE; Stably Low ($n = 5$) infants who did not protest for more than 25% of the time in either SF or RE; Dysregulated ($n = 2$) infants who protested during the SF for more than 25% of the time and continued to increase during RE; and Cry in RE only ($n = 1$) infant who only began to protest in RE.

Infant Physiology

FIGURE 1 (A–C) shows the patterns of physiologic activation for infant HR, RSA, and SC for each infant group. For infant HR, patterns of HR reflect the patterns of protest used to define each group. That is, HR was significantly correlated with infant protest for the entire sample and for all episodes ($r(35) = 0.58$, $P < 0.001$). For infant RSA, the Recovered infants showed the greatest increase in RSA from SF to RE, which together with the fact that they reduced protest from SF to RE, suggests that increases in parasympathetic tone was related to infant soothing and recovery. For infant SC, most groups (except for the infant who cried during RE only) showed a general pattern of increasing SC across episodes. The Recovered group showed the lowest mean SC levels during all episodes.

Mother Physiology

FIGURE 1 (C–F) shows the patterns of physiologic activation for maternal HR, RSA, and SC for each infant group. For maternal HR, mothers in all infant

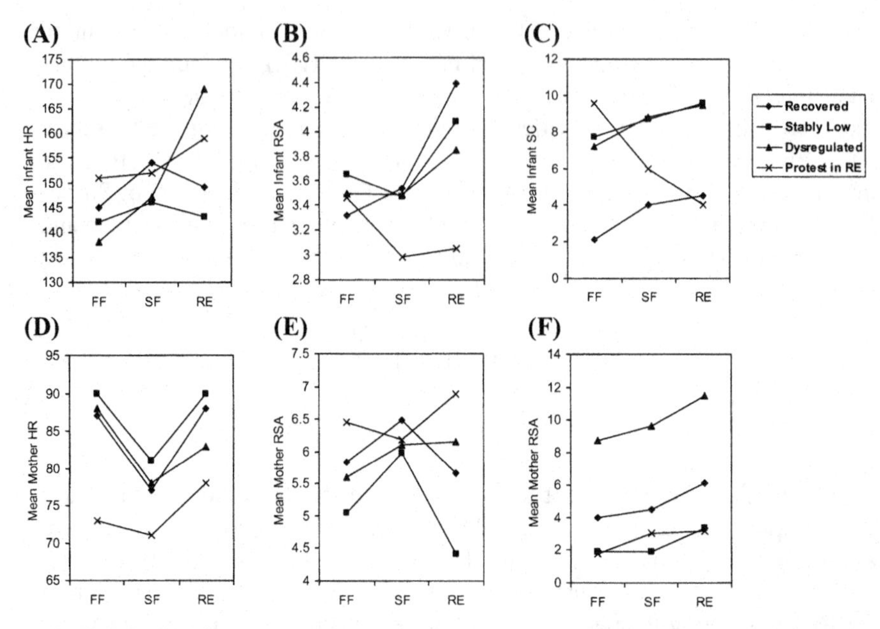

FIGURE 1. Infant (A–C) and mother (D–F) mean heart rate (HR), respiratory sinus arrythmia (RSA) and skin conductance (SC) in each episode of the Face-to-Face Still-Face by infant group.

groups showed a similar pattern of HR deceleration and acceleration consistent with the behavioral demands of the FFSF paradigm. That is, HR decelerated during the SF, which is likely due to the fact that mothers sat still during this episode. For maternal RSA, mothers in the Recovered and Stably Low groups showed a pattern of increasing RSA during the SF and decreasing during the RE. Consistent with Porges' Polyvagal theory, this suggests that mothers in these groups decreased RSA in the RE to increase the capacity to respond to the challenge of soothing their infant after the SF challenge. In contrast, mothers of the Dysregulated infants did not decrease RSA during the RE. Furthermore, in FIGURE 1 F, one can see that mothers of the Dysregulated infants had the highest mean SC levels across all episodes. These latter two findings suggest that mothers in the Dysregulated group were more physiologically anxious or at least aroused. The causal direction between maternal anxiety and infant protest behaviors during the RE is unclear, but was in part answered by looking at maternal behaviors.

Infant and Mother Behaviors during the FFSF

FIGURE 2 A–H shows the mean percentage of time for each infant and mother ICEP behavior in each infant group. Mothers of Dysregulated infants had very

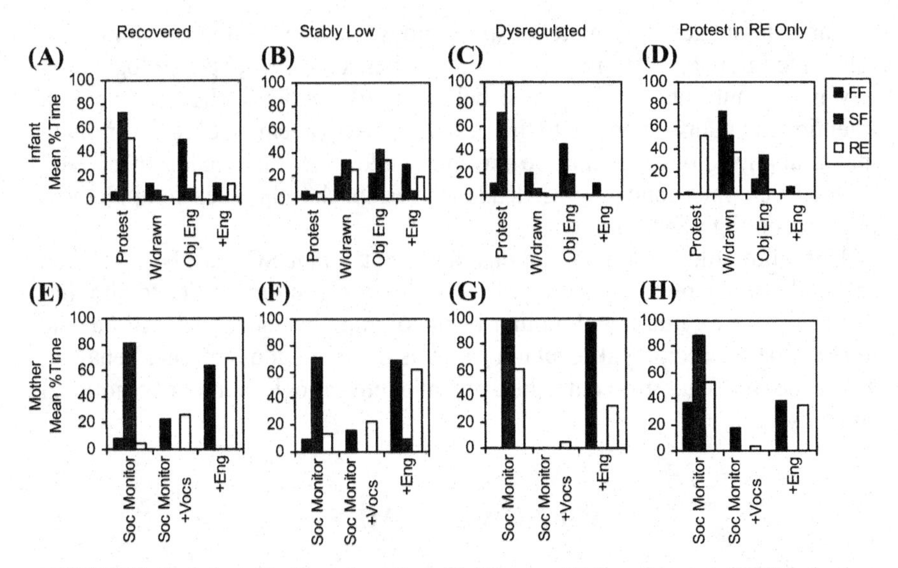

FIGURE 2. Infant (A–D) and mother (E–H) mean %time for each ICEP behavior across infant groups and by Face-to-Face Still-Face episode.

high and unmitigated levels of positive engagement with their infants during the FF play episode (FIG. 2 G) despite the fact that their infants spent most of their time disengaging from their mother (evidenced by Infant Object Engagement in FIG. 2 C). In contrast, mothers in the Recovered (FIG. 2 E) and Stably Low (FIG. 2 F) groups showed a mix of positive engagement and social monitoring, which is likely to indicate attuned and flexible behaviors responding to the infant's focus of attention. Infants in the Stably Low group (FIG. 2 B) were the only ones to show a greater proportion of positive engagement over object engagement in the FF. Furthermore, they showed very little protest during the SF and RE, and showed a mix of positive social engagement and environment engagement during the RE.

CONCLUSIONS

Results from this pilot study suggest that infants' ability to recover from the stress of the SF may be associated with RSA, which is consistent with prior research.[4] That is, increase in RSA activity after a social stressor may be related to soothing and regulation of distress. However, recovery as defined here may not be the most resilient response to a social challenge. Rather, the most resilient response may be to not become distressed at all—the Stably Low group. These infants remained physiologically calm throughout the procedure. Their mothers were also physiologically calm (according to mean SC levels) and interacted with them in a responsive manner.

Our data suggest that maternal physiology may be an important variable related to infant emotion regulation and resilience. Maternal physiologic anxiety may contribute to insensitive behaviors of mothers, who may be well intentioned but unresponsive to their infants' disengagement cues. Examining maternal physiology may thus be a useful window into maternal influences on infant development and may also lead to biofeedback techniques to supplement other parenting interventions.

This pilot study has also demonstrated that infant SC may be measured and adds to our research armory. Furthermore, given our ability to simultaneously measure infant and mother behavior and physiology we will be able to examine the reciprocal regulatory effects of infant and maternal behavior. These measures may turn out to be a potential physiologic marker of emotional empathy.

ACKNOWLEDGMENT

This study was supported by an Institutional NRSA T32 MH 16259-26 (PI: Ed Tronick; Fellow: Jacob Ham) from NIMH, the Sackler Foundation Scholarship for Research in Psychobiology from Harvard University (PI: Jacob Ham), and the Livingston Award from Harvard Medical School (PI: Jacob Ham). We would also like to thank Scott Orr, Ph.D., for his guidance in collecting and analyzing the physiologic data.

REFERENCES

1. TRONICK, E.Z. 1989. Emotions and emotional communication in infants. Am. Psychol. **44:** 112–119.
2. PORGES, S.W. 2003. The Polyvagal Theory: phylogenetic contributions to social behavior. Physiol. Behav. **79:** 503–513.
3. WEINBERG, M.K. & E.Z. TRONICK. 1999. Infant Caregiver Engagement Phases. Unpublished Manuscript. Harvard Medical School. Boston.
4. MOORE, G.A. & S.D. CALKINS. 2004. Infants' vagal regulation in the still-face paradigm is related to dyadic coordination of mother-infant interaction. Dev. Psychol. **40:** 1068–1080.

Children Survivors of the 2004 Tsunami in Aceh, Indonesia

A Study of Resiliency

YOHANA RATRIN HESTYANTI

Atma Jaya Catholic University, Department of Psychology, Jakarta, Indonesia

ABSTRACT: This exploratory study investigates factors contributing to resiliency of children in the age group of 11–15 years, survivors of the 2004 tsunami in Aceh, Indonesia, through qualitative methodology. Series of participative observation and interviews with children, parents, and local social workers were conducted. A group of 50 children from three camps of the tsunami-affected areas in Banda Aceh and Great Aceh were involved and observed through several psychosocial activities conducted in coordination with local social workers in the community. Resilient children were identified based on criteria that were developed from the context of the tsunami-affected children in Banda Aceh and Great Aceh. Six children were identified as resilient. They show absence of clinically significant levels of trauma-related symptoms as measured by Trauma Symptom Checklist for Children-A (TSCC-A). They are able to live normally, such as participate in school activities, play with friends, perform daily chores, be involved in religious activities, and develop healthy relationships with caregivers and peers. They are also perceived as cooperative in psychosocial activities. Findings in internal protective factors of these children include: strong internal motivation to recover, good heart, open to other people, high motivation to bond to religiosity, self-responsible, sense of humor, and easygoing. Contributing external factors include: support from significant others, able to do religious practice routinely, able to learn traditional dance in groups, have opportunities to be involved in structured play/psychosocial activities, and have access to natural resources for recreation, such as a river.

KEYWORDS: tsunami; child survivors; child resiliency; factors of resiliency; Acehnese children; Indonesia

Address for correspondence: Yohana Ratrin Hestyanti, Department of Psychology, Atma Jaya Catholic University, Jl. Jendral Sudirman 51, Jakarta 12930, Indonesia. Voice: +62-21-5719558; fax: +62-21-5708830.

e-mail: jo_hesty@yahoo.com

Ann. N.Y. Acad. Sci. 1094: 303–307 (2006).
doi: 10.1196/annals.1376.039

BACKGROUND

The aftermath of the tsunami in Aceh province and Nias Island, Indonesia on December 26, 2004, left approximately 167,000 people who had vanished, 190,000 homeless, and 67,000 people including children living in barracks or tents.[1] Apart from having lost families, homes, relatives, and good friends, children have to face many adversities because the process of reconstruction and recovery is quite slow. After over a year, *they still have to stay in temporary barracks and tents with a low standard of living. They also have to adapt to new neighbors and friends who came from different regions, new schools, new teachers, new composition of the families, new structure of the community, and other new living challenges. In these circumstances, children get easily bored and frustrated. They have lost control over their daily lives. Since many adults, including their parents, have no stable income, livelihood has become the most sensitive issue for these survivors.[2]

In such difficult situations, children suffered a lot of burden. Their parents did not have the time and energy left to care for them and were more likely to subject them to punishment and violent behavior.[3] Such situations made children vulnerable to long, negative, psychosocial impacts. However, even under such stressful conditions, some children have shown that they can adapt well in their daily lives. They are cheerful, able to help each other, are actively involved in intervention programs, speak confidently in front of people, and show other positive behaviors.[4] Those positive behaviors within all the adversities the children face are a sign of resiliency defined as the ability to fight back and recover from disruptive life changes. It involves processes that promote the ability to "struggle well" and overcome difficulties within significant adversities after trauma.[5]

OBJECTIVES OF THE STUDY

This brief study aimed to: (1) identify the concept of resiliency in the Acehnese community, (2) identify resilient children among child survivors, and (3) examine factors contributing to child resiliency. 1

METHODS

This is an exploratory study that employs observations and interviews involving children and their significant others (guardians or parents, local social workers). Around 117 children in the age group of 11–15 years from three camps in Lambaro Skep, Jantho, and Tanjong, located in Banda Aceh and Great Aceh areas were approached and observed. Among those, 50 children

*The period of the study was from January to February, 2006.

were routinely and actively involved in psychosocial activities that were held by a researcher's team in coordination with local social workers working for Care International Indonesia. To enable the researcher to study the community deeply, we had to concentrate on the ongoing psychosocial activities.

These preliminary findings were based on interviews with 6 children, 6 parents, 3 social workers, 1 teacher, 2 focus group discussions with parents, and 5 focus group discussions with local social workers. Those data were supported by participative observation of the interaction between children and researcher's team on psychosocial activities and other occasions in daily living and self-reports on the Trauma Symptom Checklist for Children without sexual concern items (TSCC-A).[6]

Recruitment of these children was guided by the following criteria: (1) are tsunami survivors, (2) those that lost their homes, (3) in the age group of 11–15 years, and met at least one of the following criteria: (*a*) live in barracks or tents more than a year, (*b*) lost at least one close/significant family/relatives/friends, or (*c*) have to be relocated to other places.

Children were considered resilient if they met the above criteria and had several qualities, such as: (1) actively and routinely involved in at least one activity conducted in communities, for example, religious practices or psychosocial activities (dance or other programs), (2) considered as good or nice and not troublemakers by local social workers, parents, and peers, and (3) not demonstrating clinically significant levels of trauma-related symptoms, such as anxiety, depression, anger, posttraumatic stress, and dissociation as measured by TSCC-A without suicide item (concerning cultural boundaries).

PRELIMINARY FINDINGS

Common Trauma-Related Symptoms

Common reactions of children to disaster between the age of 11 to 15 years (preadolescence) are: rebellion in the home, refuse to undertake responsibilities, school problems (such as, absenteeism, fighting, withdrawal, loss of interest, attention-seeking behaviors), physical problems (e.g., headaches, vague pains, skin eruptions, psychosomatic complaints), loss of interest in peer social activities, decreased attention and/or concentration, anger outburst and/or aggression, increased negative and deviant behavior, and increased risk of substance abuse.[7]

Many child participants showed those reactions, but the most common trauma-related symptoms were excessive energy for aggressive behavior, rebellion against parents and adults, and increased irritability. Their drives to release the negative energy were huge, but they did not have enough and mature capacities to control it. Many of them become troublemakers in their families and communities. Other common symptoms were reduction in concentration and having difficulties in following the subjects at schools—especially for those children who do not follow additional courses outside the schools.

Resilient Children

Survivors were regarded as resilient when they were able to adapt to different adversities in their new circumstances, which obviously engendered multiple development risks.[8–10] Six children were identified as resilient, indicated by the absence of clinically significant trauma-related symptoms as measured by TSCC-A. They were able to live normal lives and participate in school activities, like playing with friends, doing daily chores, involving themselves in religious activities, and developing healthy relationships with guardians or parents and peers. They were also perceived as cooperative by local social workers, peers, and researcher's team in psychosocial activities.

Contributing Factors

Both personal and external factors dynamically contribute to resiliency.[5,8–10] This study finds that internal protective factors of these children include strong internal motivation to recover, have a good heart, open to other people, have high motivation to bond to religiosity, being self-responsible, have a sense of humor, and easygoing. Four of the above qualities were strongly demonstrated by all six children and the following three qualities were indicated by one or two children only.

The study also identified external factors, such as having support from significant others (parents, guardians, siblings, peers, or social workers). In addition, to have access or to be involved in routine religious activities seemed to help children cope with their trauma. All six children were involved in such activities. Learning and reading Quran is a socially expected behavior among children and understandably getting a lot of support in the community. Although it was a strictly observed practice before the tsunami, it is becoming problematic as many communities were torn apart. Being able to practice this tradition is highly appreciated and maintains children within the supportive structure of the community. Other external factors identified in the study were: having access or involvement in traditional rituals, especially dance in group; having access to involve in structured play; and having access to natural resources for recreation, such as a river. These external factors help children channelize their energy positively and help them to bond with peers.

IMPLICATIONS

These early findings suggest a need for warm, caring, and nonviolent relationships between adults or significant others and children, as well as individual or community supports for parents or caregivers who deal with children in facing all the adversities. The multiple-level approach that includes individual, peer, family, and community psychosocial intervention programs is highly needed, along with the consideration of a locally sensitive approach.

REFERENCES

1. THE REHABILITATION AND RECONSTRUCTION AGENCY (BRR), INDONESIA. December 2005. Aceh and Nias One Year after the Tsunami Report. Executive Summary. Retrieved from www.e-aceh-nias.org.
2. Personal communication and discussions with parents in Lambaro Skep and Jantho's camps in Banda Aceh and Great Aceh. November 2005 and January 2006.
3. Personal communication and discussions with parents and local social workers in Lambaro Skep and Jantho's camps in Banda Aceh and Great Aceh. January–February 2006.
4. Discussions with volunteers and local social workers working with child survivors of the Tsunami in Aceh. February 2005, November 2005, and January 2006.
5. WALSH, F. 2003. Family resilience: a framework for clinical practice. Family Process **42:** 1–18.
6. BRIERE, J. 1995. Trauma Symptom Checklist for Children (TSCC) Professional Manual. Odessa, FL. Psychological Assessment Resources, Inc.
7. CONSUELO, B.H. 2005. Age-related reactions of children to disaster and helpful hints to enable coping. Presented at the Tsunami Trauma Training Conference, Faculty of Psychology Tarumanegara University, Jakarta, Indonesia, April 25–27.
8. SPACCARELLI, S. & S. KIM. 1995. Resilience criteria and factors associated with resilience in sexually abused girls. Child Abuse Neglect **19:** 1171–1182.
9. LOUGHRY, M. & C. EYBER. 2003. Psychosocial concepts in humanitarian work with children. A Review of the Concepts and Related Literature. The National Academies Press. Washington, DC.
10. COVE, E., M. EISEMAN & S.J.POPKIN. 2005. Resilient Children: Literature Review and Evidence from the HOPE VI Panel Study. Final Report. The Urban Institute Metropolitan Housing and Communities Policy Center, Washington, DC.

Frontal EEG Asymmetry and Regulation during Childhood

KEE JEONG KIM[a] AND MARTHA ANN BELL[b]

[a]*Department of Human Development, Virginia Polytechnic Institute and State University, Blacksburg, Virginia, USA*

[b]*Department of Psychology, Virginia Polytechnic Institute and State University, Blacksburg, Virginia, USA*

ABSTRACT: Previous research suggests an association between frontal electroencephalographic (EEG) asymmetries and both positive and negative emotion reactivity. Specifically, right frontal EEG activation is associated with emotions of negative valence in both infants and adults, whereas left frontal EEG activation is associated with emotions of more positive valence. Relatively few studies have examined such associations in children. Moreover, research on mechanisms through which emotion reactivity is related to frontal EEG asymmetries is sparse. As one possible mechanism, we hypothesize that regulatory skills and behaviors developing rapidly during childhood play a critical role in linking frontal EEG asymmetries to emotion reactivity in children. To test the research hypothesis, 25 children were followed from early-to-middle childhood at two different points in time with a 4-year interview interval. Results show that individual variations in a number of regulatory behaviors among children are significantly associated with frontal EEG asymmetries. Our results provide support for the possibility of frontal EEG asymmetry informing the study of the development of regulation in children. The discussion of the findings is centered on potential risk for and resilience to children's emotional reactivity and regulation.

KEYWORDS: frontal EEG asymmetry; childhood regulatory behaviors; vulnerability to negative emotion

FRONTAL EEG ASYMMETRY AND REGULATION DURING CHILDHOOD

Researchers who study infants and adults have reported associations between baseline frontal electroencephalographic (EEG) asymmetries and emotion reactivity.[1–4] For instance, infants who cried in response to maternal separation

Address for correspondence: Kee Jeong Kim, Department of Human Development, 317 Wallace Hall, Virginia Polytechnic Institute and State University, Blacksburg, Virginia 24061, Voice: 540-231-4671; fax: 540-231-7012.
e-mail: keekim@vt.edu

Ann. N.Y. Acad. Sci. 1094: 308–312 (2006). © 2006 New York Academy of Sciences.
doi: 10.1196/annals.1376.040

were more likely to have right frontal EEG activation than those who did not cry in response to maternal separation.[1,2] Psychosocially healthy adults with greater relative left hemisphere frontal EEG activation at baseline reacted to positive mood elicitors with more positive affect and those with greater relative right hemisphere frontal EEG activation at baseline reported more negative emotion to negative mood elicitors.[5,6] These findings have provided crucial research evidence for some aspect of vulnerability to positive and negative emotion elicitors. In turn, these reports with healthy individuals have advanced our knowledge of psychophysiological correlates of mood disorders, such as depressive and anxious psychopathology.[7,8]

Although these studies have pointed to an important association between frontal hemisphere activation and an individual's predisposition to various emotional states, the evidence linking frontal EEG asymmetry to the *regulatory* aspects of emotion is limited. Emotional regulation involves the capacity to control emotions and to adjust emotional arousal to an appropriate level of intensity to achieve one's aims.[9] We propose that individual variations in regulatory skills may account for part of the association between emotion reactivity and frontal EEG asymmetry. It is during childhood that many regulatory skills have their foundations.[10] Indeed, children must learn various strategies for managing emotional intensity in line with social rules. A great amount of individual variation in adjustment to emotional arousal during childhood involves both competent and incompetent regulation of emotions that are displayed through complex emotional expressivity and emotion-related behaviors. Unfortunately, little is known about individual differences in emotional regulation in association with frontal EEG asymmetry during this critical period. In this investigation, we followed a group of normal children from early-to-middle childhood to examine interindividual differences in the relations between frontal EEG asymmetry and regulatory behaviors.

Fifty 8-month-old infants (28 boys) and their parents were recruited from a Southwest Virginia community for a study of the effects of emotion reactivity on infant outcome.[11] When these children were 4 years old, there were 27 of these families still living in the local area and 25 families (14 boys) agreed to participate in a preschool study.[12] When these children were 8 years of age, all 25 families were still living in the local area and agreed to participate in a follow-up study. At both the 4-year and 8-year assessments, EEG was recorded during quiet baseline. At the 4-year assessment, trained observers coded the child's skills in a variety of effortful control regulatory tasks. At the 8-year assessment, children participated in a battery of regulatory computer tasks. At both visits, parents endorsed information on their children's reactivity and regulatory behaviors via temperament questionnaires (Rothbart's CBQ and EATQ).[13,14] Parents observe their children in numerous settings and, thus, provide insight into their children's behaviors that are not readily observable in the research lab.

EEG was recorded at each age from 16 scalp locations and the analyses reported here focused on 6–9 Hz power for the left and right medial frontal leads (F3, F4). Young children have a dominant frequency between 6 and 9 Hz. Eyeblink and movement artifact were removed from the recording and power values calculated and normalized. Frontal EEG asymmetries were calculated using the formula *right EEG 6–9 Hz power (F4)–left EEG 6–9 Hz power (F3).* Lower EEG power values at one hemisphere indicate greater brain activation at that hemisphere relative to the other hemisphere. For instance, greater left hemisphere frontal activation means lower left hemisphere EEG power values relative to the right hemisphere values. Thus, a positive symmetry value indicates left frontal EEG asymmetry (left hemisphere activation) and a negative asymmetry value indicates right frontal EEG asymmetry (right hemisphere activation).

Our analyses showed that frontal EEG asymmetries were related to a number of regulatory dimensions during childhood. Examining the data from a cross-sectional perspective, higher levels of parent-reported impulsivity at the age of 4 years were associated with right frontal asymmetry ($r = -0.52$; right frontal asymmetry is a negative value). In addition, children at 4 years who were better able to regulate peak distress or excitement (parent-reported falling reactivity and soothability) were more likely to present with greater left frontal asymmetry ($r = 0.63$; left frontal asymmetry is a positive value). At 8 years of age, high levels of parent-reported surgency were associated with right frontal asymmetry ($r = -0.63$). Thus, parent-reported regulatory skills (i.e., regulating peak distress) were associated with left frontal asymmetries, whereas difficulties with regulation (i.e., impulsivity, surgency) were associated with right frontal asymmetries.

Focusing on the longitudinal analyses, higher levels of parent-reported impulsivity at 4 years of age were associated with right frontal asymmetry when the children were 8 years old ($r = -0.47$). Moreover, higher levels of parent-reported low intensity pleasure in children at age 4 were associated with right frontal asymmetry at age 8 ($r = -0.72$). Children who are high in low intensity pleasure prefer quiet activities, avoiding what might be novel and fearful situations. There was also a longitudinal association between observed regulatory behavior in the research lab setting at the age of 4 years and EEG asymmetry measured at 8 years of age. Children who exhibited a higher level of controlled behavior to delay of gratification at 4 years (Kochanska's Bow task) were more likely to show left frontal asymmetries at age 8 ($r = 0.43$).[15] These longitudinal associations are intriguing in that they each suggest that 4-year behavior is correlated with 8-year frontal EEG asymmetry.

Our results provide support for the possibility of frontal EEG asymmetry informing the study of regulation in children. We found right frontal asymmetry associated with less than optimal regulatory behaviors and left frontal asymmetry with more favorable regulatory skills. These findings extend our knowledge of neurobiological patterns associated with various emotion behaviors. It is not only emotional reactivity, as shown in previous research, but also the capacity to manage reactivity that may be affected by neurobiological patterns inherent in the individual children. It should be noted, however, that exhibiting specific patterns of frontal EEG asymmetries in early childhood does not necessarily portend either difficulties or ease in developing important regulatory abilities. There is evidence for change in frontal EEG asymmetries in young children across the first 4 years of life, along with behavioral changes in temperament-related behaviors.[16] Future studies need to address continuity and discontinuity in physiological patterns reflecting emotional disposition and regulatory skills and behaviors.

To our knowledge, the present investigation provides some of the first research evidence for potential risk and resilience with respect to developing regulatory abilities in childhood. Frontal EEG asymmetries were related to variations in emotion regulatory behaviors among children in cross-sectional and longitudinal analyses.

REFERENCES

1. BELL, M.A. & N.A. FOX. 1994. Brain development over the first year of life: relations between EEG frequency and coherence and cognitive and affective behaviors. *In* Human Behavior and the Development Brain. G. Dawson & K. FISCHER, Eds.: 314–345. Guilford. New York.
2. DAVIDSON, R.J. & N.A. FOX. 1989. The relation between tonic EEG asymmetry and ten-month-old infant emotional responses to separation. J. Abnorm. Psychol. **98:** 127–131.
3. DAVIDSON, R.J. & A.J. TOMARKEN. 1989. Laterality and emotion: an electrophysiological approach. *In* Handbook of Neuropsychology. F. Boller & J. Grafman, Eds.: 419–441. Elsevier. Amsterdam, The Netherlands.
4. HAGEMANN, D. *et al.* 2005. The latent state-trait structure of resting EEG asymmetry: replication and extension. Psychophysiology **42:** 740–752.
5. DAVIDSON, R.J. 1995. Cerebral asymmetry, emotion and affective style. *In* Brain Asymmetry. R.J. Davidson & K. Hugdahl, Eds: 361–387. MIT Press. Cambridge, MA.
6. WHEELER, R.E. *et al.* 1993. Frontal brain asymmetry and emotional reactivity: a geological substrate of affective style. Psychophysiology **30:** 82–89.
7. ALLEN, J.B. *et al.* 2004. The stability of resting frontal electroencephalographic asymmetry in depression. Psychophysiology **41:** 269–280.
8. DIEGO, M.A. *et al.* 2001. CES-D depression scores are correlated with frontal EEG alpha asymmetry. Depress. Anxiety **13:** 32–37.
9. SROUFE, L.A. 1998. Emotional Development: the Organization of Emotional Life in the Early Years. University Press. Cambridge, UK.
10. CALKINS, S. 2004. Early attachment processes and the development of emotional self-regulation. *In* Handbook of Self-Regulation: Research, Theory, and Applications. R.F. Baumeister & K.D. Vohs, Eds.: 324–339. Guilford. New York.

11. BELL, M.A. 2006. Tutorial on electroencephalogram methodology: EEG research with infants and young children. *In* Handbook of Developmental Neuropsychology. D.L. Molfese & V.J. Molfese, Eds.: Erlbaum. Mahwah, NJ. In press.
12. WOLFE, C.D. & M.A. BELL. 2004. Working memory and inhibitory control in early childhood: contributions from electrophysiology, temperament, and language. Dev. Psychobiol. **44:** 68–83.
13. ROTHBART, M.K. *et al.* 2001. Investigations of temperament at three to seven years: the children's behavior questionnaire. Child. Dev. **72:** 1394–1408.
14. ELLIS, L.K. & M.K. ROTHBART. 2001. Revision of the early adolescent temperament questionnaire: presented at the 2001 biennial meeting of the society for research in child development. Minneapolis, MN, April.
15. KOCHANSKA, G. *et al.* 2000. Effortful control in early childhood: continuity and change, antecedents, and implications for social development. Dev. Psychol. **36:** 220–232.
16. FOX, N.A. *et al.* 2001. Continuity and discontinuity of behavioral inhibition and exuberance: psychophysiological and behavioral influences across the first four years of life. Child. Dev. **72:** 1–21.

Violence and Delinquency, Early Onset Drug Use, and Psychopathology in Drug-Exposed Youth at 11 Years

LINDA L. LAGASSE,[a,b] JANE HAMMOND,[c] JING LIU,[a,b]
BARRY M. LESTER,[a,b] SEETHA SHANKARAN,[d] HENRIETTA BADA,[e]
CHARLES BAUER,[f] ROSEMARY HIGGINS,[g] AND ABHIK DAS[c]

[a]*Brown Medical School, Providence, Rhode Island, USA*

[b]*Women & Infants Hospital of Rhode Island, Providence, Rhode Island, USA*

[c]*Research Triangle Institute International, Research Triangle Park, North Carolina, USA*

[d]*Wayne State University School of Medicine, Detroit, Michigan, USA*

[e]*University of Tennessee at Memphis, School of Medicine, Memphis, Tennessee, USA*

[f]*University of Miami School of Medicine, Miami, Florida, USA*

[g]*National Institute of Child Health and Human Development, Bethesda, Maryland, USA*

ABSTRACT: In this first study of violence and resilience in 517 youth exposed to cocaine and other drugs during pregnancy, we identified specific links between four types of violence and delinquency, drug use, and psychopathology in early adolescence. Further, positive and interpersonal attributes promoted resilience in the face of exposure to violence and other risks. This study provides new evidence for the impact of violence as well as resilience against disruptive forms of psychopathology and behavior.

KEYWORDS: prenatal drug exposure; cocaine; violence; preadolescence; delinquency; early drug use; psychopathology; resilience

INTRODUCTION

Violent experiences may increase vulnerability to maladaptive behavior in youth already at risk due to prenatal drug exposure, poverty, and parental mental illness.[1–4] Positive personal and interpersonal attributes may reduce the impact

Address for correspondence: Linda L. LaGasse, Brown Center for the Study of Children at Risk, Women and Infants Hospital, 101 Dudley Street, Providence, RI 02905. Voice: 401-453-7629; fax 401-453-7646.
e-mail: Linda_Lagasse@brown.edu

Ann. N.Y. Acad. Sci. 1094: 313–318 (2006). © 2006 New York Academy of Sciences.
doi: 10.1196/annals.1376.041

of violence hence promote resilience. Poor outcomes may be associated with specific types of violence as well as specific resilience-promoting attributes. In this first study of violence and resilience in youth exposed to cocaine and other drugs during pregnancy, we examine the impact of four types of violence (community, domestic, violent friends, history of child abuse) on the prevalence of delinquency, early drug use, depression, and disruptive disorders during early adolescence. We test these effects in the context of protective factors thought to lower incidence of negative outcomes including positive relationships with others[5–7] and effortful control.[8]

We hypothesize that specific types of violence increase the likelihood of specific maladaptive behavior. Further these relationships are observed over and above the effects of prenatal drug exposure, poverty, parental mental illness, and male gender. We further hypothesize that personal and interpersonal competences, in particular positive relatedness to others and effortful control, reduce the prevalence of specific maladaptive behavior despite exposure to violence and other risk factors. The findings from this study can provide insight into the pattern of factors that promote specific maladaptive behavior as well as those that buffer high-risk youth despite violent encounters.

METHOD

Participants

This study is part of the longitudinal Maternal Lifestyle Study[9,10] of developmental outcomes related to prenatal exposure to cocaine and other drugs in more than 1,000 youth assessed from birth to 11 years (in progress). The 517 youth included in this study have completed the 11-year assessment with no missing data on longitudinal measures. Across the sample, 44% were prenatally exposed to cocaine, 8% to opiates, 61% alcohol, 54% tobacco, and 23% marijuana. Recruited postnatally at four sites (Detroit, Memphis, Miami, Providence), 19% of the youth were $\leq$32 weeks gestational age at birth, and 52% were males. The sample is 83% Black, 68% below the federal poverty line, 85% on Medicaid with 85% single mothers and 40% without a high school degree.

Types of Violence

Community violence was measured by the Survey of Community Violence and Things I Have Seen and Heard (8 and 9 years, 20% highest total score, all else). *Domestic violence* was measured by caretaker report of physical or sexual abuse (4 to 10 years, any/none). *Violent friends* was measured by report of any violent activities by friends on Things My Friends Have Done (9 to 11 years, any/none). *History of child abuse* was measured by report of physical or sexual abuse involving child protective services (1 month to 10 years, any/none).

Vulnerability Factors

Prenatal exposure to cocaine or opiates was determined by postpartum maternal report or positive toxicology from meconium (any/none).[11] *Parental psychiatric symptoms* were measured by the Brief Symptom Inventory (9 years, range 0–3.5, unit change SD = 0.48). *Low SES* was measured by the Hollingshead Scale, category V (9–11 years, any/none). *Male gender* was recorded from the hospital medical chart (yes/no).

Measures of Protective Factors

Relatedness to others was measured by seven indicators of positive relationships and prosocial behavior to teachers, parents, friends, and peers on the Relatedness Questionnaire, Teacher Relationship Questionnaire, Teacher Observation of Child Adaptation, and Quality of Child's Friendship (8 to 10 years, count of scores above 20%, range 0 to 7, unit change = 1). *Effortful control* was measured by the inhibitory control and attentional focusing scales from the Child Behavior Questionnaire (4 and 6 years, range 1.23 to 2.91, unit change is SD = 0.28).

Measures of Outcomes

Crimes against people, *School delinquency*, and *General delinquency* were measured by Things You Have Done (11 years, any/none). *Any drug use* was measured by report of tobacco, alcohol, and illicit drug use on Things You Have Done (8 to 11 years, any/none). Symptoms of *Depression* (>5 symptoms, all else), diagnosis of either *Conduct Disorder or Oppositional Deviance Disorder* (CD/ODD) (yes/no), and diagnosis of *Attentional Deficit Hyperactivity Disorder (ADHD)* (yes/no) are derived from the Diagnostic Interview Schedule for Children (11 years).

Data Analysis

Mixed model regression analysis (GLIMMIX) was applied to each outcome. All models are adjusted for site effects. Results are reported as odds ratios and confidence intervals.

TABLE 1. Significant effects of risk and protective factors on maladaptive behavior at 11 years

	Maladaptive behavior, Odds ratio (95th % confidence interval)						
Risk factors	Crimes against people	School delinquency	General delinquency	Early drug use	Depression	ADHD	ODD/CD
Community violence	1.7 (1.1–2.8)			3.2 (1.3–9.1)			
Violent friends	3.7 (2.3–6.1)	2.0 (1.2–3.3)	3.8 (2.4–6.1)				
Domestic violence							2.2 (1.1–4.8)
History of child abuse					2.1 (1.1–4.0)		
Prenatal exposure to cocaine/opiates							
Parental psychiatric symptoms					1.7 (1.4–2.2)	1.4 (1.1–1.9)	1.5 (1.1–1.9)
Low SES	1.7 (1.1–2.7)		1.7 (1.1–2.7)				2.2 (1.1–4.3)
Male	1.8 (1.2–2.9)	2.2 (1.3–3.5)	2.1 (1.3–3.2)				
Protective factors							
Positive relatedness to others		0.8 (0.7–0.9)			0.8 (0.7–0.9)		0.7 (0.6–0.9)
Effortful control	0.7 (0.6–0.9)		0.7 (0.6–0.9)			0.5 (0.3–0.7)	0.6 (0.4–0.8)

RESULTS

Results are shown in TABLE 1. Community violence was associated with increased crimes against people ($P = 0.042$) and early drug use ($P = 0.012$), but all forms of delinquency were associated with having violent friends (all P's < 0.01), while depression was promoted by history of physical or sexual abuse ($P = 0.036$), and CD/ODD was more likely if exposed to domestic violence ($P = 0.038$). ADHD was not associated with any type of violence. Parental psychiatric symptoms were associated with increased depression ($P < 0.001$), ADHD ($P = 0.008$), and ODD and CD ($P = 0.003$). Low SES predicted increased crimes against people ($P = 0.031$), general delinquency ($P = 0.027$), and diagnosis of ODD or CD ($P = 0.020$). All forms of delinquency were associated with male gender (all P's < 0.01). Prenatal exposure to cocaine or opiates showed no direct effects on maladaptive behavior. Positive relatedness to others and effortful control independently reduced the incidence of CD/ODD ($P = 0.024$, $P = 0.001$, respectively) with relatedness also reducing the incidence of school delinquency ($P = 0.018$) and depression ($P = 0.010$), and effortful control reducing the incidence of crimes against people ($P = 0.011$), general delinquency ($P = 0.005$), and ADHD ($P < 0.001$).

DISCUSSION

Specific types of violence increased poor outcomes (except ADHD) over and above drug exposure, poverty, and parental mental illness. Violent friends increased all forms of delinquency. Community violence further increased the likelihood of violent crimes as well as early drug use. Experiencing physical or sexual abuse from 1 month to 10 years was associated with depression while witnessing domestic violence from preschool to 10 years was associated with ODD or CD. Characteristics underlying resilience differed by outcome. Adolescents who can exert effortful control were less violent and delinquent, and less likely to have ADHD, ODD, CD. Adolescents with positive relationships showed less school-specific delinquency (truancy, suspension), depression, ODD, or CD.

Observed links between the types of violence, resilience-promoting characteristics, and specific maladaptive behavior provide new evidence for the impact of violence on high-risk youth. Strength-based interventions should take into account the youth's unique history of exposure to violence as well as facilitate the development of personal and interpersonal attributes that may buffer its impact.

REFERENCES

1. BINGENHEIMER, J.B., R.T. BRENNAN & F.J. EARLS. 2005. Firearm violence exposure and serious violent behavior. Science **308:** 1323–1326.

2. BOLGER, K.E. & C.J. PATTERSON. 2001. Pathways from child maltreatment to internalizing problems: perceptions of control as mediators and moderators. Dev. Psychopathol. **3:** 913–940.
3. BROOKMEYER, K.A., C.C. HENRICK & M. SCHWAB-STONE. 2005. Adolescents who witness community violence: can parent support and prosocial cognitions protect them from committing violence? Child Dev. **76:** 917–929.
4. HERRERA, V.M. & L.A. MCCLOSKEY. 2001. Gender differences in the risk for delinquency among youth exposed to family violence. Child Abuse Neglect **25:** 1037–1051.
5. BOROWSKY, I.W., M. IRELAND & M.D. RESNICK. 2002. Violence risk and protective factors among youth held back in school. Ambulatory Pediatrics. **2:** 457–484.
6. RESNICK, M.D. 2000. Protective factors, resiliency, and healthy youth development. Adol.Med. **11:** 157–164.
7. EISENBERG, N., T.L. SPINRAD, R.A. FABES, *et al.* 2004. The relations of effortful control and impulsivity to children's resiliency and adjustment. Child Dev. **75:** 25–46.
8. SMITH, P., B.R. FLAY, C.C. BELL & R.P. WEISSBERG. 2001. The protective influence of parents and peers in violence avoidance among African-American youth. Mat. Child Health J. **5:** 245–252.
9. BAUER, C.R., S. SHANKARAN, H. BADA, *et al.* 2002. The maternal lifestyle study: drug exposure during pregnancy and short-term maternal outcomes. Am. J. Obstet and Gynecol. **186:** 487–495.
10. LESTER, B.M., E.Z. TRONICK, L. LAGASSE, *et al.* 2002. The maternal lifestyle study: effects of substance exposure during pregnancy on neurodevelopmental outcome in 1-month-old infants. Pediatrics **110:** 1182–1192.
11. LESTER, B.M., M.A. ELSOHLY, L.L. WRIGHT, *et al.* 2001. The Maternal Lifestyle Study: drug use by meconium toxicology and maternal self-report. Pediatrics **107:** 309–317.

Explorations of Coping Strategies, Learned Persistence, and Resilience in Long-Evans Rats

Innate versus Acquired Characteristics

KELLY G. LAMBERT,[a] KELLY TU,[a] ASHLEY EVERETTE,[a]
GENNIFER LOVE,[a] ILAN McNAMARA,[b] MASSIMO BARDI,[b]
AND CRAIG H. KINSLEY[b]

[a]*Department of Psychology, Randolph-Macon College, Ashland, Virginia, USA*

[b]*Department of Psychology, University of Richmond, Richmond, Virginia, USA*

ABSTRACT: In the current investigation, predispositions for coping styles (i.e., passive, flexible, and active) were determined in juvenile male rats. In subsequent behavioral tests, flexible copers exhibited more active responses. In another study, animals were exposed to chronic stress and flexible coping rats had lower levels of corticosteroids. Focusing on the acquired nature of coping strategies, rats receiving extensive training in a task requiring them to dig for food rewards (i.e., *effort-based rewards*) persisted longer in a challenging task than control animals. Thus, the results suggest that both predisposed coping strategies and acquired behavioral experience contribute to resilience in challenging situations.

KEYWORDS: resilience; coping; effort-based rewards; learned persistence

INTRODUCTION

Although the stress response is adaptive for overcoming acute stressors, it can lead to the emergence of stress-related disease when stress becomes chronic.[1,2] Recent research suggests that an individual's day-to-day coping strategies may also be an important factor in the genesis of stress-mediated diseases such as depression.[3–5] Consequently, the development of animal models for the investigation of coping responses may be a valuable approach for the identification of neurobiological factors serving as potential buffers against

Address for correspondence: Kelly G. Lambert, Ph.D., Department of Psychology, Randolph-Macon College, Ashland, VA 23005. Voice: 804-752-4717; fax: 804-752-4724.
e-mail: klambert@rmc.edu

Ann. N.Y. Acad. Sci. 1094: 319–324 (2006). © 2006 New York Academy of Sciences.
doi: 10.1196/annals.1376.042

the onset of stress-related mental illness. In the current investigation, predispositions for coping styles were determined in juvenile male Long-Evans rats so that the consistency of these coping profiles could be determined in subsequent behavioral and hormonal assessments.[3]

Recent research also suggests that animals' response strategies upon exposure to less intense novelty stress may yield important information about physical and neurobiological health (i.e., stress-resilience[6,7]). For example, one study demonstrated that rats exhibiting higher levels of exploratory behavior upon the introduction of a novel object had lower levels of novelty-induced corticosteroid secretion and lived approximately 30% longer lives than their inhibited counterparts.[6] Considering these findings, an animal's response in a challenging novel task may provide important information about the persistence of an animal's responses in novel situations—providing additional information about the animal's stress-resilience and predisposition toward anxiety-related disorders. Although past research has suggested that diminished associations between directed effort and outcomes (i.e., stimulus–response associations) may lead to nonresponsiveness, similar to the behavior observed in depression (i.e., learned helplessness[8]), there is little research investigating the complementary hypothesis that repeated experience strengthening stimulus–response associations may provide a buffer against mental illnesses such as depression. Considering that the brain's motor circuit, the basal ganglia, shares extensive connections with the nucleus accumbens, a structure known for its involvement in pleasure and reward, the final experiment in this series of studies explored the utility of an animal model of *effort-based rewards* to determine if such training would lead to enhanced persistence, or *learned persistence*, in subsequent challenging tasks.

EXPERIMENTS AND RESULTS

Experiment 1: The Persistence of Innate Coping Characteristics

Coping strategies were examined in 30 male Long-Evans rats (23 days old) by gently restraining them on their backs for 1 min and recording the number of times each animal tried to escape. Subsequently, animals were assigned to either a passive or active category based on their responses. A second back-test was conducted 1 week later and the animals were assigned to their final coping group: passive (received a passive score on both tests); active (received an active score on both tests); or flexible (received a passive score on one test and an active score on the other test). Each coping category was comprised of 10 animals. A one-way ANOVA was conducted to determine the effect of coping strategy on several ecologically relevant stress tests including exposure to a small clip on their tail (to simulate a bug bite), a predator odor, a novel toy stimulus, and, finally, exposure to an open field. Flexible animals attempted to remove the clip from their tails more than either the passive or active groups ($P < 0.01$ and 0.03, respectively; see FIG. 1A); in addition, the flexible group contacted the novel toy stimulus more than the passive copers ($P = 0.013$; see

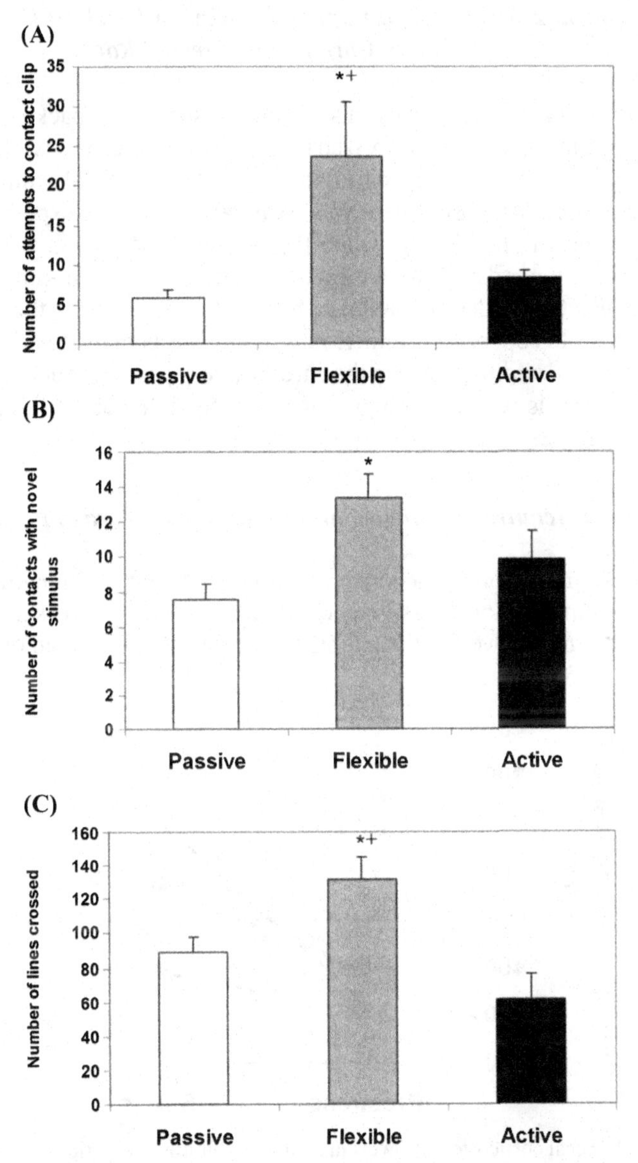

FIGURE 1. Performance of passive, flexible, and active rats exposed to a tail-clip (**A**), a novel toy stimulus (**B**), and an open field environment (**C**). *denotes statistical significant difference from passive animals; + denotes difference from active animals; bars represent s.e.m. values (see the EXPERIMENTS and RESULTS section for details).

FIG. 1B). In the open-field test, the flexible animals were more active than both the passive and active copers ($P = 0.03$ and 0.002, respectively; see FIG. 1C). No differences were observed in the predator odor test.

Experiment 2: Influence of Coping Strategy on Levels of Fecal Corticosterone in Chronically Stressed Rats

A total of 24 male Long-Evans rats were assessed in the backtest (as described in Experiment 1) and categorized into passive, active, or flexible groups ($n = 8$ each group). After being housed in activity wheels, fecal samples were collected to assess corticosterone levels. Animals were then exposed to the activity-stress paradigm[2] during which the rats were housed in the activity wheels and fed 2 h per day. After 4 days of activity-stress, fecal samples were once again collected for determination of corticosterone levels. In the prestress period, the flexible copers had significantly lower levels than the passive animals ($P = 0.04$); in addition, during the chronic stress phase, the active copers' corticosterone levels was 170% higher than the flexible copers' levels ($P = 0.05$). See FIGURE 2.

Experiment 3: Acquired Coping Characteristics and Learned Persistence

A total of 16 male Long-Evans rats were matched for "emotionality" in an open-field test and randomly assigned to either a control or a worker group of rats. During the next 5 weeks, the animals were trained daily in an open field

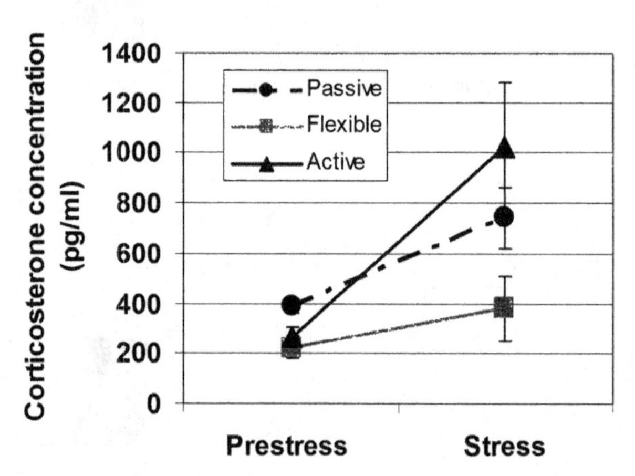

FIGURE 2. Fecal corticosterone levels in animals exhibiting the various coping strategies assessed prior to a chronic stressor and during the chronic exposure to activity-stress. In the prestress condition, flexible copers had lower levels of corticosterone than passive copers; in the stress condition, flexible copers had lower levels than their active coping counterparts (see the EXPERIMENTS and RESULTS section for details).

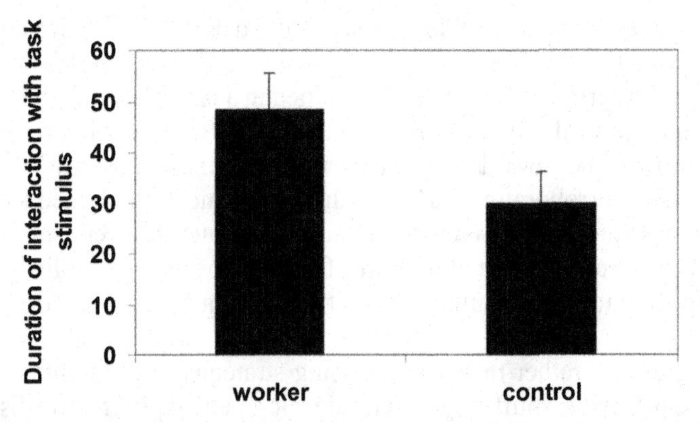

FIGURE 3. Rats trained to work for Froot Loop rewards in the digging task interacted with the novel challenge task longer than the animals that received the rewards independent of directed effort (see the EXPERIMENTS and RESULTS section for details).

apparatus with corncob bedding placed on the floor. Control animals were given the reward of four small pieces of Froot Loops regardless of physical effort expended in the training session whereas the worker rats were trained to dig for Froot Loops and received the reward only as a consequence of their physical effort. Following the 5 weeks of training, a persistence test was administered to the animals by exposing them to a novel manipulandum task for 3 min. This task consisted of a ventilated plastic cat toy with a bell and Froot Loop placed inside requiring the animals to overcome their anxiety related to the novel ball and bell and persist with their efforts to try to solve the problem of removing the Froot Loop from the stimulus. The duration of attempts to remove the Froot Loop was recorded. A one-way ANOVA indicated that the worker group of rats spent significantly more time with the challenging object than the control group ($P = 0.04$; one-tailed test). See FIGURE 3.

DISCUSSION

The present series of studies provides preliminary evidence that coping strategies are persistent across various stress assessments. Specifically, the backtest, adapted from a model used with piglets,[9] provided a means to characterize the rat pups as active, passive, or flexible copers. Interestingly, upon exposure to subsequent acute stressors, the flexible copers were the most responsive. In Experiment 2, the various coping strategies were assessed in a chronic stress paradigm (i.e., the activity-stress paradigm). Prior to the commencement of the stress paradigm, the flexible copers had lower corticosterone levels than the passive animals; further, during the chronic stress, the flexible copers exhibited lower levels of stress hormones than the active copers. Considering the toxic effects of prolonged durations of elevated stress hormones, these data suggest that the flexible copers exhibited the most adaptive response to stressful situations.

In the third experiment, animals were trained in a task requiring them to dig for Froot Loop rewards. When compared to animals that were not required to expend effort for the reward, the worker animals persisted longer in a novel challenge task. Corroborating earlier findings documenting learned helplessness when associations between effort and consequences were diminished, the rats in this study exhibited a form of learned persistence following extensive exposure to effort-contingent positive consequences (i.e., effort-based rewards).

In sum, flexible, rather than fixed, coping strategies may facilitate stress-resilience and provide a buffer against the development of psychiatric disorders such as anxiety disorders or depression.[10] In addition, coping responses may be modified through experience with effort-based rewards—leading to an increased sense of control over one's environment—and enhanced resilience in stressful situations.[11]

REFERENCES

1. Sapolsky, R.M. 2000. Glucocorticoids and hippocampal atrophy in neuropsychiatric disorders. Arch. Gen. Psychiatry **57:** 925–935.
2. Lambert, K.G., S.K. Buckelew, G. Staffiso-Sandoz, *et al.* 1998. Activity-stress induces atrophy of apical dendrites of hippocampal pyramidal neurons in male rats. Physiol. Behav. **65:** 43–49.
3. Koolhaas, J.M., S.M. Korte, S.F. DeBoer, *et al.* 1999. Coping styles in animals: current status in behavior and stress-physiology. Neuro. Bio. Rev. **23:** 925–935.
4. Campbell, T., S. Lin, C. DeVries & K. Lambert. 2003. Coping strategies in male and female rats exposed to multiple stressors. Physiol. Behav. **78:** 495–504.
5. Bryce, J.W., N. Walker, F. Ghorayeb & M. Kanj. 1989. Life experiences response styles and mental health among mothers and children in Beirut, Lebanon. Soc. Sci. Med. **28:** 685–695.
6. Cavigelli, S.A. & M.K. McClintock. 2003. Fear of novelty in infant rats predicts adult corticosterone dynamics and an early death. Proc. Nat Acad. Sci. **100:** 16131–16136.
7. Miaura, H., H. Qiao & T. Ohta. 2002. Attenuating effects of the isolated rearing condition on increased brain serotonin and dopamine turnover elicited by novelty stress. Brain Res. **926:** 10–17.
8. Seligman, M.E.P. & J.M. Weiss. 1980. Coping behavior: learned helplessness, physiological change and learned inactivity. Behav. Res. Ther. **18:** 459–512.
9. Schouten, W.G.P. & V.M. Wiegant. 1997. Individual responses to acute and chronic stress in pigs. Acta Physiol. Scand. **640:** 188–191.
10. Southwick, S.M., M. Vythilingam & D.S. Charney. 2005. The psychobiology of depression and resilience to stress: implications for prevention and treatment. Ann Rev Clin. Psychol. **1:** 255–291.
11. Lambert, K.G. 2006. Rising rates of depression in today's society: consideration of the roles of effort-based rewards and enhanced resilience in day-to-day functioning. Neurosci. Biobehav. Rev. **30:** 497–510.

Biobehavioral Indices of Emotion Regulation Relate to School Attitudes, Motivation, and Behavior Problems in a Low-Income Preschool Sample

ALISON L. MILLER,[a] RONALD SEIFER,[b] LAURA STROUD,[c]
STEPHEN J. SHEINKOPF,[b] AND SUSAN DICKSTEIN[b]

[a]*University of Michigan School of Public Health, Ann Arbor, Michigan, USA*

[b]*E.P. Bradley Hospital, Brown University Medical School, Providence, Rhode Island, USA*

[c]*Miriam Hospital, Brown University Medical School, Providence, Rhode Island, USA*

ABSTRACT: Effective emotion regulation may promote resilience and preschool classroom adjustment by supporting adaptive peer interactions and engagement in learning activities. We investigated how hypothalamus-pituitary-adrenal axis (HPA) regulation, cardiac reactivity, and classroom emotion displays related to adjustment among low-income preschoolers attending Head Start. A total of 62 four-year-olds completed a laboratory session including a baseline soothing video; emotion-eliciting slides/video clips, and recovery. Salivary cortisol, heart rate, and vagal tone were measured throughout. Independent coders used handheld computers to observe classroom emotion expression/regulation. Teachers rated child motivation, persistence/attention, learning attitudes, and internalizing/externalizing symptoms. Results reveal associations between biobehavioral markers of regulatory capacity and early school adjustment.

KEYWORDS: emotion regulation; reactivity; preschool; low-income; school readiness

INTRODUCTION

As early as preschool, low-income children show high rates of learning and behavior problems that can have a negative impact on classroom adjustment.[1]

Address for correspondence: Alison L. Miller, Ph.D., Department of Health Behavior and Health Education, University of Michigan School of Public Health, 1420 Washington Heights, SPHII, Room M5533, Ann Arbor, MI 48109-2029. Voice: 734-615-7459; fax: 734-615-2317.
e-mail: alimill@umich.edu

Ann. N.Y. Acad. Sci. 1094: 325–329 (2006).
doi: 10.1196/annals.1376.043

Modulating emotions and behaviors in the classroom setting is crucial for supporting the adaptive peer interactions and engagement in classroom learning activities that foster positive school attitudes and adjustment over time.[2] In addition, psychophysiological reactivity and regulation in response to stress has been postulated to be an important aspect of a child's regulatory capacity.[3,4] It is not clear, however, to what degree such different regulatory constructs are associated, and whether these aspects of regulatory ability relate differentially to child functioning in school. We address these questions in the current investigation.

In the current study, we examined relations among classroom emotion expression and regulation, psychophysiological stress reactivity and regulation, and early classroom adjustment. Specifically, we investigated how reactivity (heart rate, cortisol change) and regulation (RSA) in a laboratory task, and emotion expression and behavioral regulation as observed in the classroom setting were related. We also assessed how each of these indices of reactivity and regulation were associated with teacher ratings of school attitudes, motivation, and behavior problems. We studied these questions in a sample of low-income preschool children attending Head Start.

METHOD

Participants

Participants were 62 four-year-old children attending Head Start (45% male). Participant information was reported for both race (67% Caucasian, 13% African American, 19% biracial/other) and ethnicity (7% Latino, 93% non-Latino). Results reported here are based on a partial sample of an ongoing study of emotion processing in low-income children.

Procedure

Children were presented with emotion elicitation slides and brief video clips designed to elicit negative and positive valence and various arousal states. All stimuli were presented on a 15-inch computer monitor and children were videotaped (data not presented here). Heart rate data were recorded continuously during the session. Children provided salivary cortisol samples at initial baseline, after a soothing video, after an arousing video, and recovery. Children's teachers completed questionnaires to assess school attitudes and behavior problems. Independent observers also observed children in their classrooms during "center-time" activities to assess behavior during relatively structured play periods.

Measures

Laboratory Session

Reactivity variables were mean heart rate change from baseline to positive stimuli [HR(P)], mean heart rate change from baseline to negative [HR(N)], and mean cortisol change from baseline to negative [CORT(R)]. Regulation variables were baseline RSA [RSA(B)]; mean RSA change from baseline to positive [RSA(P)] and mean RSA change from baseline to negative [RSA(N)].

Classroom Observations

Handheld computers were used to conduct live observations (using "The Observer" software and the Psion Workabout, Noldus Technologies). Each child was observed 8 times for 10 min each. Seven mutually exclusive time-based emotion displays and dysregulation states were coded: Neutral, Positive, Mild Negative, Sadness, Anger, Emotionally Negative Dysregulation, and Neutral/Behavioral Dysregulation (e.g., highly active motor behavior).[2] Coders recorded the onset and offset of each state, yielding a continuous stream of behavior states, which were reduced to yield a proportional duration score. Coders trained until they achieved intraclass correlations of 0.80 or greater for each code (overall reliability kappa = 0.73).

Teacher Reports

Teachers completed the Preschool Learning Behavior Scale (PLBS),[5] which included Motivation (e.g., shows interest in activities), Persistence (e.g., sticks to activity as long as can be expected for this age), and Attitude Toward Learning (e.g., willing to be helped) subscales as well as Total score (0 = does not apply; 2 = most often applies). Teachers completed the Child Behavior Checklist-Teacher Report Form (CBCL-TRF)[6] to assess externalizing and internalizing.

RESULTS

Positive emotion displays in class were marginally related to increased HR in response to positive stimuli ($r = 0.23$, $P < 0.10$); sadness was marginally related to decreased HR in response to negative stimuli ($r = -0.23$, $P < 0.10$). Emotionally negative dysregulation was related to increased HR in response to negative stimuli ($r = 0.26$, $P < 0.05$), and to less cortisol reactivity ($r = -0.42$, $P < 0.05$).

TABLE 1. Correlations: observed classroom emotions/behavior, school adjustment [n = 61; TRF n = 20]

Teacher Rating	Positive	Sad	Anger	Mild neg.	Emot. dysreg.	Behav. dysreg.	Gleeful taunting	Neutral
Motivation	−0.05	−0.37*	−0.31*	−0.03	−0.53*	−0.09	.05	.16
Persistence	0.12	−0.03	−0.19†	−0.35*	−0.04	−0.25†	−.16	.02
Learning Attitude	0.00	−0.05	−0.29*	−0.27*	−0.15	−0.08	−.05	.08
Overall Learning	0.06	−0.23†	−0.31*	−0.19	−0.31*	−0.15	.03	.07
CBCL-TRF-Ext	−0.16	0.20	0.49*	0.55*	−0.02	0.19	.26	.01
CBCL-TRF-Int	−0.11	0.04	0.40*	0.18	0.44*	0.11	.30	.03

*$P < 0.05$; †$P < 0.10$.

We next examined relations between reactivity and regulation and teacher-rated school adjustment. Motivation was marginally related to increased HR in response to positive stimuli ($r = 0.23$, $P < 0.10$) and persistence marginally related to decreased HR in response to negative stimuli ($r = -0.23$, $P < 0.10$). Teacher ratings of motivation and overall learning behaviors were related to greater cortisol reactivity ($r = 0.65$ and 0.52, respectively, $P < 0.05$). We also found that negative emotion expression (particularly anger) related to motivation, persistence, learning attitudes, and behavior problems (see TABLE 1).

DISCUSSION

We observed some relations among stress reactivity (primarily heart rate) and emotion displays in the classroom setting, although on balance associations were modest. We did not find relations between regulation (RSA) and classroom displays. It may be that with regard to classroom functioning, a child's reactivity may have a greater impact than his or her baseline regulatory ability (as indexed by RSA).

More associations were found for observed classroom emotion displays and teacher-rated school adjustment than for the laboratory-based measures; among the laboratory-based measures, reactivity (vs. regulation) variables were somewhat more strongly related to teacher ratings. Specifically, cortisol reactivity was strongly related to teacher-rated motivation and overall positive learning/school attitudes, possibly suggesting that higher levels of reactivity may actually be beneficial for effective engagement in the school setting and with classroom activities. Although interesting, interpretation must be tempered by the fact that only a small subset of children (n = 20) had cortisol data; analyses are ongoing and this question will be investigated in more detail using the full sample.

Considering context (i.e., naturalistic vs. lab based) and level of assessment (i.e., observed behavioral vs. psychophysiological) is crucial when studying regulatory processes. We found that public aspects of regulation and reactivity (e.g., observed emotions in the classroom) had more to do with teachers' views of child functioning at school than did more private/internal aspects of a child's regulatory abilities as assessed in the laboratory setting. It is likely that effective emotion regulation skills at multiple levels are an important part of school readiness and may augment the effects of programs such as Head Start, which is designed to promote resilience for children living in poverty circumstances.

REFERENCES

1. Harden, B.J., M.B. Winslow, K.T. Kendziora, *et al.* 2000. Externalizing problems in Head Start children: an ecological exploration. Early Educ. Dev. **11:** 357–385.
2. Miller, A.L., K.K. Gouley, R. Seifer, S. Dickstein & A. Shields. 2004. Emotions and behaviors in the Head Start classroom: associations among observed dysregulation, social competence, and preschool adjustment. Early Educ. Dev. **15:** 147–165.
3. Blair, C., D. Granger & R.P. Razza. 2005. Cortisol reactivity is positively related to executive function in preschool children attending Head Start. Child Dev. **76:** 554–567.
4. Porges, S.W. 2001. The polyvagal theory: phylogenetic substrates of a social nervous system. Int. J. Psychophysiol. **42:** 123–146.
5. McDermott, P.A., L.F. Green, J.M. Francis & D.H. Stott. 2000. The Preschool Learning Behaviors Scale. Edumetric & Clinical Science. Philadelphia, PA.
6. Achenbach, T.M. & L.A. Rescorla. 2000. Manual for ASEBA Preschool Forms & Profiles. University of Vermont, Research Center for Children, Youth, & Families. Burlington, VT.

Additive Interaction of Child Abuse and Perinatal Risk as Signs of Resiliency in Adulthood

YOKO NOMURA, CLAUDE M. CHEMTOB, WILLIAM P. FIFER, JEFFREY H. NEWCORN, AND JEANNE BROOKS-GUNN

Mount Sinai School of Medicine, New York City, New York, USA

ABSTRACT: To find the biological basis of resilience, we exploited data from a longitudinal community-based study of 1,748 adult children, followed from birth to adulthood. Results showed that those with both abuse and perinatal problems demonstrated synergistically impaired well-being, a higher rate of school dropout, lower sense of success, and lower income. Among abused adult children (*n* = 271), we found that those without, relative to those with, perinatal problems had lower risk for adult psychopathology. An examination of the biological base of resilience could be added in a multidimensional/multifactorial model to help researchers identify ways to promote resiliency even before birth.

KEYWORDS: childhood abuse; low birthweight; preterm birth; psychopathology; resiliency

INTRODUCTION

Two separate and distinct bodies of research in perinatal trauma[1] and childhood abuse have demonstrated that early childhood trauma[2,3] has a critical and long-lasting effect on psychological outcomes. Recent evidence suggests a long-lasting influence of low birth weight (LBW) and premature birth on depression in young adulthood.[4,5] Another body of research that examined the long-term effect of early childhood abuse also demonstrated the increased risk of adult psychopathology, such as depression, substance use, delinquency, and suicidal ideation among those with a childhood history of abuse.[2,3] Both areas of research have separately attempted to elucidate the same possible biological pathway: dysregulation in the HPA-axis as a mediating condition.[6,7] Yet the two areas have never been integrated, despite the importance of taking advantage of the progress in research in each area.

Address for correspondence: Yoko Nomura, Ph.D., Child and Family Resilience Program, Mount Sinai School of Medicine, One Gustave L. Levy Place, Box 1230, New York City, NY 10029. Voice: 212-987-0335; Fax: 212-987-0177.
e-mail:yoko.nomura@mssm.edu

Ann. N.Y. Acad. Sci. 1094: 330–334 (2006). © 2006 New York Academy of Sciences.
doi: 10.1196/annals.1376.044

In this study, we aimed to integrate the two bodies of research and examine whether having two forms of trauma (perinatal risk and childhood abuse) would accelerate the risk of psychopathology in later life as compared to having only one or neither of them. Furthermore, among a subsample of those with childhood abuse ($n = 271$), we examined if those without a perinatal risk factor were more resilient than those with it.

METHOD

Subjects

About 1,748 children were followed regularly from birth through 8 years of age and were recontacted 25 years after their last assessment in young adulthood (mean age = 33). Full details of the study, sampling, and assessments can be seen elsewhere.[8]

Assessments

Birth weight, 5-min Apgar scores, and head circumference were recorded by a nurse observer at the time of delivery. Gestational age was determined by mothers' self-report of their last menstrual period and sonogram. Perinatal factors were dichotomized at a conventional, clinically significant cut-off: low birth weight (< 2,500 g), low 5-min Apgar score (< 7), small head circumference (< 32 cm), and preterm birth (< 37 weeks). The subjects' psychiatric status was assessed using the General Health Questionnaire-28 (GHQ-28).[9] Childhood history of severe abuse was measured by the Conflict Tactics (CT) scale. Those who scored above mean plus standard deviation were assigned 1 for a history of severe childhood abuse and the rest 0.[10] The subjects' quality of life, physical health, well-being, and demographics, such as income and educational attainment as adults, were based on self-report. Potential confounders include mother's income in their third month of pregnancy, mother's income at birth, mother's education at child's birth, mother's parity, mother's marital status and age, and child's age, sex, and race. All of the confounders were based on mother's self-report.

Data Analysis

Risk of psychological problems in adult offspring was evaluated using logistic regression. In subsequent analyses using a subset of those who had childhood history of abuse ($n = 271$), we examined the difference in psychosocial and demographic characteristics for signs of resiliency. We used logistic regression analysis for dichotomous outcomes and multiple regression for continuous outcomes. Potential confounders were included in all models.

RESULTS

First, in the four-group analysis (offspring with both childhood abuse and a perinatal problem, those with childhood abuse alone, those with a perinatal problem alone, and those offspring with neither), we found evidence for a synergistically increased risk of depression, suicidal ideation, and somatization. The risk of psychopathology by having both risk factors exceeded the additive risk of a perinatal problem and childhood abuse, suggesting an additive interaction. Risk of depression, suicidal ideation, and somatization among offspring with both abuse and perinatal risk increased synergistically showing clear evidence of additive interaction. For example, offspring with both abuse and preterm birth had a 10-fold ($P < 0.0001$) increased risk of depression relative to those with neither childhood abuse nor preterm birth; for those with abuse alone the increase was 3-fold ($P = 0.005$); and for those with preterm birth alone, 1.8-fold. A 10-fold increased risk for having both abuse and preterm birth should have been equal to an addition of a 3-fold increased (abuse alone) and a 1.8-fold increased (preterm birth alone) risk, had there been no additive interaction between abuse and preterm birth. The patterns were extremely similar for abuse and other perinatal problems—low birth weight, small head circumference, and low Apgar scores.

In a subsample of offspring who had abuse history, we tested whether offspring with normal perinatal outcomes (normal birth weight and normal term birth) as compared to offspring with problems had signs of resiliency. As can be seen in TABLE 1, those with optimal birth outcomes (normal birth weight and full-term birth) received more education, higher household incomes, were less likely to see doctors, and had a better quality of life.

CONCLUSIONS

Having two risk factors, that is, childhood abuse and a perinatal problem, synergistically increased the risk of psychopathology in young adulthood. Youth with both risk factors should be considered as the highest risk population. Offspring with normal birth weight and full-term birth relative to their counterparts had a significantly lower rate of psychopathology. Resiliency, as measured by educational attainment, income, and perception toward their life, was found to be significantly higher in youth with normal birth weight and full-term birth relative to those with low birth weight and preterm birth. Examination of the biological base of resilience should be added to a

TABLE 1. Characteristics among adult children who had a childhood history of abuse by birth weight and birth-term birth status as a sign of resiliency

Adult characteristics	Birth weight Normal ($n = 226$) Mean (sd)	Low ($n = 45$) Mean (sd)	Birth term Normal ($n = 226$) Mean (sd)	Preterm ($n = 45$) Mean (sd)
Education (years)	11.4 (2.3)	11.2 (2.3) *	11.4 (2.3)	11.2 (2.3)*
Household income ($)	29,770 (27,845)	19,114 (17,623)*	28,735 (26,069)	24,585 (29,550)*
Individual income ($)	15,497 (21,438)	12,190 (15,842)	15,993 (22,039)	9,596 (9,897)+
General health	5.38 (1.3)	5.14 (1.5)+	5.38 (1.3)	5.10 (1.6)+
Physical condition	5.32 (1.4)	5.09 (1.7)+	5.30 (1.4)	5.24 (1.5)+
Frequency to see a physician	4.63 (1.8)	5.39 (1.5)**	4.74 (1.7)	4.81 (1.8)*
Quality of life	5.78 (2.3)	5.59 (2.6)**	5.97 (2.3)	4.74 (2.7)

NB: General health and physical condition were measured in 7-point Likert scale (1 = terrible, 2 = unhappy, 3 = mostly dissatisfied, 4 = mixed, 5 = mostly satisfied, 6 = pleased, and 7 = delighted). Quality life was measured in 10-point Likert scale (1 = worst possible to 10 = best possible). Frequency to see a physician is based on number of visits per year. There were three cases without birth term information. + = $.10 \leq p < .05$; * = $.05 \leq p < .01$; ** = $.01 \leq p < .001$

multidimensional/multifactorial model of resiliency to help policy makers and researchers identify ways to promote resiliency even before birth.

REFERENCES

1. GRAY, R.F., A. INDURKHYA & M.C. MCCORMICK. 2004. Prevalence, stability, and predictors of clinically significant behavior problems in low birth weight children at 3, 5, and 8 years of age. Pediatrics **114:** 932–940.
2. PENZA, K.M., C. HEIM & C.B. NEMEROFF. 2003. Neurobiological effects of childhood abuse: implications for the pathophysiology of depression and anxiety. Arch. Women Ment. Health **6:** 15–22.
3. MACMILLAN, H.L., J.E. FLEMING, D.L. STREINER, *et al.* 2001. Childhood abuse and lifetime psychopathology in a community sample. Am. J. Psychiatry **158:** 1878–1883.
4. GALE, C.R. & C.N. MARTYN. 2004. Birth weight and later risk of depression in a national birth cohort. Br. J. Psychiatry **184:** 28–33.
5. THOMPSON, C., H. SYDDALL, I. RODIN, *et al.* 2001. Birth weight and the risk of depressive disorder in later life. Br. J. Psychiatry **179:** 450–455.
6. NEWPORT, D.J., C. HEIM, R. BONSALL, *et al.* 2004. Pituitary-adrenal responses to standard and low-dose dexamethasone suppression tests in adult survivors of child abuse. Biol. Psychiatry **55:** 10–20.
7. SANCHEZ, M.M., C.O. LADD & P.M. PLOTSKY. 2001. Early adverse experience as developmental risk factor for late psychopathology: Evidence from rodent and primate models. Dev. Psychopathol. **13:** 419–449.

8. HARDY, J., S. SHAPIRO, D. MELLITS, *et al.* 1999. Self-sufficiency at age 27 to 33 years: factors present between birth and 18 years that predict educational attainment among children born to inner-city families. Pediatrics **99:** 80–87.
9. GOLDBERG, D. 1978. Manual of the General Health Questionnaire. Windsor, UK: NFER.
10. STRAUS, M.A. 1979. Measuring intrafamily conflict and violence: the conflict tactics (CT) scales. J. Marriage Family **41:** 75–88.

Resilience among At-Risk Hispanic American Preschool Children

GERALDINE V. OADES-SESE AND GISELLE B. ESQUIVEL

Graduate School of Education, Division of Psychological and Educational Services, Fordham University, New York, New York, USA

ABSTRACT: This study combines cognitive (i.e., intelligence), psychosocial (i.e., inhibition, activity level, negative emotionality, emotion regulation, autonomy), and cultural–linguistic factors (i.e., level of acculturation and bilingualism) to determine patterns of resilience and vulnerability among 207 economically disadvantaged Hispanic American preschool children, from 50 early childhood classrooms, as gauged by their social competence during peer play. Person-oriented analysis yielded six distinct profiles, two profiles of which were resilient and one identified as vulnerable. Results of this study revealed within-group differences in resilience among these children and the significant role bilingualism and maintenance of the home language play in their social–emotional development.

KEYWORDS: resilience; preschoolers; temperament; bilingualism; acculturation; social competence

INTRODUCTION

This is the first study to examine resilience among economically disadvantaged Hispanic American preschool children. Based on a similar study by Mendez, Fantuzzo, and Cicchetti[1] using African American preschoolers, this study examines cognitive (i.e., intelligence) and psychosocial factors (i.e., inhibition, activity level, negative emotionality, emotion regulation, autonomy) to determine profiles of resilience and vulnerability among Hispanic American preschool children as gauged by social competence during peer play. In addition, cultural–linguistic factors (i.e., level of acculturation and bilingualism) were examined and included as potential protective factors.

Address for correspondence: Geraldine V. Oades-Sese, Ph.D., 113 West 60th Street, Room 1008, New York, NY 10023-7484. Voice: 201- 401-3003; fax: 732-463-1850.
e-mail:oadessese@fordham.edu

Ann. N.Y. Acad. Sci. 1094: 335–339 (2006). © 2006 New York Academy of Sciences.
doi: 10.1196/annals.1376.045

METHOD

Participants

Two hundred seven Hispanic American preschoolers (54.1% males; 45.9% females) ages 4- (67.6%) to 5 years old (32.4%) from 50 classrooms of two early childhood centers at an urban public school district participated in this study. Students' eligibility for reduced or free lunch indexed socioeconomic status.

Measures

The following measures were used in this study: (*a*) the *Stanford-Binet Intelligence Scales-Fifth Edition*[2] to measure nonverbal intelligence; (*b*) the *Temperament Assessment Battery for Children-Revised Teacher Form*[3] to measure Inhibition, Negative Emotionality, and Activity Level; (*c*) the *Emotion Regulation Checklist*[4] to measure emotion regulation; (*d*) the *Woodcock Language Proficiency Battery-Revised*[5] to measure oral language proficiency in English; (*e*) the *Woodcock Language Proficiency Battery-Revised Spanish Form*[6] to measure oral language proficiency in Spanish; (*f*) the Dependent/Autonomous Scale of the *Social Competence and Behavior Evaluation-Teacher Form*[7] to measure autonomy; (*g*) an adapted version of the *Short Acculturation Scale for Hispanic Youths*[8] to measure acculturation level; and the (*h*) *Penn Interactive Peer Play Scale*[9] to measure social competence observed during social play.

Procedures

Each child was individually administered an English and Spanish oral language proficiency test, and a cognitive test (in dominant language/bilingual) in separate testing sessions. Parents completed a demographic survey and acculturation scale. Teachers completed rating scales for temperament, emotion regulation, autonomy, and social competence. A cluster analysis (K-Means) was conducted to identify profiles of resilience and vulnerability followed by a multivariate analysis of variance (MANOVA) to determine if profiles differentially related to social competence during peer play.

RESULTS

Cluster analysis findings identified two resilient profiles (see Table 1): (*a*) The *Prosocial-Resilient Bilingual-English Dominant* ($n = 48$; 23%) was composed of 44% boys and 56% girls, of which 69% were 4-year-olds. This group had the highest mean score on emotion regulation and autonomy and the lowest on inhibition and negative emotionality. This group was fluent in English with some proficiency in Spanish. (*b*) The *Prosocial-Resilient Bilingual-Spanish Dominant* ($n = 37$; 18%) was composed of 46% boys and 54% girls, of which 73% were 4-year-olds. This group was the next highest on emotion regulation and autonomy, and lowest on negative emotionality. This profile was the most fluent in Spanish with some proficiency in English.

The *Active-Emotional Low Bilingual* ($n = 27$; 13%) was the most vulnerable profile composed of mostly boys (70%) than girls (30%), of which 67% were 4-year-olds. This group had the highest mean score on inhibition, negative emotionality, and active level; and lowest mean score on NVIQ, emotional regulation, and autonomy. This group scored three standard deviations below the normative mean in both languages. This group was followed by the *Acculturated Monolingual* ($n = 18$; 8.7%) composed of more boys (72%) than girls (28%), of which 78% were 4-year-olds. This group was relatively high in inhibition, negative emotionality, and activity level, and was fluent in English but negligible in Spanish.

Along the continuum between the resilient and vulnerable profiles were the Calm Limited Bilingual and the Socially Emerging Bilingual. The *Calm Limited Bilingual* ($n = 37$; 18%) was composed of 46% boys and 54% girls, of which 51% were 4-year-olds. This group was rated lowest in activity level and was limited in English and Spanish. Finally, the *Socially Emerging Bilingual* ($n = 40$; 19%) was composed of more boys (63%) than girls (37%), of which 73% were 4-year-olds. This group was similar to the Acculturated Monolingual group in temperament with slightly higher scores in emotion regulation and autonomy. This group was fluent in English with some Spanish.

Findings from the MANOVA indicated that there were significant differences among the six cluster memberships (Wilk's $\lambda = 0.41$, F (15, 550) $=$ 14.09, $P = 0.000$, partial $\eta^2 = 0.26$) for the combined dependent variables of play interaction, play disruption, and play disconnection. Univariate analysis of variance (ANOVA) indicated significant difference among the six cluster groups for play interaction, F (5, 1566) $= 33.77$, $P = 0.000$, partial $\eta^2 = 0.46$); play disruption, F (5, 1412) $= 16.39$, $P = 0.000$, partial $\eta^2 = 0.29$; and play disconnection $F(5, 1620) = 19.92$, $P = 0.000$, partial $\eta^2 = 0.33$). A Scheffe *post hoc* analysis revealed that profiles were differentially related to social competence. In terms of social competence, the two resilient profiles had significantly higher means of play interaction compared with other profiles, $P <$ 0.001. The Calm Limited Bilingual was similar in social competence with the Prosocial-Resilient Bilingual-Spanish Dominant. The Active-Emotional Limited Bilingual had a significantly lower mean of play interaction than all other clusters and significantly higher means in play disruption and disconnection, $P<0.001$. The resilient profiles had significantly lower mean scores in play disruption and disconnection, $P<0.001$. (Note: Child acculturation level was not significantly related to social competence.)

TABLE 1. Between-group differences for resilient child attribute measures

Measure	Prosocial-resilient bilingual English dominant (1) ($n = 48$)		Calm limited bilingual (2) ($n = 37$)		Acculturated monolingual (3) ($n = 18$)		Socially emerging bilingual (4) ($n = 40$)		Active-emotional low bilingual (5) ($n = 27$)		Prosocial-resilient bilingual Spanish dominant (6) ($n = 37$)	
	M	SD	*M*	SD	*M*	SD	*M*	SD	*M*	*SD*	*M*	*SD*
NVIQ	104.58	8.33	95.59	6.71	96.28	9.07	107.42	6.95	93.81	7.51	107.43	7.77
English oral language	91.71	9.48	74.14	11.59	85.00	15.05	89.43	10.92	58.07	12.37	70.97	11.45
Spanish oral language	66.77	23.51	69.08	17.97	32.17	7.38	67.15	19.73	59.81	18.87	91.35	13.83
Acculturation level	48.56	7.66	42.05	7.39	69.33	11.26	48.25	7.81	41.33	5.57	36.46	5.91
Inhibition	38.81	5.07	53.14	9.49	52.11	9.02	49.32	6.72	57.44	10.07	43.73	6.09
Negative emotionality	41.46	6.00	41.97	5.71	53.00	7.12	53.00	6.32	56.89	10.33	41.32	4.51
Activity level	46.19	6.89	42.76	4.46	55.78	7.57	54.30	7.91	59.26	9.21	46.78	7.06
Emotion regulation	58.15	2.19	49.10	3.43	43.42	3.30	46.28	3.06	37.92	3.00	56.35	2.15
Autonomy	53.04	5.30	46.68	5.89	41.83	6.51	43.00	5.64	36.22	4.73	51.05	7.69

NOTE: NVIQ has an $M = 100$, SD = 15. All other variables are T-scores with an M = 50, SD = 10.

DISCUSSION

Resilient and vulnerable profiles that emerged were consistent with the resilience literature in terms of cognitive ability, language skills, temperament, autonomy, and emotional regulation as protective factors. Levels of bilingualism emerged as contributing to the resilient profiles, consistent with the literature in second language acquisition. This study empirically validated that socially resilient preschool children were proficient in one language while gaining proficiency in a second language, while children at risk showed minimal proficiency in either language. In addition, children who were monolingual English (but exposed to Spanish at home) were also at risk.

REFERENCES

1. Mendez, J.L., J. Fantuzzo & D. Cicchetti. 2002. Profiles of social competence among low income African American preschool children. Child Dev. **73:** 1085–1100.
2. Roid, G.H. 2003. Stanford-Binet Intelligence Scales, Fifth edition. Riverside. Itasca, IL.
3. Martin, R.P. & R. Bridger. 1999. The Temperament Assessment Battery for Children-Revised: Manual. School Psychology Clinic Publishing. Athens, GA.
4. Shields, A. & D. Cicchetti. 1997. Emotion regulation among school-age children: the development and validation of a new criterion Q-sort scale. Dev. Psychol. **33:** 906–916.
5. Woodcock, R.W. 1991. Woodcock Language Proficiency Battery-Revised. Riverside. Itasca, IL.
6. Woodcock, R.W. & A.F. Muñoz-Sandoval. 2004. Woodcock-Muñoz Language Survey-Revised comprehensive manual. Riverside. Chicago, IL.
7. LaFrenière, P.J. & J.E. Dumas. 1995. Social Competence and Behavior Evaluation: Preschool edition (SCBE). Western Psychological Services. Los Angeles, CA.
8. Barona, A. & J.A. Miller. 1994. Short Acculturation Scale for Hispanic Youth (SASHY): a preliminary report. Hisp. J. Behav. Sci. **16**: 155–162.
9. McWayne, C., Y. Sekino, V. Hampton & J. Fantuzzo. 2002. Manual: Penn Interactive Peer Play Scale: Teacher and Parent Rating Scales for Preschool and Kindergarten Children. University of Pennsylvania. Philadelphia, PA

Pathways of Adaptation from Adolescence to Young Adulthood

Antecedents and Correlates

JELENA OBRADOVIĆ, KEITH B. BURT, AND ANN S. MASTEN

Institute of Child Development, University of Minnesota, Minneapolis, Minnesota, USA

ABSTRACT: This study examines longitudinal change using a person-centered approach to differentiate patterns of adaptive functioning from adolescence to adulthood. Data are drawn from a 20-year longitudinal study of competence and resilience in the lives of 205 school children (29% minority). Results indicate five distinct pathways of adaptation: (1) low-declining, (2) low-improving, (3) middle-improving, (4) middle-declining, and (5) consistently high. The study also compares the five groups on childhood risks and resources, and on longitudinal assessment of competence and adversity. Interestingly, the most dramatic changes in pathways of adaptation occur during the period of emerging adulthood.

KEYWORDS: adaptation; competence; risk; adversity; resilience

INTRODUCTION

Studies of developmental processes indicate that adaptive and maladaptive behaviors are both continuous and prone to lawful change over time.[1] Prior adaptation predicts future success or failure in developmental tasks, and yet dramatic "turning points" occur, often during transitions or life-altering experiences.[2] Most longitudinal studies of continuity and change in adaptation have used variable-centered approaches to chart negative changes and outcomes. This study examines longitudinal change in adaptation using a recently developed person-centered methodology and indices of positive development to differentiate adaptive patterns from adolescence to adulthood.

METHODS

Participants were drawn from a 20-year longitudinal study of competence and resilience.[2–4] This study employs data collected on 202 school children

Address for correspondence: Jelena Obradović, M.A. Institute of Child Development, University of Minnesota, 51 East River Road, Minneapolis, MN 55455. Voice: 612-625-1308; fax: 612-624-6373. e-mail: obra0005@umn.edu

Ann. N.Y. Acad. Sci. 1094: 340–344 (2006). © 2006 New York Academy of Sciences.
doi: 10.1196/annals.1376.046

(113 girls, 29% minority) during childhood (ages 8–12 years; T1), adolescence (ages 14–19 years; T2), emerging adulthood (ages 17–23 years; T3), and young adulthood (ages 28–36 years; T4). During the three follow-up waves, two clinicians independently rated participants' global adaptation on a 7-point scale (1 = very poorly adjusted, 4 = average, 7 = very well adjusted) based on information collected in Status Questionnaires on various domains of participants' functioning. For each round of data collection, indicators of developmentally salient domains of competence were created using multiple informants (i.e., self, parent, clinical ratings) and various methods (i.e., surveys, interviews, and assessments). A more detailed description of competence indicators can be found in prior publications.[2,3] Childhood family socioeconomic status (SES) was assessed using the Duncan Socioeconomic Index, while the measure of parenting quality (PQ) reflected the clarity and consistency of parental expectations and rules, as well as parental warmth and support. In emerging adulthood, two interviewers rated participants on the reality of their goals and on their persistence and commitment to those goals on a 5-point scale. In young adulthood, self-worth was assessed using the Perceived Competence Scale.[5] Indices of family and community adversity exposure were created by averaging two independent 7-point ratings (1= low, 4 = moderate, 7 = catastrophic) of cumulative stressful life events during childhood, adolescence, and emerging adulthood based on life history charts.[6]

Analyses were conducted using semiparametric mixture modeling, designed to approximate the overall sample distribution of global adaptation scores by a mixture of two or more homogenous latent distributions using SAS PROC TRAJ.[7] We used the Bayesian Information Criterion (BIC), which balances parsimony and model fit, to compare the improvement of the models' explanatory power at each step. BIC was used to determine the number of adaptation groups that best reproduce the sample data. Group differences on antecedents and correlates were examined with analysis of variance (ANOVA) and Mann–Whitney tests.

RESULTS AND DISCUSSION

Examination of fit statistics revealed that five groups best represented the sample data ($2^*\Delta$BIC [4 vs. 5] = 5.58; $2^*\Delta$BIC [5 vs. 6] = −12.62). More specifically, five distinct pathways of adaptation emerged: (1) low-declining, (2) low-improving, (3) middle-improving, (4) middle-declining, and (5) consistently high (see FIG. 1). Interestingly, the most dramatic changes in pathways of adaptation occurred during emerging adulthood. TABLE 1 shows the number of participants assigned to each group and their demographic characteristics.

The results of ANOVA and Tukey–HSD *post hoc* tests are shown in TABLE 2. Adolescent and emerging adulthood measures of competence in age-salient domains, especially academic competence, tracked global adaptation pathways.

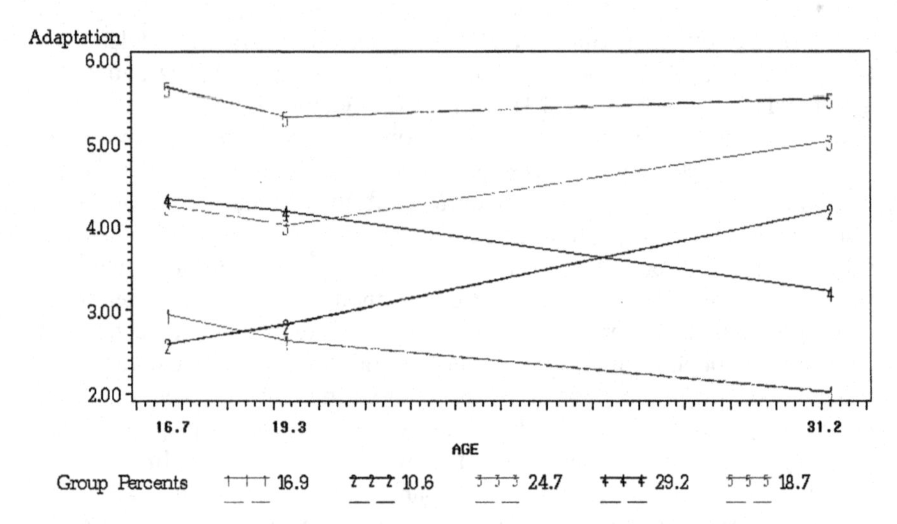

FIGURE 1. SAS PROC TRAJ solution: Mean adaptation scores by trajectory grouping and age.

Indices of childhood, adolescence, and emerging adulthood competence did not discriminate the groups that diverged after T3 (groups 1 vs. 2, and groups 3 vs. 4). Thus, we examined other factors to distinguish these group trajectories. The low-declining group 1 was the most disadvantaged group in terms of childhood risk and resources, with the highest family adversity, percentage of single parents and minority children, and the lowest SES, IQ, and PQ. Group 1 also had significantly higher exposure to community adversity at T3 than all other groups. In contrast, the low-improving group 2 did not face as many risks. They struggled in a school context but by young adulthood found a way to excel in parenting, social conduct, and work competence. Meanwhile, the middle groups differed in their "reality of goals" ($M_3 = 4.3$, $M_4 = 3.9$) and "commitment and persistence" ($M_3 = 3.6$, $M_4 = 3.1$) in emerging adulthood, with the middle-declining group 4 exhibiting significantly lower levels than the middle-improving group 3, according to Mann–Whitney planned comparisons ($P < 0.05$). While participants in group 4 appeared to fail to adapt to the newly salient tasks of young adulthood, the late bloomers in group 3 seized

TABLE 1. Global adaptation groups: number of participants and childhood demographic characteristics

	1	2	3	4	5	Total
N	35	18	46	65	38	202
Girls	60%	72%	67%	40%	58%	56%
Minority	43%	22%	35%	28%	16%	30%
Single parent	57%	33%	37%	34%	29%	38%

TABLE 2. Mean differences in competence, adversity, and childhood resources across group membership

	1	2	3	4	5	*F*-test
Childhood						
Family adversity	5.70^{a}	5.14^{ab}	4.53^{b}	4.62^{b}	4.55^{b}	4.12**
Community adversity	1.59	1.69	1.59	1.87	1.61	*ns*
Family SES	31.49^{a}	44.06^{ab}	41.08^{a}	40.34^{a}	57.89^{b}	8.91***
Parenting quality (PQ)	-0.60^{a}	-0.23^{ab}	-0.12^{ab}	-0.02^{b}	0.86^{c}	13.38***
IQ	-0.53^{a}	-0.35^{a}	-0.05^{a}	-0.00^{a}	0.75^{b}	9.62***
Academic competence	-0.45^{a}	-0.30^{a}	-0.11^{a}	-0.16^{a}	0.92^{b}	13.31***
Social competence	-0.15	-0.05	-0.01	-0.06	0.35	*ns*
Conduct competence	-0.58^{a}	-0.15^{abc}	0.12^{bc}	0.01^{b}	0.54^{c}	6.80***
Adolescence						
Family adversity	5.60^{a}	5.79^{a}	5.13^{ab}	5.00^{ab}	4.82^{b}	3.53**
Community adversity	3.13	2.73	2.72	2.29	2.42	*ns*
Academic competence	-0.80^{a}	-1.13^{a}	−0.06^{b}	0.15^{b}	1.01^{c}	33.61***
Social competence	−0.38^{a}	−0.45^{a}	−0.04^{a}	0.03^{a}	0.59^{b}	5.65***
Conduct competence	−.93^{a}	−0.78^{a}	0.06^{b}	0.32^{b}	0.48^{b}	16.57***
Emerging adulthood						
Family adversity	4.57	4.25	4.03	4.36	3.95	*ns*
Community adversity	3.11^{a}	1.83^{b}	2.14^{b}	2.11^{b}	2.00^{b}	3.77**
Academic competence	-1.13^{a}	-0.89^{a}	0.29^{b}	0.07^{b}	0.94^{c}	45.76***
Social competence	-0.79^{a}	-0.40^{ab}	−0.04^{b}	0.14^{b}	0.81^{c}	16.47***
Conduct competence	-0.80^{a}	-0.56^{a}	0.14^{b}	0.12^{b}	0.59^{b}	13.10***
Young adulthood						
Academic competence	-1.09^{a}	-0.45^{ab}	-0.06^{b}	-0.01^{b}	1.07^{c}	33.70***
Social competence	-0.78^{a}	0.24^{b}	0.22^{b}	-0.07^{b}	0.35^{b}	6.95***
Conduct competence	-1.08^{a}	0.01^{b}	0.40^{b}	-0.02^{b}	0.37^{b}	14.53***
Romantic competence	-0.57^{a}	-0.13^{ab}	0.52^{b}	-0.33^{a}	0.43^{b}	10.41***
Work competence	-0.97^{a}	-0.05^{bc}	0.36^{cd}	-0.24^{b}	0.73^{d}	19.53***
Parenting competence	-1.17^{a}	0.17^{bc}	0.53^{c}	-0.22^{b}	0.69^{c}	18.87***
Self-worth	2.44^{a}	2.88^{ab}	3.36^{c}	2.86^{b}	3.50^{c}	22.78***

NOTES. IQ: composite of Vocabulary and Block Design subscales of the Wechsler Intelligence Scales for Children–Revised (WISC-R); Superscripts indicate significant group differences; $^{*}P < 0.05$; $^{**}P < 0.01$; $^{***}P < 0.001$.

opportunities in the transition to adulthood to succeed in new domains of parenting, work, and romantic competence. The consistently high group 5 stood out as distinctive from the other groups in childhood, with high competence (academic, conduct) and resources (PQ, IQ). This group exhibited significantly higher academic and social competence than all other groups in adolescence and emerging adulthood, but by young adulthood the middle-improving group 3 caught up with group 5 on all competence measures except for cumulative academic attainment.

This study shows that childhood exposure to risks and lack of resources, as well as subsequent inability to plan for and achieve newly salient tasks of young adulthood, can undermine adaptation over time. It underscores the importance of the developmental period between emerging and young adulthood, which appears to be a window of both opportunity and vulnerability. Interestingly, gender seems to play a role in this period of transition. The improving groups,

groups 2 and 3, had higher percentages of females, while the middle-declining group, group 4, had the highest percentage of males. Given that high adversity youth appeared in all groups, diverse pathways of resilience and maladaptation could be further differentiated in larger samples. Future studies using this analytic strategy would benefit from larger samples and more frequent assessments.

REFERENCES

1. RUTTER, M., J. KIM-COHEN & B. MAUGHAN. 2006. Continuities and discontinuities in psychopathology between childhood and adult life. J. Child Psychol. Psychiatry **47:** 276–295.
2. MASTEN, A.S., *et al.* 2004. Resources and resilience in the transition to adulthood: continuity and change. Dev. Psychopath. **16:** 1071–1094.
3. ROISMAN, G.I., *et al.* 2004. Salient and emerging developmental tasks in the transition to adulthood. Child Develop. **75:** 123–133.
4. MASTEN, A.S., *et al.* 2005. Developmental cascades: linking academic achievement, externalizing and internalizing symptoms over 20 years. Dev. Psychopath. **41:** 733–746.
5. Harter, S. 1982. The perceived competence scale for children. Child Develop. **53:** 87–97.
6. GEST, S.D., M. REED & A.S. MASTEN. 1999. Measuring developmental changes in exposure to adversity: a life chart and rating scale approach. Dev. Psychopath. **11:** 171–192.
7. NAGIN, D.S. 1999. Analyzing developmental trajectories: a semiparametric, group-based approach. Psychol. Methods **4:** 139–157.

Relational and Academic Components of Resilience in Maltreated Adolescents

KHUSHMAND RAJENDRAN AND LYNN VIDEKA

School of Social Welfare, University at Albany, Albany, New York, USA

ABSTRACT: This study examines the components of resilience in adolescents (aged 11–15 years; $n = 816$) who were referred to the child welfare system for maltreatment. Data from a national probability study of children and families in the child welfare system showed that adolescents faced a number of risk factors like maltreatment, poverty, and exposure to violence in the community. Social competence, academic achievement, and a sense of relatedness to caregiver were fit in a structural equation model as components of latent resilience. Social competence and the quality of relationship with a caregiver were strongly linked to latent resilience.

KEYWORDS: competence; resilience; psychological resilience; adolescents; maltreatment; abuse; child welfare; sexual abuse; physical maltreatment; neglect; violence; stressors; risks; academic competence; social competence; relationship with parent; closeness to caregiver

INTRODUCTION

Resilience has been conceptualized either as the presence of competence in situations of risk[1,2] or as a group of protective characteristics in the individual or family.[3] The current study integrates both protective processes and competent adaptation as components of resilience in high-risk populations.

It is based on data from the National Survey of Child and Adolescent Well-being (NSCAW), the first national probability survey of children who were investigated by Child Protection Services (CPS) between October 1999 and December 2000.[4] The study sample was adolescents aged 11–15 years who resided with a permanent caregiver and attended school (unweighted $n = 816$). A total of 58% of the population was female. Half of their primary caregivers were White (51%); 27% Black; 17% Hispanic; 4% American Indian; and 1% Asian.

Resilience is competence in the presence of significant stressors. An assessment of possible stressors was conducted using weighted analysis in SPSS 13.

Address for correspondence: Lynn Videka, University Hall 307B, 1400 Washington Ave., Albany, NY 12222. Voice: 518-956-8170; fax: 518-956-8175.
e-mail: kr7039@albany.edu

Ann. N.Y. Acad. Sci. 1094: 345–349 (2006). © 2006 New York Academy of Sciences.
doi: 10.1196/annals.1376.047

TABLE 1. Stressors experienced by adolescents referred to child protective services

Stressor	Category	Estimated n (%)	Standard Error (%)
Maltreatment	Neglect: failure to provide/supervise	1,27,900 (37.1)	29,628.54 (5.3)
	Physical maltreatment	1,44,254 (29.8)	20,891.35 (3.2)
	Sexual maltreatment	62,095 (12.8)	14,223.85 (2.4)
	Emotional	27,802 (5.7)	6,790.57 (1.5)
	Other	30,627 (6.3)	14,372.7 (2.9)
Family Income	Less than $9,999 per annum	1,07,932 (22.3)	22,820.3 (4)
	$9,999–$15,000 per annum	98,120 (20.3)	16,584 (2.6)
Dependents on income	4–5 persons	1,97,533 (40.8)	34,521 (6)
	6 or more persons	1,02,180 (21)	28,149.7 (0.6)
Exposure to Violence	Saw a person arrested at home	1,74,517 (36)	32,239 (5.9)
	Involved in a gang fight	33,047 (6.8)	10,909.5 (2)
	Threatened with gun or knife	42,747 (8.9)	22,552 (4.5)

One of the most compelling stressors in the current sample may be a history of abuse and/or neglect. Maltreatment can be a constant source of stress, [5] and can affect the cognitive, social, and emotional development of children. Sexual abuse was reported in 13% of the population. A total of 37% were referred for neglect or failure to provide; 30% for physical abuse; 6% for emotional abuse; and the same number (6%) were reported for other forms of maltreatment like exploitation, moral, or educational. This study also showed the presence of other risk factors like poverty and violence in the home and community (see TABLE 1).

RESILIENCE ASSESSMENT

Child self-report, performance, and caregiver reports were used in 10 observed measures of three latent constructs—social competence, academic achievement, and sense of relatedness to caregiver—to fit a structural equation measurement model. A list of measures is referenced in FIGURE 1. The study hypothesized that three latent constructs would be components of resilience.

MODEL FIT

The model was fit in AMOS 5 by fixing the variance of the higher order factor to 1.0; that is, by treating it as a standardized latent variable. A variety of indices of model fit were evaluated. The overall chi-square (34.57, $P = 0.096$, 25 df) and other fit indices Root Mean Square Error of Approximation [RMSEA] = 0.038; Probability of Close fit [PCLOSE] = 0.719, and Comparative Fit Index

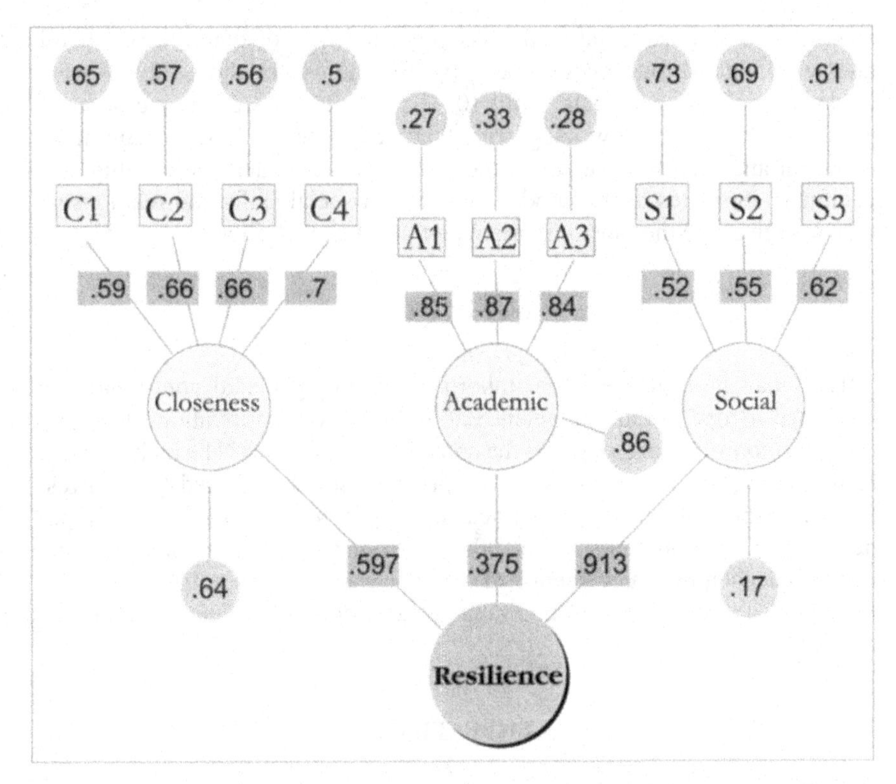

FIGURE 1. Components of Resilience. Measures used: Closeness to caregiver,[4] C1 = Autonomy, C2 = Involvement, C3 = Emotion, C4 = Structure; Academic/cognitive, A1 Woodcock-Johnson Reading,[8] A2 Woodcock-Johnson Math,[8] A3 K-BIT Cognitive;[9] Social Competence, S1 Parent Report on child social skills,[10] S2 Loneliness social dissatisfaction scale,[11] S3 School engagement.[4]

[CFI] = 0.981) did not suggest points of ill fit. FIGURE 1 shows the standardized parameter estimates for the structural coefficients.

To deal with possible effects of non-normality, a bootstrap estimate of the complete, nonmissing data was taken. This alternate model (chi-square = 35, P = 0.06, Generalized Fit Index [GFI] = 0.989, CFI = 0.993, RMSEA = 0.026, Standardized Root Mean Square Residual [SRMR] = 0.028, no theoretically meaningful modification indices) was found to be comparable to the Full Information Maximum Likelihood [FIML] missing data model.

All path coefficients were statistically significant. The largest path coefficient was the one between social skills and resilience. Every 1 standard deviation increase in resilience was associated with social skills improving by 0.91 standard units, academic skills improving by 0.38 units, and closeness to the caregiver increasing by 0.60 units. Social skills accounted for 83% of the variance in resilience. Closeness to the caregiver accounted for 36% of the variance and academic skills accounted for 14% of the variance. Error rates were highest for academic skills (0.86), followed by those for closeness to caregiver (0.64) and social skills (0.17). The residuals of the measures of academic ability were low, suggesting that though they did not explain much of the variance in resilience, they were good measures of academic ability. The parameter estimates in this model suggest that social skills and relationship with caregiver are the most important components of resilience.

DISCUSSION

This analysis brings out the importance of interpersonal contributors to resilience. Broad social competence as well as a quality relationship to the caregiver contributed strongly to the construct of resilience. The path between resilience and academic ability was surprisingly small, and needs to be investigated further. It is possible that academic skill is not a very large component of resilience in this sample. Other researchers have also found the link between academic achievement and resilience small or insignificant.[6,7] This finding also underlines the importance of assessing multiple components of resilience.

LIMITATIONS

This study includes only an unweighted analysis of children referred to the child welfare system in a certain time frame and so may not be truly representative of all abused and neglected children. It also does not look at larger systemic or community contributors to resilience, nor does it measure the persistence of resilience over time. Though global risk is established, a more comprehensive study needs to include interactive effects and effects of intensity of risk on resilience.

REFERENCES

1. Masten, A.S., J.J. Hubbard, S.D. Gest, *et al.* 1999. Competence in the context of adversity: pathways to resilience and maladaptation from childhood to late adolescence. Dev. Psychopathol. **11:** 143–169.
2. Flores, E., D. Cicchetti & F.A. Rogosch. 2005. Predictors of resilience in maltreated and nonmaltreated Latino children. Dev. Psychopathol. **41:** 338–351.
3. Wolin, S. & S. Wolin. 1995. Resilience among youth growing up in substance-abusing families. Pediatr. Clin. N. Am. **42:** 415–427.
4. Dowd, K., S. Kinsey, S. Wheeless, *et al.* 2004. National Survey of Child and Adolescent Well-Being (NSCAW) Combined Waves 1–4. Data File Users Manual General Release Version. National Data Archive on Child Abuse and Neglect. Ithaca. New York.

5. Masten, A. & J.D. Coatsworth. 1998. The development of competence in favorable and unfavorable environments: lessons from research on successful children. Am. Psychol. **53:** 205–220.
6. Cicchetti, D., F.A. Rogosch, M. Lynch, *et al.* 1993. Resilience in maltreated children: processes leading to adaptive outcomes. Dev. Psychopathol. **5:** 629–647.
7. Carle, A.C. & L. Chassin. 2004. Resilience in a community sample of children of alcoholics: its prevalence and relation to internalizing symptomatology and positive affect. J. Appl. Dev. Psychol. **25:** 577–595.
8. Woodcock, R.W., K. McGrew & J. Werder. 1994. Mini-Battery of Achievement (MBA). Riverside Publishing Company, Chicago.
9. Kaufman, A. & N. Kaufman. 1997. Kaufman Brief Intelligence Test (K-BIT): Expressive Vocabulary, Definitions, and Matrices. American Guidance Service, Inc. Circle Pines, MN.
10. Gresham, F.M. & S.N. Elliott. 1990. Social Skills Rating System. American Guidance Service, Inc. Circle Pines, MN.
11. Asher, S. & V. Wheeler. 1985. Children's loneliness: a comparison of rejected and neglected peer status. J. Consult. Clin. Psychol. **53:** 500–505.

Using Protective Factors in Practice

Lessons Learned about Resilience from a Study of Children Aged Five to Thirteen

VALERIE B. SHAPIRO AND PAUL A. LEBUFFE

Institute of Clinical Training and Research, Devereux Foundation, Villanova, Pennsylvania, USA

ABSTRACT: There are many advantages of using resilience as a framework to guide the screening, assessment, and promotion of social–emotional health in children. This article reviews which individual attributes are most important for the resilience of elementary school-age children, as primarily determined by the positive attribute's ability to discriminate between typically developing children and those with disciplinary, mental health, and/or special education referrals or services. This research lends itself to a practical framework to scientifically measure and utilize individual social–emotional strengths for the purposes of fostering resilience in all children.

KEYWORDS: resilience; protective factor; assessment; social–emotional; DESSA; strength; devereux; screen; prevention

The use of the constructs of resilience and within-child strengths to guide the practice of assessment and intervention in education and child psychology is a relatively new approach. As a consequence, the literature discussing strength-based approaches at the practice level is sparse and often anecdotal. The lack of empirical direction for the practical use of resilience in educational and treatment planning exists despite the President's New Freedom Commission on Mental Health[2] stating that the transformation of the mental health delivery system relies on our ability to focus on the consumer's ability to cope with life's challenges, facilitate recovery, and build resilience. The gap between mandate and practice was further emphasized when the strength-based perspective was incorporated into law when the Individuals with Disabilities Education Improvement Act (IDEIA)[3] reauthorization regulations were adopted in July 2005. The revision requires that strengths be considered in the development of an Individualized Education Plan (IEP), that positive behavior supports be

Address for correspondence: Valerie B. Shapiro, 444 Devereux Drive, Villanova, PA 19085. Voice: 610-542-3115; fax: 610-542-3132.
e-mail: VShapiro@Devereux.Org

Ann. N.Y. Acad. Sci. 1094: 350–353 (2006). © 2006 New York Academy of Sciences.
doi: 10.1196/annals.1376.048

used in school settings, and that a greater emphasis be placed on prevention services, allowing school systems to use up to 15% of their federal money for early intervention instead of for traditional special education services or out of district placements. The spending of this early intervention money is required to be for scientifically based behavioral and academic interventions that make use of technologically sound assessments. Many advantages of strength-based practice have been articulated, and by mandate, strength-based practices have been "adopted." But is the field ready to use individual strengths in a scientifically and technologically sound manner?

To initially investigate this hypothesized disparity, 40 client files were randomly selected in March 2003 from three different mental health service programs, including a wrap-around program for children with developmental disabilities, a special education day treatment program for children with social skills deficits and affective disorders, and a residential treatment setting for boys with oppositional defiant and conduct disorders. Upon reviewing each child's current and previous treatment plans, assessments, educational reviews, and IEP, a combined 329 statements of strengths were found. Statements ranged from ones that seemed irrelevant to his or her mental health (e.g., "well nourished" "motivated to have cyst treated") to those that seemed like potential assets to recovery (e.g., "likes to be around others" "enjoys drawing") and to those that actually seemed like potential concerns (e.g., "likes to be clean—4 showers/day"). Other strength-statements seemed entirely inappropriate (e.g., "adjusts well to tranquil environment," "light-skinned"). These exploratory findings led to a thorough review of the literature and a series of focus groups with multidisciplinary professional teams to determine what strengths are theorized to promote well-being. After generating a list of 765 uniquely phrased potential within-child protective factors, we collapsed similar content and operationalized the items resulting in a set of 156 potential strength statements. We then devised an empirical study to determine the degree of clinical utility that exists for the hypothesized characteristics.

METHOD

To empirically investigate the relationship between the 156 theorized strengths and children's actual social and emotional well-being, a contrasted group study was designed. Parents and teachers provided ratings of the observed frequency of 156 positive behaviors in children who had either already been identified as having significant social and emotional problems ($n = 86$) or who had not been so identified ($n = 322$). The criteria used to determine an "identified" child/adolescent was the presence of one or more of the following: a referral to the office for aggressive or violent behavior during the academic year, a referral to a mental health professional for an evaluation regarding emotional/behavioral problems during this academic year, treatment by a mental health professional for emotional/behavioral problems during the academic year, a program or plan developed to manage his/her behavior problems, a psychiatric diagnosis, or special education services for emotional/behavioral problems.

Data were collected on 408 children in kindergarten through seventh grade attending 35 schools and after-school programs in 26 states. The children comprised a diverse sample and included Black ($n = 67$, 16%), Latino ($n = 61$, 14%), and socioeconomically disadvantaged children ($n = 68$, 16%). Teachers provided 58% of all ratings and parents provided the rest. The data collection form asked them to indicate on a 5-point Likert scale ranging from "never" to "very frequently" how often they had observed the 156 strengths in the past 4 weeks. Informants were also given the opportunity to indicate that the item was unclear, or that they felt the item did not apply to the child being rated.

RESULTS

A multistage data analysis plan was used to reduce the initial pool of 156 potential strengths to a more manageable, useful, reliable, and valid pool of strengths. As a first step in the analysis, those items that were frequently marked as unclear, does not apply, or left blank, were eliminated. The items with the highest percentages of unclear ratings were, "look for deeper meaning in daily routines" (7%), and "delay gratification" (6%). A larger percentage of informants, especially teachers, indicated that certain items were not applicable. These items included, "participate in religious activities" (22%), "recycle or do something to help the environment" (12%), and "spend time on a hobby" (10%).

The next criterion applied to the potential strengths was the ability of the item to differentiate between the identified and nonidentified samples. In addition to t-tests, effect sizes (d-ratios) were also examined. Those items where the mean scores differed significantly and were separated by at least half a standard deviation ($d \geq 0.50$) were retained. Only 7 of the original 156 items did not differentiate significantly between the two groups. In addition, only 30 items had effect sizes of less than half a standard deviation. Examples of items that did not differentiate included, "participate in after school or community activities," "show talent in athletics, the arts, or in a technical/mechanical area," and "engage in cultural activities or traditions."

The third step was to examine the corrected item-total correlations. Very few items were eliminated on this basis. Fourth, item raw scores were correlated with the student's age, gender, and race. To avoid strengths that seemed biased across these dimensions, 10 additional items were eliminated. As a final step, redundant or very similar items were eliminated. These five steps winnowed the pool of potential strengths from 156 items to 81 items. Using a discriminate analysis function, these 81 strength-based items correctly classified children based on their referral status in 87.6% of all cases, demonstrating that strength-based indicators can empirically predict well-being.

DISCUSSION AND CONCLUSIONS

This study advances our knowledge of within-child strengths in many ways. First, it provides a comprehensive review of our existing knowledge about within-child strengths. Second, it investigates which strengths have contextual validity to both parents and teachers. Third, it explores which of these strengths differentiate between students already identified with significant emotional and behavioral disorders and those who are not. Interestingly, some of the strengths that are widely recognized in the literature as protective were not validated through this study. This was most strikingly the case for items related to religion and spirituality. Further studies will scrutinize this 81 item-set through a larger and more diverse sample of student behavior, organize the content into scales, and will explore how the empirically validated strengths lend themselves to intervention planning and progress monitoring. Such findings will be utilized to design practical, strength-based tools for educators and mental health professionals to use data to support the social and emotional development of children with disabilities, identify students at risk for emotional and behavioral problems, and to promote the resilience of all children.

REFERENCES

1. LeBuffe, P.A. & V.B. Shapiro. 2004. Lending "strength" to the assessment of preschool social-emotional health. The California School Psychologist **9:** 51–61.
2. New Freedom Commission on Mental Health. 2003. Achieving the Promise: Transforming Mental Health Care in America, Final Report. DHHS Pub. No. SMA-03-3832. Rockville, MD.
3. CFR Parts 300, 301, and 304 Proposed Rule. 2005. Federal Register. Vol. 70: 118. Office of Special Education and Rehabilitative Services, Department of Education. Washington, DC.

Prenatal Cocaine Exposure

Cardiorespiratory Function and Resilience

STEPHEN J. SHEINKOPF,[a,b] LINDA L. LAGASSE,[a,b]
BARRY M. LESTER,[a,b] JING LIU,[a,b] RONALD SEIFER,[a,c]
CHARLES R. BAUER,[d] SEETHA SHANKARAN,[e] HENRIETTA BADA,[f]
ROSEMARY HIGGINS,[g] AND ABHIK DAS[h]

[a]*Brown Medical School, Providence, Rhode Island, USA*

[b]*Women and Infants Hospital of Rhode Island, Providence, Rhode Island, USA*

[c]*E. P. Bradley Hospital, East Providence, Rhode Island, USA*

[d]*University of Miami School of Medicine, Miami, Florida, USA*

[e]*Wayne State University School of Medicine, Detroit, Michigan, USA*

[f]*University of Tennessee at Memphis, School of Medicine, Memphis, Tennessee, USA*

[g]*National Institute of Child Health and Human Development, Bethesda, Maryland, USA*

[h]*Research Triangle Institute, Rockville, Maryland, USA*

ABSTRACT: Cardiac vagal tone (VT) was studied as a resilience factor in children prenatally exposed to cocaine and nonexposed controls (n = 550). A cumulative risk index was derived and used to classify children as high versus low risk. VT was measured during mildly stressful observations at 1 and 36 months of age. Children were classified as having consistently high, consistently low, or fluctuating VT. Risk and VT interacted to predict adaptive behaviors. For high-risk children, low VT was related to higher ratings of adaptive behaviors. This finding suggests that regulatory functioning, as indexed by VT, may be a protective factor in prenatal CE.

KEYWORDS: prenatal drug exposure; cocaine; cumulative risk; children; vagal tone; heart rate variability; developmental outcome

INTRODUCTION

Children with prenatal cocaine exposure (CE) are at risk for poor developmental outcomes. However, prenatal drug exposure occurs in the context of

Address for correspondence: Stephen Sheinkopf, Brown Center for the Study of Children at Risk, Women and Infants Hospital, 101 Dudley Street, Providence, RI 02905. Voice: 401-453-7640; fax: 401-453-7639.
e-mail: Stephen_Sheinkopf@brown.edu

Ann. N.Y. Acad. Sci. 1094: 354–358 (2006).
doi: 10.1196/annals.1376.049

multiple risk factors, and the effects of CE on development appear to be both subtle and highly variable.[1,2] Yet the variable manner in which prenatal CE confers risk offers an opportunity to study mechanisms that either potentiate or ameliorate risk in this population. Identifying such processes of risk and resilience will allow for a more precise description of pathways to competence and disturbance in prenatal CE and may offer insights into such processes in other populations of children.

Prenatal CE may impact children's capacity to regulate affect, behavior, and cognition in the face of environmental demands.[3] This regulatory framework also suggests processes that may serve to buffer children from the effects of risk factors that coalesce with CE. In the present study, we used cardiorespiratory measures, including vagal tone (VT), as an index of children's regulatory capacity. High resting levels of VT are thought to index a readiness to respond to the environment, whereas task-related reductions in VT are seen to reflect children's reactivity and engagement with the environment under nonthreat stress conditions.[4] Thus, lower VT during attention-demanding conditions reflects adaptive mechanisms of self-regulation that support responses to environmental demands.[5] We examined VT as a potential protective factor in a cohort of children with and without prenatal CE. We hypothesized that high degrees of risk in infancy would predict negative outcomes in the preschool period. We predicted that low task-related VT (reflecting attention-related modulation of VT) would predict positive developmental outcomes even in the presence of high degrees of risk.

METHOD

Participants

Participants were drawn from a sample of 1,388 children from the Maternal Lifestyle Study (MLS), a large-scale longitudinal study of children with prenatal CE (cocaine with or without opiates; $n = 658$) and non-CE controls ($n = 730$). Prenatal exposure to other substances (i.e., alcohol, nicotine, and cannabis) varied but was allowed in both groups. The sample was 77% Black, 16% White, 6% Hispanic, and 1% Other. There were roughly equal numbers of boys (52%) and girls (48%).

Risk Measurement

A subset of measures from birth to 12 months was chosen and formed the basis of a cumulative risk index. These included prenatal substance exposure (cocaine, opiates, alcohol, nicotine, and cannabis), poverty, low SES (Hollingshead score), caregiver psychopathology and depression, parenting stress, risk for child abuse, caregiver instability, poor home environment, domestic violence, child abuse or neglect, and single parent status. From these measures,

16 items were each dichotomized to reflect high versus low risk and summed to create a cumulative risk index ($\alpha = 0.68$).

Outcome Measures

Measures of developmental outcome were administered in the preschool period and included the Wechsler Preschool and Primary Scales of Intelligence, Revised (WPPSI-R) at 54 months, the Vineland Scales of Adaptive Behavior at 36 months, and the Child Behavior Checklist (CBCL) at 36 months. Together these measures allowed for an assessment of cognitive abilities, behavioral competence, and behavioral disturbance.

Physiologic Measurement and Data Analysis

ECG recordings were acquired during an infant exam[6] at 1 month of age and during a toy interaction task at 36 months of age. VT was derived from the ECG time series using the algorithm by Porges.[7] Children were classified as high or low risk by a median split of the cumulative risk score. Similarly, the sample was split into those with high versus low VT during the 1- and 36-month physiologic measurements. Based on these values, children were classified as having consistently high VT (high stable), low VT (low stable), and fluctuating VT rankings (unstable) during the task conditions. Because reductions in VT during attention-demanding tasks are generally thought to reflect adaptive mechanisms,[4,8] it was expected that low VT during tasks would predict positive outcomes. From this source sample, children were included in analyses if they had valid VT data at ages 1 and 36 months ($n = 550$). Hypothesis testing used a 2×3 factorial analysis of variance ANOVA (Risk $\times$ VT Stability).

RESULTS

Results are illustrated in FIGURE 1. High-risk children had lower 54-month full-scale IQ scores than the low-risk children ($P < 0.001$). There was a marginal effect of VT stability on IQ ($P = 0.08$), with the low-stable group having somewhat higher IQ scores than the high-stable and unstable groups. There was not a significant interaction between VT stability and risk groupings. On the CBCL, high-risk children had higher total behavior problems at 36 months ($P < 0.001$). Neither VT stability nor the interaction term had a significant effect on CBCL scores. In the area of adaptive behaviors (our competence measure), high-risk children had lower Vineland total scores than low-risk children ($P < 0.001$). The main effect of VT stability was not significant, but the interaction between VT stability and risk classification did reach statistical significance ($P = 0.02$). Follow-up analyses revealed that high- and

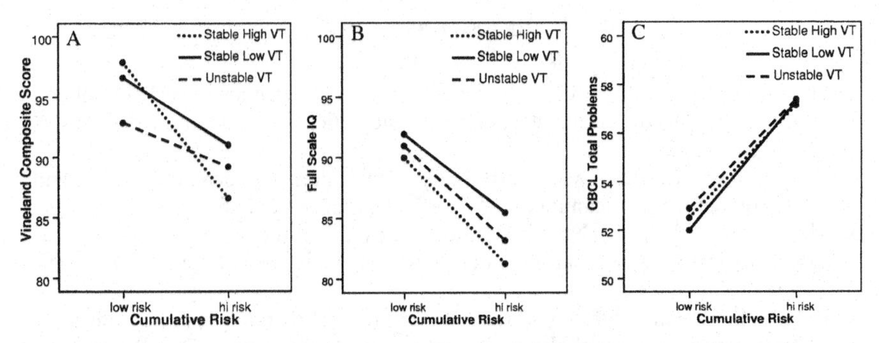

FIGURE 1. Effects of cumulative risk on developmental outcomes for children with consistently high and low vagal tone, and inconsistent levels of vagal tone during tasks at 1 and 36 months of age. Outcomes include adaptive behaviors (**A**), cognitive ability (**B**), and caregiver-rated problem behaviors (**C**).

low-stable VT groups did not differ from each other within those children classified as low risk. In contrast, within the high-risk children, the low-stable group had significantly higher Vineland total scores than the high-stable group ($P = 0.04$). The unstable group did not differ significantly from either of the stable VT groups.

DISCUSSION

Our analyses indicated that cumulative risks in the first year of life predicted poor developmental outcomes in the preschool period, including lower IQ, lower adaptive behaviors, and more behavior problems. However, the relationship between early risk and later outcome was in part dependent on whether children demonstrated consistent evidence for physiologic regulation during attention-demanding situations. Most notably, the impact of cumulative risk on adaptive abilities, our measure of behavioral competence, was dependent on the degree to which children showed consistently low VT during tasks at age 1 and 36 months. Consistently low VT during attention-demanding activities appeared to moderate the impact of cumulative risk. More specifically, children with lower VT during tasks, indicative of active regulation in response to environmental demands, showed higher levels of adaptive behaviors even for children with high cumulative risk scores. This finding is consistent with theory linking reduced VT during tasks to adaptive regulation. Low VT during tasks may reflect regulatory capacities that serve to buffer the effects of pre- and postnatal risk factors on later developmental outcomes. In other words, VT in this context appears to serve as a resiliency factor in high-risk children. The specificity of these results to adaptive behaviors suggests that such regulatory capacity is important for the display of complex adaptive skills in children's natural environments.

REFERENCES

1. FRANK, D.A. *et al.* 2001. Growth, development, and behavior in early childhood following prenatal cocaine exposure: a systematic review. J. Am. Med. Assoc. **285:** 1613–1625.
2. LESTER, B.M., L.L. LAGASSE & R. SEIFER. 1998. Prenatal cocaine exposure and child outcome: the meaning of subtle effects. Science **282:** 633–634.
3. MAYES, L.C. 2002. A behavioral teratogenic model of the impact of prenatal cocaine exposure on arousal regulatory systems. Neurotoxicol. Teratol. **24:** 385–395.
4. PORGES, S.W. *et al.* 1996. Infant regulation of the vagal "brake" predicts child behavior problems: a psychobiological model of social behavior. Dev. Psychobiol. **29:** 697–712.
5. PORGES, S.W. 1995. Cardiac vagal tone: a physiological index of stress. Neurosci. Biobehav. Rev. **19:** 225–233.
6. LESTER, B.M., E.Z. TRONICK & T.B. BRAZELTON. 2004. The neonatal intensive care unit network neurobehavioral scale procedures. Pediatrics **113:** 641–667.
7. PORGES, S.W. 1986. Respiratory sinus arrhythmia: physiological basis, quantitative methods, and clinical implications. *In* Cardiorespiratory and Cardiosomatic Psychophysiology. P. Grossman, K. Janssen, and D. Vaitl, Eds: 101–115. Plenum Press. New York.
8. CALKINS, S.D. 1997. Cardiac vagal tone indices of temperamental reactivity and behavioral regulation in young children. Dev. Psychobiol. **31:** 125–135.

Neighborhood Risk and the Development of Resilience

ELLA VANDERBILT-ADRIANCE AND DANIEL S. SHAW

Department of Psychology, University of Pittsburgh, Pittsburgh, Pennsylvania, USA

ABSTRACT: The purpose of the study was to advance our understanding of resilience by studying multiple protective factors associated with positive adjustment among an ethnically diverse sample of 310 low-income boys followed prospectively from ages 1.5 to 12 years, using neighborhood quality to define risk status. The results indicated that child and family protective factors measured in early childhood were all significantly associated with positive adjustment at 11 and 12 years of age. However, these results were qualified by risk level, such that parent–child relationship quality was only significantly related to positive outcomes in the context of low levels of risk.

KEYWORDS: resilience; neighborhood risk; protective factors

INTRODUCTION

The study of resilience provides information on conditions under which established risk factors do not result in negative outcomes.[1] Such research can inform theories of psychopathology and guide intervention and policy efforts to improve the lives of children at risk for maladaptive outcomes. Despite growing interest in resilience, research is limited by few prospective, longitudinal studies examining multiple aspects of risk, protective factors, and competence.[2]

This study aims to advance our understanding of resilience by studying multiple protective factors associated with competence among an ethnically diverse sample of 310 low-income boys followed prospectively from ages 1.5 to 12 years. Child and family factors (e.g., child IQ, emotion regulation, nurturant parenting, parent–child relationship quality, and marital quality) measured in early and middle childhood were expected to be positively associated with child adjustment in early adolescence. However, it was expected that mean levels of neighborhood risk would moderate this relationship, such that the

Address for correspondence: Ella Vanderbilt-Adriance, Department of Psychology, University of Pittsburgh, 4425 Sennott Square, 210 S. Bouquet St., Pittsburgh, PA 15260. Voice: 412-624-8738; fax: 412-624-8991.
e-mail: elv4@pitt.edu

Ann. N.Y. Acad. Sci. 1094: 359–362 (2006). © 2006 New York Academy of Sciences.
doi: 10.1196/annals.1376.050

protective factors would be more strongly associated with positive adjustment in the context of high neighborhood risk.

METHODS

Participants in this study were part of the Pitt Mother and Child Project, an ongoing longitudinal study of risk and resilience in urban, low-income boys.[3] In 1991 and 1992, 310 infant boys (6–17 months) and their mothers were recruited from Allegheny County Women, Infants, and Children (WIC) Nutrition Supplement Clinics. At the time of recruitment, the sample was predominantly European and African American (53% and 36%, respectively), and the mean per capita income was $241 per month. Two-thirds of the mothers in the sample had 12 years or less of education, and consequently much of the sample could be considered high risk due to their low SES. Target children and their mothers were seen for home and/or lab assessments at ages 1.5, 2, 3.5, 5, 5.5, 6, 8, 10, 11, and 12 years, involving a variety of questionnaire and observational measures. Beginning at the age of 6 years, teachers also filled out several questionnaires on child adjustment.

Child protective factors included IQ (brief version of the WPPSI-R[4] at the age of 5.5 years) and emotion regulation (composite of observed anger subtracted from behavioral distraction during a waiting task[5] at the age of 3.5 years). Family factors included parent–child relationship quality (composite of the openness and conflict factors of the Adult-Child Relationship Scale[6] at ages 5 and 6 years), maternal nurturance (HOME[7] observational ratings at the age of 2 years), and marital quality (composite of scores on the Marital Adjustment Test[8] at ages 1.5, 2, and 3.5 years). Adversity was established at the community level, using 1990 and 2000 census data to determine neighborhood risk over time; neighborhood risk scores at the assessments from ages 1.5 to 10 years were averaged for each participant. Positive child adjustment at 11 and 12 years was determined by subtracting youth self-reported antisocial behavior (Self-Report of Antisocial Behavior[9]) from a composite of mother- and teacher-rated social skills (Social Skills Rating System[10]).

RESULTS

A series of Pearson correlations were computed to assess direct associations between child and family protective factors and positive child adjustment. In line with hypotheses, child IQ, nurturant parenting, parent–child relationship quality, and marital quality were all positively associated with child adjustment at 11 and 12 years (rs $= 0.16$ to 0.36, Ps < 0.05); emotion regulation was a nonsignificant trend ($r = 0.13$, $P < 0.10$).

To examine whether mean neighborhood risk from ages 1.5 to 10 years moderated the relationship between protective factors and positive child outcome in early adolescence, a series of hierarchical regressions were computed. In each regression equation, the centered protective factors were entered in the first step, followed by centered neighborhood risk and finally the interaction between the protective factor and neighborhood risk. Significant interactions were explored following procedures described by Aiken and West,[11] in which simple slopes were calculated at one standard deviation below and one standard deviation above the mean for neighborhood risk. Only one significant interaction was found among the five protective factors tested. Parent–child relationship quality interacted with neighborhood risk ($B = -0.20$, $P < 0.05$), such that high levels of parent–child relationship quality were more strongly associated with positive child adjustment in the context of low levels of neighborhood risk ($B = 0.67$, $P < 0.001$) than in the context of high levels of neighborhood risk ($B = 0.29$, $P < 0.01$).

DISCUSSION

Results from the current study suggest that child IQ, nurturant parenting, and marital quality act similarly across levels of neighborhood risk, such that children with high levels of these protective factors, relative to those with low levels, are more likely to have positive outcomes in early adolescence. Contrary to predictions, however, parent–child relationship quality appeared to be more strongly related to positive outcomes in the context of lower rather than higher levels of neighborhood risk. This suggests that once neighborhood risk reaches a certain threshold, having a good relationship with a parent is not sufficient to counteract the negative effects of multiple stressors. Thus in addition to promoting protective factors in children at risk, this study points to the importance of reducing the level of risk that children are exposed to in the first place.

Future studies should examine whether these same findings hold for girls and for boys and girls living in rural and suburban contexts. Second, the current study used a measure of neighborhood risk that collapsed individual variability over time. It would be interesting to examine whether using a dynamic representation of neighborhood risk over time (e.g., trajectories) would yield similar results.

ACKNOWLEDGMENTS

The Pitt Mother and Child Project (PMCP) has been supported by grants to Daniel Shaw from the National Institute of Mental Health (MH 46925 and MH 50907).

REFERENCES

1. MASTEN, A.S. 2001. Ordinary magic: resilience processes in development. Am. Psychol. **56:** 227–238.
2. MASTEN, A.S. *et al.* 1999. Competence in the context of adversity: pathways to resilience and maladaptation from childhood to late adolescence. Dev. Psychopathol. **11:** 143–169.
3. SHAW, D.S. *et al.* 2004. Hierarchies and pathways leading to school-age conduct problems. Dev. Psychopathol. **16:** 483–500.
4. WESCHLER, D. 1989. Weschler Preschool and Primary School of Intelligence–Revised. Psych Corp. San Antonio, TX.
5. MARVIN, R.S. 1977. An ethological-cognitive model for the attenuation of mother-infant attachment behavior. *In* Advances in the Study of Communication and Affect: Vol. 3. The Development of Social Attachments. T.M. Alloway *et al.* Eds: 25–60. Plenum. New York.
6. PIANTA, R.C. *et al.* 1995. The first two years of school: teacher-child relationships and deflections in children's classroom adjustment. Dev. Psychopathology **7:** 295–312.
7. CALDWELL, B.M. & R.H. BRADLEY. 1984. Home observation for measurement of the environment. U of Arkansas. Little Rock. AR.
8. LOCKE, H.J. & K.M. WALLACE. 1959. Short marital-adjustment and prediction tests: their reliability and validity. Marriage Fam. Living. **21:** 251–255.
9. ELLIOTT, D.S. *et al.* 1985. Explaining delinquency and drug use. Sage. Thousand Oaks, CA.
10. GRESHAM, F.M. & S.N. ELLIOTT. 1990. Social skills rating system manual. Am. Guidance Serv. Circle Pines. MN.
11. AIKEN, L.S. & S.G. WEST. 1991. Multiple Regression: Testing and Interpreting Interactions. Sage. Thousand Oaks, CA.

Association of Direct Exposure to Terrorism, Media Exposure to Terrorism, and Other Trauma with Emotional and Behavioral Problems in Preschool Children

YANPING WANG,[a] YOKO NOMURA,[a] RUTH PAT-HORENCZYK,[b] OSNAT DOPPELT,[b] ROBERT ABRAMOVITZ,[c] DANIEL BROM,[b] AND CLAUDE CHEMTOB[a]

[a]*Mount Sinai School of Medicine, New York City, New York, USA*

[b]*Israel Center for the Treatment of Psychotrauma, Herzog Hospital, Jerusalem, Israel*

[c]*Jewish Board of Family and Children's Services, New York City, New York, USA*

ABSTRACT: This study examined the differential impact of various types of trauma exposure on emotional and behavioral problems in preschool children. Participants were 95 mothers of 1- to 4-year-old children in Israel. Results suggested a differential pattern of associations between the types of trauma exposure (i.e., direct exposure to terrorism, media exposure to terrorism, and other trauma) and children's internalizing and externalizing problems. This line of research is important for the identification of risk factors and the development of effective prevention and intervention strategies to promote resilience in preschool children exposed to specific type(s) of trauma.

KEYWORDS: direct exposure to terrorism; media exposure to terrorism; other trauma; preschool children; differential associations; emotional and behavioral problems

INTRODUCTION

Significant advances have been made in research on trauma and PTSD in the recent decades. However, preschool-age children have received far less attention than adolescents and adults. Researchers have suggested differential

Address for correspondence: Claude Chemtob, Ph.D., Mount Sinai School of Medicine, Department of Psychiatry, One Gustave L. Levy Place, Box 1230, New York City, NY 10029. Voice: 212-987-0559; fax: 212-987-0177.
e-mail: claude.chemtob@mssm.edu

**Ann. N.Y. Acad. Sci. 1094: 363–368 (2006). © 2006 New York Academy of Sciences.
doi: 10.1196/annals.1376.051**

response to trauma depending on children's developmental levels.[1–5] To date, few empirical studies are available that examined preschoolers' reaction to trauma and our knowledge is still very limited about the extent of the impact of trauma exposure on various aspects of preschool children's emotional and behavioral functioning.

An emerging body of research on terrorism has identified some unique features of terrorism-induced trauma.[6] However, there is a lack of research on the differential reactions to terrorism from those associated with other types of trauma exposure. Another line of research has investigated the influence of media exposure of disaster events on children and suggested a significant correlation between media exposure and posttraumatic stress symptoms.[7–10] The association of media exposure to violence and aggressive behavior in children is also well documented.[11–13] In general, there is a lack of integration in the research literature that examines the differential effects of various types of trauma exposure. There is some evidence from the adult trauma literature that suggests differential mental health outcomes in association with different types of trauma exposure.[14] However, little is known about how preschool children may react differently to various types of trauma exposure.

This study intended to examine three types of trauma exposure (direct exposure to terrorism, media exposure to terrorism, and other trauma) and their differential effects in predicting risk of emotional and behavioral problems in preschool children.

METHOD

Participants

A total of 95 mothers of 1- to 4-year-old children in Israel participated in the study. The children included 37 girls (38.9%). The average age of the children was 33.8 months (SD = 8.9).

Measures

Demographic information was obtained on child's gender, age, birth weight, and mother's education level.

Child's history of trauma exposure was assessed using a brief terrorism exposure questionnaire for direct terrorism exposure (e.g., was present during a terrorist attack with or without injury, was near a terrorist attack, or knew someone close to the child who was injured or killed during a terrorist attack) and media exposure to terrorism (how much time the child was exposed to terrorist events through media) and an abbreviated version of the Traumatic Events Screening Inventory (TESI)[15] for other trauma (e.g., severe accident, natural disaster, violence other than terrorism, attacked by animal, having someone close to the child with severe illness or injury).

Child's behavioral and emotional problems were assessed by mother's report on the Achenbach's Child Behavior Checklist (CBCL).[16] A t-score of 60 and above was used as the cutoff to indicate clinically significant problems on the Internalizing, Externalizing, and Total Problems scales. The cutoff point of 65 and above was used for the other syndrome and DSM-IV-oriented subscales.

Data Analysis

Logistic regression analyses were conducted to predict risk of behavioral and emotional problems in children with direct terrorism exposure, media exposure to trauma, and other trauma exposure as predictors. Child's birth weight and mother's education level as potential confounders were also included in the models for statistical adjustment.

RESULTS

Descriptive Statistics

Among the 95 children, 7.4% (n = 7) had direct exposure to terrorism, 22.3% (n = 21) reportedly watched TV with terrorism contents for 5 min or more, and 48.4% (n = 46) had experienced at least one traumatic event that is not related to terrorism. The rates of behavioral problems at or above the borderline range in children across the syndrome and DSM-oriented scales on the CBCL ranged from 4.2% (Withdrawn) to 23.4% (Internalizing problems).

Logistic Regression Analyses

FIGURE 1 shows that having direct exposure to terrorism is significantly associated with increased risk of Internalizing (OR = 6.2, CI = 1.1–35.7, P = 0.04), Externalizing (OR = 12.5, CI = 2.0–79.5, P = 0.007), and Total Problems (OR = 6.3, CI = 1.1–37.2, P = 0.04) in preschool children. Direct exposure to terrorism is not significantly associated with risk of problems in other syndrome or DSM-IV-oriented scales.

FIGURE 2 indicates that preschool children who watched TV with terrorism-related contents for 5 min or more on a regular, daily basis were at increased risk of Externalizing problems (OR = 4.5, CI = 1.1–17.7, P = 0.03), being emotionally reactive (OR = 9.4, CI = 1.6–54.5, P = 0.01), sleep problems (OR = 10.1, CI = 1.4–71.1, P = 0.02), aggressive behavior (OR = 4.6, CI = 1.1–19.7, P = 0.04), and oppositional defiant problems (OR = 17.5, CI = 1.8–171.9, P = 0.01).

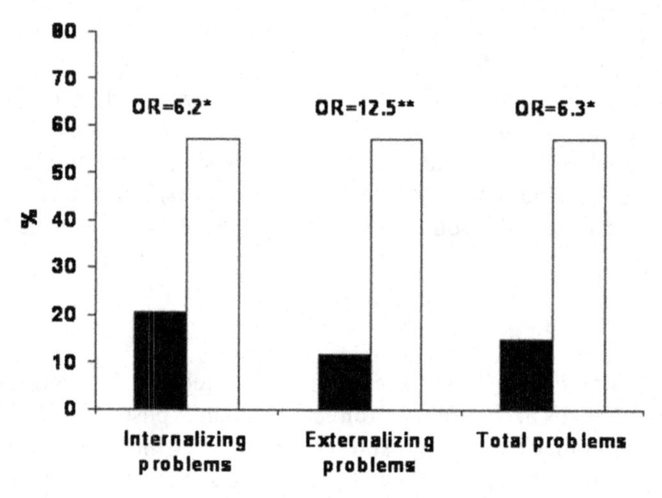

FIGURE 1. Risk of behavioral problems by direct exposure to terrorism.

FIGURE 3 shows that exposure to nonterrorism-related trauma was significantly or marginally significantly associated with increased risk of problems in the areas of anxious/depressed (OR = 4.5, CI = 0.74–27.1, $P = 0.10$), withdrawn (OR = $+\infty$, $P = 0.05$), affective problems (OR = 8.1, CI = 0.90–72.8, $P = 0.06$), and anxiety problems (OR = 10.1, CI = 0.95–106.2, $P = 0.05$).

CONCLUSIONS

This study suggested differential associations between three types of trauma exposure and emotional and behavioral problems in children age 4 years and

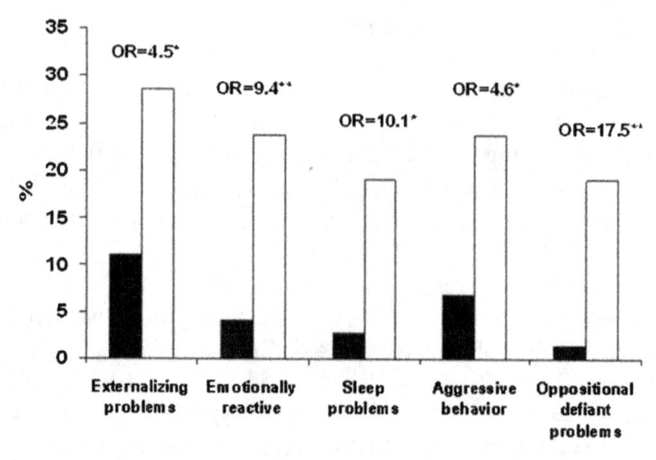

FIGURE 2. Risk of behavioral problems by media exposure to terrorism.

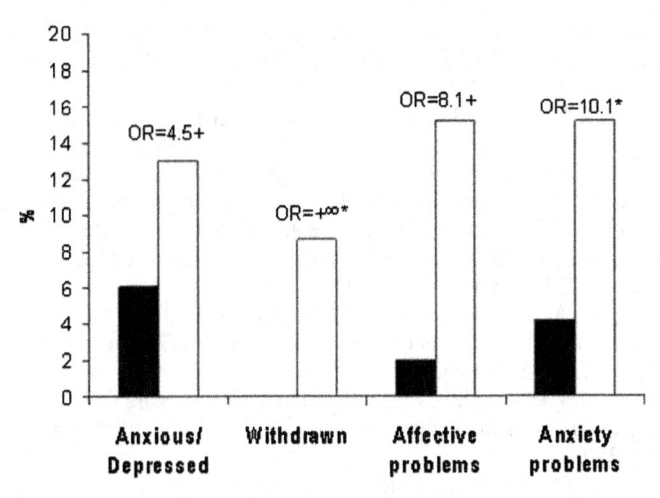

FIGURE 3. Risk of behavioral problems by exposure to other trauma.

under. More research on preschool children's reaction to various types of trauma is needed to help caregivers, professionals, and policy makers create early identification of preschool children at risk, screen and control for environmental risk factors (such as media exposure to terrorism and other traumatic events), and improve services for young children and their families with specifically tailored prevention and intervention strategies.

ACKNOWLEDGMENTS

The study was supported by The Picower Foundation, the Erna Reich Fund of UJA Federation of New York, and the Child and Family Resilience Program (Director, Claude Chemtob) at Mount Sinai School of Medicine. The authors thank Ms. Shelley Horwitz of the UJA Federation for her support of this work.

REFERENCES

1. HANFORD, H.A. *et al.* 1986. Child and parent reaction to the Three Mile Island nuclear accident. J. Am. Acad. Child Adolesc. Psychiatry **25:** 346–356.
2. OSOFSKY, J.D. 1995. The effects of exposure to violence on young children. Am. Psychol. **50:** 782–788.
3. REALMUTO, G.M. *et al.* 1992. Adolescent survivors of massive childhood trauma in Cambodia: life events and current symptoms. J. Trauma Stress **5:** 589–599.
4. TERR, L.C. 1988. What happens to early memories of trauma? A study of twenty children under age five at the time of the documented traumatic events. J. Am. Acad. Child Adolesc. Psychiatry **27:** 96–104.

5. VOGEL, J.M. & E.M. VERNBERG. 1993. Psychological responses of children to natural and human-made disasters, 1: Children's psychological responses to disasters. J. Clin. Child Psychol. **22:** 464–484.
6. FREMONT, W.P. 2004. Childhood reactions to terrorism-induced trauma: a review of the past 10 years. J. Am. Acad. Child Adolesc. Psychiatry **43:** 381–392.
7. DUGAL, H., G. BEREZKIN & J. VINEETH. 2002. PTSD and TV viewing of World Trade Center. J. Am. Acad. Child Adolesc. Psychiatry **41:** 494–495.
8. GOLDBERG, S. 1993. Violence at a distance: thinking about a nuclear threat. *In* The Psychological Effects of War and Violence in Children. L. Leavitt & N. Fox, Eds.: 231–242. Erlbaum. Hillsdale, NJ.
9. KLINGMAN, A., A. SAGI & A. RAVIV. 1993. The effect of war on Israeli children. *In* The Psychological Effects of War and Violence in Children. L. Leavitt & N. Fox, Eds.: 75–92. Erlbaum. Hillsdale, NJ.
10. PFEFFERBAUM, B. *et al.* 2000. Posttraumatic stress two years after the Oklahoma City bombing in youths geographically distant from the explosion. Psychiatry **63:** 358–370.
11. CENTERWALL, B.S. 1992. Television and violence: the scale of the problem and where to go from here. J. Am. Medical Association **267:** 3059–3063.
12. HEATH, L., L.B. BRESOLIN & R.C. RINALDI. 1989. Effects of media violence on children: a review of the literature. Arch. Gen. Psychiatry **46:** 376–379.
13. STRASBURGER, V.C. & E. DONNERSTEIN. 1999. Children, adolescents, and the media: issues and solutions. Pediatrics **103:** 129–139.
14. RODGERS, C.S. *et al.* 2004. The impact of individual forms of childhood maltreatment on health behavior. Child Abuse Negl. **28:** 575–586.
15. RIBBE, D. 1996. Psychometric review of Traumatic Event Screening Instrument for Children (TESI-C). *In* Measurement of Stress, Trauma, and Adaptation. B.H. Stamm, Ed.: 386–387. Sidran Press. Lutherville, MD.
16. ACHENBACH, T.M. & L.A. RESCORLA. 2000. Manual for ASEBA Preschool Forms and Profiles. University of Vermont, Research Center for Children, Youth, and Families. Burlington, VT.

Index of Contributors